Angels of Death

Angels of Death

Exploring the Euthanasia Underground

ROGER S. MAGNUSSON

(with contributions from Peter H. Ballis)

Yale University Press
New Haven and London

Published 2002 in Australia by Melbourne University Press and in the
United States by Yale University Press

Typeset in 11 point Sabon by Syarikat Seng Teik Sdn. Bhd., Malaysia
Printed in Australia by Brown Prior Anderson

Library of Congress Control Number: 20011099166
ISBN 0-300-09439-6 (cloth : alk. paper)
A catalogue record for this book is available from the British Library.

10 9 8 7 6 5 4 3 2 1

To mum and dad

Foreword

by The Hon. Justice Michael Kirby AC CMG

THIS IS A TROUBLING BOOK, with an upsetting title about a disturbing topic. Yet problems do not go away because we choose not to face them. Scholars have an obligation to explore topics that many in polite society would prefer to go unmentioned. Homosexuality, for example, was a topic kept in the shadows for too long. Until the wall of 'Don't ask, don't tell' was breached, society and many people had to live with falsehoods which the law reinforced.

The special value of this book is that it contributes usefully to the debate about the response of our society and its laws to assisted death. It does so by going beyond verbal analysis, by which clever people express their opinions. It surveys real life experiences of people involved in the 'euthanasia underground'. It is one thing to talk about great principles, whether found in holy texts or in modern statements of fundamental human rights. It is quite another to explore, in dialogue with doctors, nurses, patients, lovers and families, the largely hidden world in which patients in extremis are sometimes helped to die with dignity.

It is natural that the law should be concerned about the death of human beings. Death is the antithesis to life, which is the precondition to consciousness, essential to the enjoyment of liberty and the pursuit of happiness. Even the most primitive legal systems provide rules, supported by sanctions, against terminating human life. Many societies still punish attempted suicide. Although this is no longer an offence in Australia, assisting or encouraging another to attempt to commit suicide is an offence in five jurisdictions. Yet if the information contained in this book is, even in part, a true reflection of what is happening, we are facing another instance where the law is apparently being honoured in the breach as well as in the observance.

Some will draw the inference that the answer to this disclosure is a more vigorous enforcement of the law against anyone who assists, or attempts to assist, to end the life of a patient, even one with an incurable condition who wants to die. Others will read this book and infer that the present lack of 'quality control' demands that we face reality, introduce strict legal protections, impose proper procedures and expel amateurs and 'cowboys' from the assisted suicide business. Still others will find the whole topic so complex, puzzling and painful that they will prefer to ignore it. But the point that Dr Magnusson makes is that to ignore the issue is, effectively, to accept the realities that were long suspected, but which this book now documents.

In a sense, it was the advent of HIV/AIDS that demanded a book of this kind. Hospital practices in relation to terminating life support, hospice practices of inducing coma and death by palliative injections, and terminal decisions by mostly elderly patients could earlier usually pass unnoticed. But it was the arrival of AIDS, with its profound impact on a large cohort of young people (mostly homosexual men) that presented the new dimension to the euthanasia debate that is a chief focus of this book. These were people, often already alienated from the law, their families and society, who wanted to take control of their last moments of life. There are powerful passages in this book that illustrate the awful circumstances of the close of life of many such people, rejected by their genetic family but loved for whom they are by others, determined to support them on their last journey. There is a tragic irony in the fact that some of those who oppose assisted death most vehemently are amongst the most intolerant of the rights of such patients to live with dignity according to their nature. HIV/AIDS has thus presented a new dimension to the euthanasia debate. If for no other reason, this book is to be welcomed because it explores that issue.

The most valuable aspect of Dr Magnusson's analysis is that he avoids dogmatic adherence to the camp of absolute opposition to, or of uncompromising support for, legislation to permit and regulate the rights of terminally ill patients who choose to die. He does not disguise the powerful points made by each side of the debate. He does not pretend that the issue can be simply handed over to opinion polls which regularly show a majority of respondents in favour of a facilitating law of some kind. He does not disguise his anxiety about instances of 'botched' 'mercy killings'. He acknowledges the importance of the symbolism of the law and of health care ethics that remain committed to the defence of human life.

To some extent, modern medication and palliative care, as described in the book, bypass the need, for many people, of physician-assisted suicide. The 'break-through-dose' of morphine, administered to ease intolerable pain, will hasten death, as those who administer it well know. Yet the debate addressed in these pages will not go away. Relief of pain is not the only consideration. Many readers will agree with the opinion of Justice Brennan of the Supreme Court of the United States in the *Cruzan* Case, quoted in the closing chapter: 'Dying is personal. And it is profound. For many the thought of an ignoble end, steeped in decay, is abhorrent'.

People of this persuasion will see the effective power to control the end of one's life as the ultimate expression of personal autonomy, inherent in human dignity. Opponents will view it as defiance of God's will or as a bad signal that enhances the power of doctors and families over vulnerable patients. All of the main arguments are laid before the reader. Whilst Dr Magnusson offers his own opinion, he acknowledges that it is 'tinged with some uncertainty'. I suspect that that will be the conclusion of many who reflect, without dogma, upon the puzzles and dilemmas uncovered here.

What is to be done? Like Dr Magnusson, I will leave to the reader the privilege of finding the correct conclusion. But after this book, the debate will never be quite the same.

High Court of Australia, Canberra, 2001

Contents

Tables

Figure

Acknowledgements

THIS BOOK HAS BENEFITED from the generosity and input of many people. It was a real pleasure to be able to collaborate on aspects of the project with a longtime friend, (Professor) Harry Ballis, whose advice on methodology was crucial, and whose influence permeates well beyond the sections we co-wrote. Over many a cappucino in Lygon Street, Melbourne, or sprawled in front of the log fire in his living room in the Gippsland foothills, we argued about the data, co-wrote papers, and were genuinely moved as we tried to come to grips with the themes from these confronting and brutally frank stories. I'd like to thank Christine Ballis, who was a gracious host to me on many weekends at the 'Ballis palace', as well as Sarah, Peter, and Harry's colleagues at Monash University: Ian Hamilton, Lyle Munro, Parimal Roy and Steve Russell.

Laura Cherubin transcribed many of the interviews I recorded, and was an integral part of this project from the beginning. I am grateful for her friendship. More recently, Lisa Stapledon kindly assisted with transcription, and Myra Cheng provided valuable research and administrative assistance as the writing neared completion.

There are many, many people who assisted me by organising interviews, providing leads, introductions, references and encouragement, hosting seminar visits, or who took the time to discuss issues with me. Thank you Donald Abrams, Nerida Bates, (Professor) Peter Baume, Belinda Bennett, Peter Bruce, Tom Carter, Colleen Cartwright, Martine Cornelisse, (Professor) David Currow, Peter Doyle, (Professor) Julie Gerberding, Roger Hunt, Helga Khuse, Stephen Jamison, Marek Jantos, Vicki King, Kay Koetsier, Kris Larson, Graham Lister, (Professor) Eric Magnusson, Jennifer McGaugh, Marilyn McMurchie, Michael Moore, (Professor) Derek Morgan, (Professor) Ronald Numbers, Walt Odetts, Marshall Perron, Bruce

Parnell, Andrew Pethebridge, (Professor) Beverley Raphael, (Professor) Jan Remmelink, Darren Russell, Christopher Ryan, Sally Shute, (Professor) Peter Singer, (Professor) George Smith, Rodney Syme, (Professor) Bill Thompson, Eric Timewell, Bernadette Tobin, (Professor) Jim Walter, and (Professor) Gerald Winslow. There are many others.

I'd like to acknowledge the collegiality and help I gained from discussions and from reading the work of fellow researchers into assisted death, particularly (Professor) John Dombrink and Dr Dan Hillyard from the School of Social Ecology at the University of California (Irvine) (how can Harry and I ever forget Laguna beach?!), (Professor) John Griffiths from the University of Groningen, and Russel Ogden from Simon Fraser University in Vancouver, whose pioneering experiences researching HIV/AIDS assisted death made history. Back in Sydney, thank you Bridget Nguyen-Ngoc, for preparing Figure 9-1, and a very affectionate thank you to Meghan Haire, who read through the entire manuscript, and was a constant source of encouragement and cheer.

The progress of the project benefited from grants on several occasions. In particular, I acknowledge grants from the Faculty Infrastructure Fund, Faculty of Law, The University of Melbourne, and from the Australian Research Council small grants scheme. Margaret McAleese, Carolyn Kearney and Michelle Daly from the Law library, The University of Sydney, provided excellent assistance locating materials. I thank also the human research ethics committees of the University of Melbourne and the University of Sydney, for recognising the value of research into 'underground' phenomena, and showing that ethical research into assisted death, using a qualitative methodology, is possible.

Brian Wilder, former director of Melbourne University Press, backed up his early faith in the project with a contract it has taken me several years to fulfil! In his later role as mentor and commissioning editor he gave valuable advice and a sense of perspective. I was well served by John Meckan, director, MUP, on many occasions. Dr Janet McCalman came very highly recommended, and I am grateful for her reader's report, with its careful blend of encouragement and good advice. I am in awe of Wendy Sutherland, who edited the manuscript, and whose attention to detail was matched with kindness and tact. As this book travelled along the production line I have dealt in particular with Melissa Mackey (Publishing Co-ordinator), Teresa Pitt (Commissioning Editor), Gabby Lhuede (Pro-duction Controller—thanks Gabby!), and Deborah Clark (Marketing Manager). I am grateful to you all for your hard work, patience and good humour.

Justice Michael Kirby of the High Court of Australia is known internationally for his advocacy of a rational, compassionate approach to the challenges of HIV/AIDS. His vision for the role of law in responding to complex human issues, including tragedies, has been an inspiration to me (and not only me) for many years. I am honoured that Justice Kirby has written the foreword to this book.

I am unable to cite the real names of the interviewees I spoke to, but I am deeply grateful to them for sharing their experiences with candour and honesty: their testimony is the heart and soul of this book and I hope I have given voice to some of the intensity and anguish of their bedside experiences. Thank you Amanda, Anne, Bill, Bob, Butch, Chris, Damian, Dean, Dianne, Donald, Emma, Erin, Gary, Gay, Gordon, Harry, Harvey, Helen, Jane, John, Joseph, Josh, Kerry, Kyle, Liz, Margaret, Marjorie, Mark, Martin, Merril, Michelle, Nola, Paula, Peter, Ria, Richard, Robert, Russell, Ruth, Sam, Stanley, Stephen, Tara, Terri, Tim, Tom, Tony, Warren, Zane.

Introduction

IT WAS A COLD WINTER AFTERNOON, and I was sitting in an interview room in John's shopfront premises, drinking coffee from an exquisite china cup. John is a funeral director. He is a warm and charming middle-aged man who has lived through well over a decade of AIDS, yet still retains a sharp, dry wit, and a sense of the absurd. We had been talking for nearly an hour, and my dictaphone was running.

'Would you say that there is an informal network out there?' I asked, 'a euthanasia underground?'

'I would certainly say that', he said. 'In fact at one stage the group was given the nickname the "Angels of Death" '.

'Angels of Death', I repeated.

'Yes', he said, 'an informal network of people who co-operate together in order to facilitate euthanasia'.

'And it has no formal existence apart from the fact that those people who are involved know of one another?'

'That's right', he said; 'it's just that simple'.

This is a book about the 'euthanasia underground'. It reports on the experiences of health care workers in Australia and the United States who have been intimately involved in caring for people with AIDS. It presents and analyses first-person accounts of involvement

in assisted suicide and euthanasia, and seeks to contextualise interviewees' involvement in assisted death within the broader context
of palliative care. These are the stories of the 'angels of death'. In
telling them, my intention is to explore that secret part of the medical and nursing professions that few will ever talk about, and about
which the public knows very little.

The findings presented in this book are derived from 49 detailed, face-to-face interviews which I carried out over a three-year
period with a wide variety of health professionals, principally in
Sydney, Melbourne and San Francisco. A small number of interviews were also carried out in Canberra and Brisbane. Each interview was conducted on a pseudonymous basis, and interviewees
were also invited to respond to a substantial questionnaire. The aim
of the study was to investigate the attitudes and practices of Australian and American health care workers towards assisted suicide
and euthanasia, especially within HIV/AIDS health care contexts.
How is assisted death actually practised within health care settings?
What are the issues that surround the making of such a momentous
decision? How do health carers justify their attitudes and actions in
this area?

The issues that emerge from these interviews have important
implications for the debate about assisted dying. The euthanasia
debate will not go away. In 1995 and 1994 respectively, legislatures
in the Northern Territory, and in Oregon, enacted legislation legalising assisted death. These experiments faced resistance. In Australia,
Commonwealth legislation repealed the *Rights of the Terminally Ill
Act* in 1996. As this book goes to press, Oregon's initiative, the
Death with Dignity Act, faces ongoing attacks in Congress, and possibly from the Bush administration. But despite the desire by some
groups to declare victory in the 'war against euthanasia', the moral,
legal, and policy challenges are far from over.

The legalisation of assisted death illustrates a marked trend in
liberal, western democracies towards the 'privatisation' of the body.
The body has moved 'from being a public object, the focus of a
broader vision of human dignity, to being an object of purely individual expression and concern'.[1] Some groups, pre-eminently the
Catholic Church, argue that the trend towards greater autonomy
and private rights, as reflected in a so-called 'right to die', will lead

to the progressive dismantling of the community, which can only cheapen the value of human life. Others see in the right to die a long-awaited advance in the struggle for freedom and dignity.

No one has the right to foreclose debate on issues of such importance and complexity. At the same time, it is important for debate to be fuelled by knowledge rather than conjecture. Extravagant claims, and 'rhetorical bogeymen'[2]—the usual suspects in this debate—flourish in a knowledge vacuum. It is important, therefore, to penetrate the wall of silence to discover the reality of assisted suicide and euthanasia in our society, and to face up to the social costs of the current policy of prohibition. This book provides a window into illicit euthanasia practice, thanks to the frankness of health carers who shared their feelings and attitudes, and gave detailed, self-incriminating accounts of their involvement.

A summary of the methodology and recruitment strategy used in this study can be found in the Appendix. All interviews were conducted on a pseudonymous basis, in accordance with a written protocol approved by the Human Research Ethics Committee of the University of Melbourne. In most cases, interviewees either volunteered to be interviewed after hearing of the study during public presentations which I gave, or were recommended by their colleagues to be involved. These twin strategies facilitated contact with a broad range of health carers, at a variety of levels of seniority, from shift-worker nurses, to physicians with international reputations. No 'master list' of interviewees was retained, thus preserving anonymity and encouraging frankness during the interview. Table 0-1 sets out the occupational categories of the interviewees.

Table 0-1: Occupational categories of interviewees	(n=49)
Doctor (includes psychiatrists)	19
Nurse	17
Therapist (Psychologist/Counsellor)	7
Community Worker	5
Other (Funeral Director)	1

While the legalisation of assisted death has become a matter of widespread community debate, there is a surprising lack of interview-based research into current euthanasia practices.[3] While survey-based studies can monitor trends in attitudes and actions, they do not facilitate a detailed exploration of the processes that operate at the bedside, and the social and emotional milieu within which assisted suicide and euthanasia are practised. Similar criticisms have been made of survey studies in their failure to capture the 'contextualised' nature of nurses' *attitudes* towards euthanasia, and the fact that those attitudes are 'grey', rather than 'black and white'.[4]

Testimony that cuts both ways

The interview findings presented in this book cut both ways. Advocates of euthanasia law reform should not be fooled into thinking that the debate is *only* about the issue of self-determination, which can be appropriately resolved by a law authorising medically-supervised killing under controlled conditions. The interview data demonstrate nothing if not the complexity of end-of-life issues, the subtle conflicts of interest that arise at the bedside, the cry for death as a mis-expression of other unresolved needs, and the fundamental ambivalence toward assisted death expressed both by patients, as well as many of those who participate in it.

If euthanasia is to be legalised, then this study supports a muscular, pro-regulatory model for achieving this. A law which merely decriminalised physician-assisted death would simply perpetuate the *laissez-faire* environment which the policy of prohibitionism has already helped to create. Politicians should not jump on the bandwagon of perceived public approval (an unlikely prospect in face of the effective alliance between churches and medical bodies), but should recognise the challenge involved in creating guidelines that will ensure that assisted death remains 'voluntary, regulated, and . . . an option of last resort'.[5]

Conversely, opponents of euthanasia law reform should be disabused of the notion that the law's prohibition of compassionate killing is effective in protecting vulnerable patients. Prohibition drives assisted death underground. At present, health care workers who perform euthanasia determine the conditions for their own involvement. Secret euthanasia, without appropriate regulation, raises many disturbing issues (see Chapters 10 and 11). Some of the experiences recounted in this book either cry out for those prosecutions which the policy of prohibition has failed to deliver, or for the safety valve of a protocol permitting assisted death in carefully defined circumstances, thereby educating the medical profession and protecting patients from incompetence and recklessness.

The purpose of this book is therefore to expose the social practices, relationships, and networks that constitute 'underground' euthanasia. I hope also to demonstrate the complexity of the euthanasia issue, and in the process to capture some of the passion, pathos and bitter-sweetness of those bedside moments, as health professionals care for patients in the midst of pain, bodily decay and existential anguish.

Testimony that speaks for itself

This book presents the results of an independent study that was carried out without funding or collaboration from either right to die or right to life societies. Ethics approval was first obtained from The University of Melbourne Human Research Ethics Committee and, subsequently, from The University of Sydney Research Ethics Committee. I began the study with no fixed views either for or against euthanasia. The experience, together with Harry Ballis, of analysing and discussing the interview data led me initially to conclude that there was an overwhelming case for the legalisation of euthanasia, albeit within a statutory framework containing appropriate safeguards.

Continuing reflection, however, has tempered this sense of confidence with concern about the potential, barely tangible risks of legalisation: the spectre of quiet demises, of people—disappointed with their lives—trying to leave early so as not to be a burden. *Sydney Morning Herald* columnist Richard Glover may be right to suggest that a legalised euthanasia regime would encourage self-effacing people—eager to conserve the family silver, and to spare their loved ones the agony of waiting—to consider killing themselves as one of the options for their medical care.[6] It is possible that this happens anyway, even in the absence of legislation. Any responsible euthanasia law must ensure that great care is taken to assess and protect those who lose their sense of identity and personal value at the end of life. Opponents of legislation, for various reasons, will argue that no such law can be framed.

This study largely adopts a harm minimisation approach to euthanasia policy. An important policy question raised by the data is whether the prospect of those quiet, outwardly-autonomous yet disempowered deaths outweighs the indignities of the current, unregulated euthanasia market. Much of the policy debate has been built on the fear of a future gone horribly wrong. Politicians and the medical profession are reluctant to face up to the here-and-now of illicit euthanasia, and there has been little research into the processes involved. Many participants in the public debate hold deeply entrenched positions which render evidence and research superfluous.

Although my own support for legalisation is tinged with some uncertainty, I am confident that the interview findings will tell their own story, and that readers will form their own conclusions. The intention behind this book is not to produce a manifesto but to inject new perspectives into the euthanasia debate. Ultimately, there is only one place to start constructing a humane and responsible social policy: with those who are dying, those who care for them, and those who for whatever reason, choose to become 'angels of death'.

1

Who would do such a thing?

We don't . . . know what the unspoken ethics are, the unspoken
rules, the guidelines the doctors or people are using at present to
make those decisions.

Associate Professor Elaine Thompson, 24 August 1995[1]

Who performs illegal euthanasia? Who would do such a thing? This
chapter introduces five 'euthanisers': three doctors, a nurse and
a psychologist—real men and women who live in cities along
Australia's east coast, or in the San Francisco bay area. My aim is to
present some of the anecdotes, personalities and personal philosophies that emerged from the interviews, and so to communicate a
sense of the material which makes up the present study.

One advantage of an interview-based approach is that it provides the opportunity to explore issues in depth, and to clarify attitudes and specifics of involvement. Importantly, interviewees raised
issues one would not have thought to include in any questionnaire.
But most of all, the interview created a space for interviewees to tell
their stories. Under assurances of anonymity, these stories give us
unprecedented access to the world of illicit euthanasia.

Introducing Gary

Standing in stark contrast to media stereotypes of euthanasia advocates as obsessed, marginal zealots, Gary displays the cool confidence

of a successful, middle-class doctor. Cosmopolitan and cappuccino-drinking, Gary is an articulate crusader whose bravado is tinged with cynicism for the medical establishment. What motivates him, I wondered?

'I'm not [a] hit-man', he said, as we sat talking during his lunch-time in a small, windowless treatment room in a busy, inner city sur-gery. 'Once I've got the needle in their arm, they can still change their mind at any time, till they're unconscious. I always give them ample opportunity to take it out, but every single one who's got so far as to set a date [has gone through with it].'

'It's almost a sense of relief for [the patient], once they've made the decision . . . a huge weight is lifted—they know that their suffer-ing is going to be finished soon.' 'It's not an unpleasant procedure if it's done well, it's quick, they just float out of it, and they *stop*.'

In Gary's experience it is usually the patient who raises the topic of euthanasia, although Gary was one of several doctors who admitted to raising the issue themselves early on in the relationship in order to discover the patient's views.

'This guy . . . had Kaposi's Sarcoma', said Gary, describing one of half a dozen euthanasia episodes we discussed during the inter-view. 'He'd [had] several courses of chemotherapy and they were just not effective anymore . . . his face had swollen up, he was in a lot of pain . . . and so we'd sort of agreed on the time, [although] when I went around there he was already unconscious.'

'His lover, his mother, his sister, three or four friends . . . were all looking after him', said Gary, 'taking it in turns. [He'd] told me, and he told his lover and his mother that if he did slip into uncon-sciousness . . . he wanted to be finished quickly, he didn't want to hang around, and so with his family around, we—we did it'.

Gary explained that the presence of the family at the bedside caused some difficulties, 'the least of which was actually getting into the guy because there were all these people sort of clambering over him'.

'You might inject the wrong arm?' I asked.

'Yes', he said, with a laugh. 'I still had to find a bit of him that wasn't being grabbed by someone.'

'He would have died within the next four or five days', said Gary. 'This took a minute or two; to me that does not seem to be a huge problem [he pauses] since *it's hastening things up only a little in the scheme of things.*'

In many ways, this candid observation sums up Gary's personal philosophy of euthanasia.

At a number of points during the interview, Gary digressed and began to reflect more generally about the nature of his clientele. 'Most of the ones I've done, the people haven't had any real religious beliefs, and most of them seemed to regard it as a bit of an adventure, I suppose; they haven't done death yet! [he laughs]. They've done everything else, they've got nothing to look forward to, here's their death coming, they don't seem particularly afraid of it, it's quite surprising, *I think I would be.*'

'I did one a couple of weeks ago', said Gary, 'with a nurse. I picked her up at her house, [and we] drove to the [patient's home]'. 'He'd just had his 28th birthday. We were alone in the room together, but his mother, father, brother, priest, were all there, sort of outside, and as we finished him off, there must have been three or four carloads of people arrived: friends and relatives and family.'

While Gary and the nurse were preparing the lethal injection, another community nurse arrived. 'We didn't want her to know about it so we had to sort of hide and wait . . . and then the priest arrived and he didn't seem to want to leave, I think he'd settled in for the day, he was having cups of tea and a bit of a chat to the nurse' [laughter].

Did the priest suspect something, I asked?

'I don't think he was a real clever priest', said Gary. 'I think he might have suspected something.'

'[So] while the mother and the father distracted the priest, the nurse and I sort of went into the bedroom and had a chat [to the patient]', Gary explains. 'The nurse asked him to—she'd sent a request up with someone six months earlier about Tattslotto numbers and nothing had happened yet—so she asked him to (when he got up to heaven) to ask the big guy about the numbers that she'd been waiting on. He said he'd relay that message for her . . . he [said he] was going to take control of things [up there]'.

'It was all done in a fairly . . . light-hearted manner', said Gary. 'He was well aware of what was going to happen, so we injected him, and it only took a few minutes, he died, we left the room, the father went in . . . the brother . . . then the priest went in and gave him the last rites.'

Despite the humour and the crisp, effective intervention on this occasion, Gary had also been involved in a number of highly distressing 'botched jobs' (see Chapter 10).

'I get sad', said Gary, 'I get depressed; it's not nice to kill someone, it's not an easy thing to do [although] it does get easier with time—after doing several, that's easier than the first couple.'

Gary is a 'revisionist' doctor (see Chapter 6), who challenges traditional perceptions of the doctor's professional role and argues that euthanasia should be seen as an act of medical care. 'The Medical Board would probably not take a great view of the fact that I've killed quite a few patients', he says, 'but they're all frumps, and they're not operating in the real world'.

Introducing Jane

Of all the doctors interviewed in this study, none outshines Jane as an unconventional and uncompromising patient's advocate. An early advocate of combination therapy, Jane spoke with enthusiasm about protease inhibitors, and how she believes they have turned HIV into a manageable condition for many patients. Behind the enthusiasm lies a history of relentlessly pursuing drug companies for compassionate access to new drugs. Jane freely admitted to stealing substantial quantities of drugs from hospital fridges, and attributes the good health of her patients to their early and sustained access to new drugs. When morphine, Tegretol (carbamazepine) and other pain-relieving drugs were not effective in controlling intractable nerve pain in one patient with lymphatic cancer, Jane turned to amphetamines. 'We were actually buying street speed and . . . putting his speed doses in his dosette box every day', she says.

Jane admitted to subverting a number of drug trials involving her patients in an effort to assist them. For example, she had occasionally used blood serum to infect a patient with an opportunistic infection if this was a requirement for accessing a promising new drug and if her patient had been placed on the placebo arm of the trial. She also gave diuretics to her patients and sent them to the tropics for a few weeks to lose weight so that they could come within the weight loss criteria for accessing new treatments.

Although protease inhibitors had slowed down Jane's involvement in euthanasia in the period preceding interview, Jane estimated she had been involved in 50–60 deaths: 'probably one a month' for 'three years', and before that at a lesser rate. Like Gary, Jane had a policy of initiating discussion of euthanasia early on in her relationship with the patient. Jane didn't feel comfortable if the patient decided upon euthanasia 'at a point in their life when they had a whole lot of other issues going on'. She preferred to know that the patient had had 'that view the entire way through, including when they were really well'.

As with some of the other gay interviewees, Jane felt a unique sense of kinship with gay men and women with the virus. Unusually, though, she made no attempt to cordon off her private life from her professional one: 'I treat most of my closest friends'. Jane ridiculed the 'cute' idea that 'there is a line that you actually cross' between professional and personal involvement: 'I just reject the whole notion of professionalism, I think'.

After a 'botched attempt' early in her career, when a patient awoke 14 hours after taking 'at least five times the lethal dose of at least four drugs', Jane has followed a policy of remaining with the patient throughout the euthanasia process. Unfortunately, this is far from standard practice.

For Jane, euthanasia is a 'professional procedure', 'the final part of taking care of a patient'. 'You've got to give certainty . . . it has to be something . . . you can guarantee. The last part of someone's life for me [is] the most critical part of their life; making that perfect is the most critical thing that you can do for them.'

Jane gave several examples of the bedside dynamics of euthanasia, admitting that there had been some 'very twisted episodes'. She had one patient with 'nightmare veins', 'virtually every vein in his body was stuffed'. The boy had previously taken home a 'kit' of needles and medications from Jane's surgery, because 'he wasn't sure when he would decide that he wanted to go'. 'He had everything at his house, [but] then he couldn't find them when he decided that this was actually going to be the end.'

Having driven out to the patient's home (he was 'one of the few boys I knew who lived outside of the inner city'), Jane then had to drive back through the rain to her surgery for more butterfly needles. She arrived back at the patient's house to find him outfitted 'in this white wedding dress'. It was 'one of his award-winning designs and he [had] decided that this [was] what he was going to be buried in'. He was saying that 'everything else [had] just been a dress rehearsal', and now he was 'Aunt Always', and 'don't get any blood on the lace'. 'It was a very twisted night', Jane recalls.

There would be few people better placed than Jane to observe the impact of AIDS, and euthanasia, upon the gay community. At the last euthanasia death she attended, Jane estimated that *everyone else present had personally been involved in 'five, maybe ten' deaths themselves*. 'Partly it's the [gay] community taking care of its own, and partly it's what you see when you've got one disease that hits into one community . . . within one geographic area.'

Jane concedes that the comments and reactions to death within the gay community may well be unique. The last time she was involved in euthanasia was with a boy who had 'designed his whole funeral . . . he wanted a whole lot of candles all over the church'. After the death, Jane rang one of his friends who was aware of the funeral arrangements. The friend joked that 'his sense of timing was always bad'. The previous week had been the AIDS candlelight vigil and 'if he'd done it last week . . . there would have been candles all over the park . . . we could have just gone down [to] the park and [taken] them'.

Comments like that would be considered obscene, in another context, I suggested.

'Yeah, but not in this community', said Jane, 'it's the way they deal with it . . . we thought it was hysterical . . . if you talk to intensive care staff, they do exactly the same thing . . . anyone who is dealing with [death] on a constant basis . . .'

During the interview, I explored how Jane copes with the stresses of HIV practice, and her extensive involvement in euthanasia. Initially, the stress of participating in euthanasia would 'really wipe me out . . . I would . . . finish with them and just cry for hours'. For Jane, the loss of friends, loss of patients, and the loss to her community are inextricably linked.

Jane considers herself 'lucky' to have several friends who also 'have a high community profile'. 'We have this sort of unwritten agreement that we all fall apart together', she says. 'We never do it in public . . . it would always be . . . at one of our places . . . it tends to be an all night affair . . . it tends to involve, you know, lots of different sorts of substances and lots of music . . . It can often go for an entire weekend.'

'I don't make sense of it anymore', says Jane. 'I used to sort of, you know, try and understand it, [but] I don't anymore: it just happens. For me the important stuff is to try and make sure that this is a real decision for the [patient]; that it's a valid decision for them.'

Introducing Kyle

Kyle is one of the quiet achievers of this study, a general practitioner who has built euthanasia into an aspect of professional practice, and developed a philosophy around it. '[My] approach to management of any disease is [that] the patient is a co-manager', he says. 'I'm here to advise, to educate and to offer options, but all decisions have to be made by the patient themselves.'

As a medic in Vietnam, Kyle practised assisted death 'out of necessity'. 'We got hit one night and had four major burns. It was obvious that two would not survive even in the best of conditions and our chances of getting more than two out in the middle of the monsoons was very questionable, so we opted to send two out by helicopter, barely got them out, and then I euthanised the other two with large doses of morphine.'

Was the compassionate killing of dying troops on the battlefield considered a legitimate part of emergency medicine, I asked?

'It was a practice that was not discussed', says Kyle. 'You had to make the decision, you had to triage . . . if somebody was unsalvageable, then they were no longer expected to spend days of suffering . . .'

Kyle emphasises that it wasn't as if 'all of a sudden I sneak up on somebody, pounce on a vein if I can find one on a 95% burned body, and say 'Goodbye!' These [were] patients that were screaming for relief and there was absolutely no way that we could get them to any kind of advanced care and even if we could, they would not have survived'.

Faced with this decision, Kyle placed himself in the position of the patient. 'What would I want done to me? How would I want to be treated?' 'It's pretty straightforward for me', he says. 'It's not a big issue that causes a lot of internal debate.'

Having been 'open about assisted death' as a result of his experiences in Vietnam, Kyle found that when AIDS came along, he was naturally sympathetic to patients who wanted to choose assisted suicide. 'There is a similarity between the battlefield and HIV . . . you're at the end of the line and you can't move the patient to a higher level of care [or offer them] a different approach.' 'I've always believed [that] quality of life is an issue that only the individual can really measure. I cannot measure pain . . . I cannot measure loss of vanity . . . suffering . . . depression . . . End-of-life issues are more than just taking a breath and a heartbeat . . . I think people should always be able to make their own decisions and I think it makes a stronger society when people have to assume that responsibility.'

During the interview, Kyle outlined the three-step approach he has developed for screening patients who want an assisted death. First, he explores with the patient their own personal philosophy of death, what death will mean for them, and what impact it will have on their partner, family and friends. Kyle needs to make sure that the patient is 'at peace with death', and doesn't see it as 'something awesome or frightening or spooky'. 'AIDS has taught us that many people have been able to accept death in a very quiet, serene way.'

Secondly, Kyle likes to explore the philosophy and feelings of the patient's immediate support group: those who are likely to be involved in the euthanatic procedure. Kyle likes the death to be discussed openly so that when the procedure is performed it will not be perceived as 'clandestine or secretive or . . . negative'. 'I have to be convinced that everybody is in agreement [and that this] is what they want.'

Health workers are divided in the extent to which they involve others in planning the euthanasia event. Many prefer to limit the procedure to the patient and a partner, or perhaps one or two close family members. The more who are aware of it, the higher the risks for the doctor. A number of interviewees reported withdrawing from a planned procedure because the patient had advertised it widely and injudiciously.

The third part of Kyle's pre-death counselling process focuses on how the procedure itself will be accomplished. 'If you're offering assisted death to someone you have to have the methodology', says Kyle. 'Early on I let it be known that I myself will only provide the tools and that I will not be involved in doing the actual procedure.'

Later on in the interview, Kyle explained this position. 'I'm an adviser', he said. 'I'm an educator, I'm a person that gives options. In my population, we do not depend on . . . professional care givers to . . . perpetrate the assisted death. In Vietnam, I had no choice, I had to push the syringe.' With AIDS, however, Kyle limits his involvement to writing prescriptions, advising on preparations, and educating the patient how the drugs might best be ingested, whether rectally, through the bloodstream, or mixed in yoghurt.

Kyle points out that the community of HIV care givers is 'fairly tight'. 'It reminds me again of wartime medicine', he says, 'where the hours are long, the responsibilities are immense, the stresses are unbelievable, and as such we've come together because we've often been isolated by our colleagues'.

In contrast to some of the doctors interviewed in this study, Kyle's style is particularly low key. He is well integrated into his community, and it provides full camouflage. 'I have trouble with the Kevorkian approach to things', says Kyle, who believes that people suffer from the sensationalism that accompanies Kevorkian's methods. Assisted suicide is a 'planned treatment' and 'a matter of trust', rather than 'a rubout, or a wipeout or a knockout. I see this not as a means of snuffing out life but of making life more comfortable . . . I'm very much at peace with this, it's not an issue that I go home and struggle with afterwards.'

Introducing Erin

You know, I worked in an ICU [intensive care unit] and the advanced medical technology that we [used on] some of these people was *harmful*, you know . . . We kept them alive, [the] respirator was blowing air into them, you know, sixteen breaths a minute but the alarm was going off every three minutes and they were . . . uncomfortable and being suctioned and tormented . . . I was *doing harm*, you know. And for the first time I took those [ethics] principles back out and really looked at them, as a care giver . . . but also trying to understand what the patient was going through.

The active involvement of nurses in euthanasia is one of the neglected aspects of the euthanasia debate. The seeds of Erin's involvement, like that of other nurses who participated in this study, lies in witnessing suffering patients.

Erin crossed the boundary for the first time while nursing in a Catholic hospital in another State. 'We had a patient that came in a number of times', recalls Erin, 'a revolving-door pulmonary patient [who] . . . just didn't have good lungs and would catch a pneumonia at the drop of a hat . . . He asked me to help him die . . . He said "Do you know what it's like to be on a respirator?" He'd been on [one], intubated a number of times. He said "Do you know what it's like, do you know the terror I have when I try to go to sleep at night . . .?" '

'They found he had TB', says Erin, 'so everybody was wearing masks and . . . he said "Is this quality of life?" '

Although traumatic, this case was a turning-point. After a long period of soul-searching, Erin came to the conclusion that medical ethics are all 'very nice in theory', but—as he put it—'*it's not the stuff that's dealing with the folks in bed, you know*'.

'As it turned out I helped him', says Erin, explaining how he killed the patient by placing the cardiac monitor on standby and then turning off the oxygen. 'I didn't sleep for a week', he reports.

Erin's interview was unusually long, conducted over cans of soda from the bar fridge of my hotel room. It provided a fascinating insight, however, into the world of deception that permeates the euthanasia underground, and the central role that nurses play within it. Erin detailed the ways in which nurses co-operate to subvert hospital procedures when assisting bedridden inpatients to die, and how doctors are manipulated into creating a 'paper chain' which justifies the prescription of drugs which patients can stockpile and later take as an overdose (see Chapter 9).

Erin self-identifies as a gay man, a spiritual person and a Catholic, but one who is confused and contemptuous of his church's approach to issues of life and death. He recalls an occasion when the ethics committee of a Catholic hospital created a task force to look into the issue of pain control. Erin, who was a Catholic brother at the time, was a member of the task force, which was directed to report back to the ethics committee. The task force moved too far, however, by including the book *Final Exit*, by euthanasia advocate Derek Humphry, within the scope of its research, and by creating a package of materials for committee members to read and discuss. The plan was for the members of the ethics committee to meet to discuss the materials the task force had collated. At the time this was to occur, however, the chair of the ethics committee abruptly intervened and dissolved the meeting, thanking the members of the task force and 'patt[ing] us on the head', but saying that these things could not be discussed.

At various points during the interview, discussion turned back to the Catholic church. If the church believes condoms are wrong in the 'straight community' because they will be used as contraceptives, then why does it frown on condoms in the gay community, where no issue of contraception is involved, and where they save lives? 'I'm sorry', said Erin, loudly and aggressively, in interview, 'but I'm a person on the street and that fucking doesn't make sense!'

He went on to explain that while working in a Catholic hospital clinic, although unable to hand out condoms he 'sure as hell' clipped out the addresses from the backs of AIDS brochures and gave directions to his clients.

I found this admission intriguing. It illustrates the little rebellions that individuals wage from within the system, motivated by compassion, and 'dissident' values. Within clinics and hospitals, from recent graduates to the internationally renowned, health carers are quietly subverting the taboos of the old moral order, including the taboo on assisted death. As Erin's interview illustrates, religious institutions are not exempt.

At the time of interview, Erin had been living for less than twelve months in the city where I met him. Despite this, he had already managed to participate in euthanasia on four occasions:

procuring medication, counselling the euthanatic procedure, and administering medication.

'I believe in life', says Erin, explaining that he didn't like to be thought of as 'an angel of death'. It's just that 'death is one of the options', albeit an option Erin likes to discuss early on during clients' illness, while they are 'alert and orientated and running pretty stable'. Erin warns that western medicine, in trying to heal the patient, actually causes harm. In contrast, 'the native American style is that the healer will first consider [whether] the patient need[s] to be healed before they act . . .'

Introducing Mark

> He had gotten kind of deaf, and clearly had trouble walking up and down the stairs, it was pain[ful] but he liked to follow me around the house so if I went upstairs he liked to follow me and sometimes I would look back and he'd be halfway up the stairs kind of standing there and I could see that he was trying to regain himself and make it the rest of the way up. So I finally took him to the [doctor] and I said 'I think maybe he is really in too much pain', *I mean it's not him any-more* . . . he should really be put out of his suffering, and that's what we did.

In the passage above, Mark, a clinical psychologist, is talking about his 14-year-old poodle, that was put down by a vet. He uses the story of his poodle, however, to illustrate his attitude towards euthanasia. 'Killing someone who is suffering . . . is in the service of decency and respect', he said as we sipped coffee in his spacious living room.

Do you have any deep moral objections to euthanasia if you feel it is appropriate within the patient's own value system, I ask him?

'I don't . . . have any deep ones, I don't even have any shallow ones', he replied.

The interview with Mark ended as it had begun: with a discussion of Mark's role as a therapist for patients with AIDS. When a patient reaches the end and wishes to discontinue treatment, this causes 'a lot of anxiety in the physician, and his [*sic*] inclination is to abandon a patient who makes him feel like that'. An issue which 'always comes up' in psychotherapy is the 'patient's experience of [their] physician withdrawing from them'. 'If a psychologist did that it would be illegal, it's called *abandonment*, you can't abandon someone when they're hopeless', but physicians are not, as a group, 'particularly psychologically insightful'.

Ultimately, Mark justifies his involvement in euthanasia on the basis that he is filling the role that doctors shouldn't have vacated in the first place. 'A physician should follow a patient out to the end in a supportive way . . . that *ought* to be a physician's role; I end up there by default', he says.

The sheer drama of Mark's middle-of-the-range euthanasia career (at the date of interview he had been involved on five or six occasions), makes his interview one of the most colourful of the study. A typical example was his account of 'Carlos' and 'Danny'. Both men had AIDS. Danny and Carlos were lovers, and Danny was also Mark's patient.

Carlos had intractable abdominal pain: 'they couldn't treat it, he was using narcotics for months and months [and] was confined to bed' in 'absolute misery'. Carlos talked with Danny about the possibility of suicide, and they agreed that if this was what Carlos wanted, then Danny would support him. Not long after, Carlos ingested 7500 milligrams of Seconal (secobarbital), and drank a third of a bottle of vodka.

Twenty-four hours later Carlos was still alive, although comatose, and Danny called me up in a panic, Mark recalls. Danny dragged the telephone over closer to Carlos' bed. 'I could hear [that] he sounded very brain damaged just from the sound of the breathing', said Mark. Danny was frightened and wanted to call '000', until Mark reminded him that if an ambulance arrived, Carlos would end up in hospital on life-support.

'Well I'm going to put a plastic bag over his head and tie it around his neck', said Carlos, and that's what he did.

Later in the day, Mark came around to their home, and called Carlos' doctor to report the death.

'Does it look like natural causes, no monkey business or anything?' asked the doctor.

'No', Mark replied.

'That's what I thought', said the doctor.

The Coroner's office was informed, and not long after the police 'literally burst into the house, knocked down the front door, spent the whole day there fingerprinting things in the house'.

Over the next 12 months, Danny's own health deteriorated, and Danny's parents came to live with him to assist in his care. Danny reached the point where he had set a date for his own death. Mark rang Danny's doctor—the same man who had been Carlos' doctor—to request a prescription of insulin to assist in Danny's death. The doctor refused. '"There's nothing in the medical chart that justifies [insulin]", he said and I could tell that it was very painful for the doctor to say this', Mark recalls.

Danny had become 'kind of demented' by this time, drifting in and out, and Danny's mother implored Mark for help. Mark had another conversation with Danny ('I just wanted the confidence again'), reassuring himself that euthanasia really was Danny's wish. 'He said he was very grateful that I would help because his mother was upset and he was concerned about how upset she was.'

Mark found a bottle of potassium chloride 'in a linen closet in the hall', and explained to Danny that 'a sufficient quantity would cause a heart attack'. He asked Danny whether he preferred to be awake or sedated when he took his overdose.

Mark sedated Danny with Valium and then injected him in the leg. 'He had a very severe arrhythmic episode which I later realised was the effect of the potassium chloride which [was] probably suppressed by the Valium', said Mark. 'There is not a whole lot of literature on this stuff.'

A second injection under the arm worked instantaneously.

At this point in the interview, Mark interjected that 'this is actually a strange story', and explained that by then it was 8 o'clock at night and that he had left his car outside Danny's home, with the parking lights on. 'While I'm upstairs giving him the first injection the doorbell rings, and it's a policeman, and he says: "I'm just stopping because someone's left their lights on in the car out the front", and the mother said: "Oh, that's alright, my son's *doctor* is here, he's just left his car out there"'.

After Danny had died, Mark called a cremation service, which sent two men over, at 'about midnight'. Both men wore green sportscoats.

The sportscoats were 'forest green' and each looked like he was wearing the other one's blazer, Mark recalls. One very tall, heavy guy was wearing a blazer with the sleeves well above the wrist, and the other 'tiny little guy' was wearing a coat with the sleeves almost covering his fingers. They arrived in an unmarked Japanese pick-up truck, completely unmarked, showed their credentials and then they began to wrap the body in linen 'in a very respectful, elegant kind of way'.

The two men helped Danny's mother dress the body. 'It was one of the most painful things I've ever seen', said Mark. 'She wanted to change his clothes and dress him in a T-shirt and some clean clothes, and when we rolled [the body over] all the blood had settled in his posterior so it looked like a huge bruise and she said: "Oh my God, now what's wrong with him?" I said: "well, he's dead, this is what happens when the blood settles, it's not circulating", and then she started laughing, and she said: "you know, just to see one more thing wrong with my son, it's unbearable to me"'.

While the two men from the cremation service were wheeling the body away, two police cars came screeching up to the house. 'One guy gets out of each car, and they're sort of running towards us . . . with their hands on their guns', Mark recalls. And here were 'these two guys with their blazers on, with this body, and the cop who's out in front says: "so what's going on here?" And the little guy says: "well, this is a man who is an AIDS patient who died at home", and he sort of gestured over his shoulder at me and said: "that's his doctor"'.

'So the cop says to me: "What's going on here, doc?" I said, "well just as the guy told you, 'Mr Jones' was an AIDS patient who died at home, these people are from [a cremation service] and are removing the body", and the cops said: "OK doc, thanks a lot", and they got back in their cars and left.'

'I have no idea what it was about', Mark admitted to me in interview. 'There was something about the car out the front . . . that bothered them . . . I have a Mercedes, so my speculation at the time was that they [thought]: well either this is a doctor or a drug dealer and it's probably a drug dealer.'

An interesting feature of this account, and of others that Mark told, is that he was represented, and indeed represented himself, *as a doctor*. Under any criteria for eligibility to participate in euthanasia within a legalised, statutory framework, Mark—a clinical psychologist with no medical qualifications—would be *ineligible*. Nevertheless, in an environment where doctors 'abandon' their patients, Mark *becomes* the doctor, fulfilling the role that doctors have abdicated. It is interesting to note that this even extended to signing Danny's death certificate. Mark's interview provides a timely reminder that illicit euthanasia is not only performed by doctors, but by lovers and family members of the deceased, assisted by a variety of health professionals, as well as therapists, community workers, and even funeral directors.

Despite their differences, Gary, Jane, Kyle, Erin and Mark have one thing in common. In different ways—some quietly, some loudly—they are dismantling old taboos and struggling to create new notions of decency. Some kill with unease and guilt, others with a clear conscience. Some carry it out with polished professionalism, within an integrated philosophy of care; others don't even try anymore to make sense of it all. These actions do not take place in a social vacuum, but against the background of the euthanasia debate, and the subtle erosion of the sanctity of life ethic. Chapters 2–4 will examine the social and legal context of the debate about assisted death, before returning to the interviewees in Chapter 5.

2

Doctors who kill

I have no problem with it morally or ethically and quite frankly I couldn't give a damn what the law says.

Dr Dave Moor, who claims to have helped four to five people die per year for the past thirty years.[1]

He would have died within the next four or five days . . . instead of it taking a day or two . . . this took a minute or two; to me that does not seem to be a huge problem since it's hastening things up only a little in the scheme of things.

Gary, General Practitioner

In March 1995 seven Melbourne doctors went public on the front page of *the Age* newspaper in an open letter to the Premier of Victoria, admitting to having performed euthanasia, and calling for the introduction into Parliament of the assisted suicide legislation advocated by the Voluntary Euthanasia Society.[2] Referring to the legal prohibition upon euthanasia, the doctors wrote:

> It cannot be right to tolerate this totally unsatisfactory situation, where it is a matter of chance whether patients will receive the treatment which they so desperately seek and where it must be only a matter of time before some doctor is prosecuted by the state for following the dictates of his [*sic*] conscience.[3]

Despite calls for their prosecution,[4] and accusations of 'making heroes of themselves',[5] investigations by the Victoria Police and the Medical Practitioners' Board of Victoria were abandoned for lack of evidence.[6] The 'Melbourne 7' went on to win the Victorian Voluntary Euthanasia Society's 1995 community service award.

The action by the 'Melbourne 7' is but one of many examples which illustrate an increasing resistance among sections of the medical profession to 'play dumb' about their involvement in euthanasia. Doctors such as Jack Kevorkian and Timothy Quill in the United States, Nigel Cox in England, and Philip Nitschke and Rodney Syme in Australia have come to embody the growing protest against the laws that criminalise assisted suicide and euthanasia.

Euthanasia is the debate that won't go away. It flares intermittently, dies down, but always returns. This chapter traces some recent episodes in the ongoing history of open defiance by doctors of the law. Although there is no one terminology for talking about assisted death, there is nevertheless wide consensus about the terms used below. In the United States the debate has tended to focus on physician-assisted suicide (PAS). Assisted suicide encompasses such actions as intentionally prescribing or making available a lethal quantity of drugs, assisting a patient to take a lethal overdose by preparing a cocktail of drugs, or accessing a vein. In Australia the debate has focused more broadly on active voluntary euthanasia (AVE). In contrast to assisted suicide, the primary actor in a case of voluntary euthanasia is the doctor or health carer, who intentionally causes the death of the terminally ill person by direct action, such as a lethal injection, at the patient's request. Although euthanasia involves killing, the term tends to be used to refer specifically to killing that is motivated by an intention to relieve the burden of disease of injury.

England: Adams and Cox

Despite the imprisonment of Jack Kevorkian in 1999, doctors are rarely punished for their involvement in assisted death. Back in 1956 an English general practitioner, Dr John Adams, was tried for murder at the Old Bailey. Adams had injected 2.6 grams of heroin and 2.6 grams of morphine into Mrs Morrell, an 81-year-old stroke patient. Adams' case was not helped by massive publicity revealing that, at his encouragement, elderly patients had frequently left him gifts, instead of paying his fees (which attracted heavy rates of tax). Mrs Morrell had, in fact, signed a will leaving Dr Adams a chest containing silver, and Adams had falsified cremation certificates by claiming he was not a beneficiary under her will.[7]

The Adams case is notable for the principle of 'double effect' which emerged from Justice Devlin's summing-up to the jury. This principle, now widely accepted in common law countries,[8] provides that if the doctor's purpose in administering potentially lethal drugs to a terminally ill patient is to relieve pain and distress, such treatment will be lawful, even if it has the incidental or secondary effect of shortening life.[9] Such a principle is vital for the provision of adequate, compassionate palliative care. The jury acquitted Dr Adams of murder, although he was fined heavily for a variety of lesser offences and barred from practising for three years.[10]

While morphine has therapeutic properties which relieve pain and distress, no argument based on 'double effect' was available to Dr Nigel Cox, an English rheumatologist who was convicted of attempted murder on 19 September 1992. Cox's patient was 70-year-old Lillian Boyes, who had suffered acute rheumatoid arthritis for 20 years. Mrs Boyes had 'developed ulcers and abscesses on her arms and legs, a rectal sore penetrating to the bone, fractured vertebrae, deformed hands and feet, swollen joints, and gangrene from steroid treatment'. She 'howled and screamed like a dog' when anyone touched her.[11] Five days before her death, Mrs Boyes pleaded for an injection to end her life. Three days later, Dr Cox wrote in her notes: 'She still wants out and I don't think we can reasonably disagree'. Eventually he injected Mrs Boyes with two ampoules of potassium chloride, and recorded this in the notes. Mrs Boyes died peacefully within minutes; the cause of her death was recorded as bronchopneumonia, and her body was cremated.[12]

The case came to light when a Roman Catholic relief nurse read the notes and reported the matter to hospital authorities, who informed the police. In the absence of a body, and the risk in asking a jury to convict for murder (which carries a mandatory life sentence in Britain), Cox was charged with attempted murder. As Sir Harry Ognall, the presiding judge, later remarked, the principal strength of

an English jury is that it will frequently say 'To hell with the law—
to convict this person would not be fair'.[13] Nevertheless, Justice
Ognall rejected the argument that Cox's intention in injecting lethal
quantities of a drug which lacked any analgesic properties was to
relieve pain, rather than to kill. A distressed and crying jury found
Cox guilty, and Justice Ognall, declaring that Cox had 'betrayed his
unequivocal duty as a physician',[14] imposed a 12 months suspended
prison sentence.

The United States: Quill and Kevorkian

In 1988 the *Journal of the American Medical Association (JAMA)*
published a first-person account of euthanasia by a gynaecology resi-
dent rotating through a large private hospital. The doctor was called
out in the middle of the night to attend a 20-year-old patient who
was dying from ovarian cancer. She had unrelenting vomiting caused
by a sedating alcohol drip, her breathing was laboured, and she had
not eaten or slept in two days. 'It was a gallows scene', the doctor
wrote, 'a cruel mockery of her youth and unfulfilled potential. Her
only words to me were "Let's get this over with"'.[15]

The doctor retreated to the nurses station, reflecting that 'The
patient was tired and needed rest. I could not give her health, but
I could give her rest'.[16] He instructed a nurse to draw up 20 mg of
morphine sulfate, which he injected into the patient. He watched as
the woman relaxed, her breathing rate slowed, then stopped. He
concluded the article: 'It's over, Debbie'.

Publication of this account caused a thunderstorm of protest.[17]
Four medical ethicists wrote: 'This is, by his own account, an impulsive yet cold technician, arrogantly masquerading as a knight of
compassion and humanity'.[18] The *JAMA* editor, defending the charge
that 'he knowingly publicises a felony and shields the felon',[19]
argued that:

> I believed it was time for the euthanasia debate to be held on the pages
> of a peer-reviewed medical journal. Such discussions should not be
> confined to whispers in doctors' dressing rooms and hallways and
> such actions covered up easily because the autopsy has become a
> vanishingly rare procedure in many hospitals, hospices, and nursing
> homes . . .[20]

The *JAMA* editor's hopes for more open and frank debate in the medical literature are slowly being realised. An important contributor to that debate is Timothy Quill. In 1991, as a 41-year-old intern from Rochester, New York, Quill published an article about his leukemia patient, Diane, in the *New England Journal of Medicine*. Diane had refused aggressive treatment, and asked Quill for a prescription of barbiturates to help her to commit suicide. Quill writes:

> I wrote the prescription with an uneasy feeling about the boundaries I was exploring—spiritual, legal, professional and personal. Yet I also felt strongly that I was setting her free to get the most out of the time she had left, and to maintain dignity and control on her own terms until her death.[21]

As agreed, Diane met with Quill one last time before she took her life. 'When we met', he writes,

> it was clear that she knew what she was doing, that she was sad and frightened to be leaving, but that she would be even more terrified to stay and suffer. In our tearful goodbye, she promised a reunion in the future at her favorite spot on the edge of Lake Geneva, with dragons swimming in the sunset.[22]

Two days later, Diane said her final goodbyes to her husband and son, and asked them to leave her alone for an hour. When they returned, they found her dead on the couch, covered in her favourite shawl. Quill certified the cause of death as acute leukemia 'to protect all of us, to protect Diane from an invasion into her past and her body, and to continue to shield society from the knowledge of the degree of suffering that people often undergo in the process of dying'.[23]

Following publication of his article on 'Diane', the Rochester District Attorney declined to prosecute Quill on the basis that without a body, no crime could be proved. However, an anonymous tip later revealed the true identity of 'Diane', and investigators traced her body to a community college, where it had been stored for dissection.[24] Quill appeared before a Grand Jury, which refused to indict him.[25] Assisted by the Seattle-based organisation, 'Compassion in Dying', Quill has since been involved in litigation before the

Supreme Court seeking (unsuccessfully) to overturn a New York State law prohibiting assisted suicide.[26] Elsewhere, Quill and others have also proposed criteria for physician-assisted suicide within the wider context of compassionate palliative care.[27]

Quill's account of Diane's experience was published in order to present an alternative to Kevorkian-style suicides.[28] Quill has emerged as a critic of Kevorkian, observing of the latter that 'suicide is the sole basis for the relationship he has with his patients, and that is frightening'.[29] Quill has critics of his own, including the Catholic ethicist Edmund Pellegrino, who argues that if assisted suicide is legalised, there will be a subtle shift from 'awaiting the patient's decision and readiness, to subtle elicitation of a request for death'.[30]

While Quill continues his practice as a physician in Rochester, Jack Kevorkian is serving a 10–25-year sentence for second-degree murder in a Michigan State prison. Few can be unaware of the cat-and-mouse game that Kevorkian, a retired, Detroit-based pathologist, played with the criminal justice system throughout the 1990s.

Although no stranger to controversy in bioethics debates, Kevorkian's notoriety took a new turn when on 4 June 1990 he drove Janet Adkins, a 54-year-old mother of three with recently diagnosed Alzheimer's disease, to a suburban campsite where she committed suicide in the back of Kevorkian's rusty Volkswagen van.[31] Janet's husband, meanwhile, waited at a nearby hotel. Before this, Kevorkian had scouted south-eastern Michigan in vain for a clinic, church or funeral home which would allow him to supervise suicides on its premises.[32] Adkins had read about Kevorkian in *Newsweek*, and had seen him on television six weeks earlier, discussing his 'suicide machine'. Her suicide troubled Hemlock Society founder Derek Humphry, who said 'It's not death with dignity to have to travel 2,000 miles from home and die in the back of a camper'.[33]

The principle behind Kevorkian's suicide machine was simple. Kevorkian inserted an intravenous line into the patient, connecting this to a saline solution. It was then up to the patient to turn a switch which allowed thiopentone sodium to enter the bloodstream, producing unconsciousness, and, after a short period of time, a lethal solution of potassium chloride.

Kevorkian was charged with first degree murder after Adkins' death,[34] although the charge was dismissed because Michigan did not have, at that time, any law prohibiting assisted suicide.[35] Temporary legislation was enacted in February 1993, but was ignored by Kevorkian, who attended his seventeenth assisted suicide on 4 August 1993, after the new law took effect. On this occasion, Kevorkian picked up Thomas Hyde, a 30-year-old landscaper with Lou Gehrig's disease, drove him into a parking space behind Kevorkian's apartment, and fixed a mask over Hyde's face. Although Lou Gehrig's disease causes the eventual loss of all motor function, Hyde could still move his left hand, which he used to remove a clip, thus starting the flow of carbon monoxide gas.[36] Kevorkian began using carbon monoxide poisoning as a method of achieving suicide after his licence to practise medicine in Michigan was revoked in 1991, thus making it impossible to buy or prescribe the drugs needed for his 'suicide machine'.

When he was charged under the new law for assisting Hyde's suicide, Kevorkian told reporters 'I welcome going to trial. It isn't Kevorkian on trial . . . It's your civilisation and society'.[37]

Kevorkian violated the terms of his bail by assisting in further suicides, vowing to go on a hunger strike if jailed. Patient number 19 was Merian Frederick, a 72-year-old woman with Lou Gehrig's disease. With his Volkswagen van impounded, this suicide took place, for the first time, in Kevorkian's own home. Kevorkian's modest apartment, above a shop selling plaster gargoyles, in a building scheduled for demolition, was less than a block from police headquarters. On the morning of Frederick's death, in a highly publicised episode, Kevorkian ate breakfast at a local pancake house (a single scrambled egg, ham, toast and coffee) while Kevorkian's lawyer, Geoffrey Fieger, told the press 'You may well be looking at his last meal. Jack's going to jail. He will not post bond'.[38]

Kevorkian was charged following Frederick's death, and jailed after refusing to post the $50 000 bond. Acting on his previous threats, Kevorkian began a hunger strike, taking only water, fruit juice and vitamins. 'The gauntlet is down', said Fieger. 'It is ending now. Either this immoral law ends or Dr Kevorkian's life does.'[39]

Nearly three weeks later, Kevorkian walked free after a judge reduced his bail and it was paid by a supporter. While Kevorkian was in jail, Michigan's law banning assisted suicide had been declared unconstitutional, but another judge ruled that Kevorkian must still face trial for his role in Thomas Hyde's suicide.

At the Hyde trial, Kevorkian admitted that he knew about the Michigan statute that made assisted suicide a felony, but added, 'laws like that have been passed throughout history, mainly in the dark ages'.[40] Nevertheless, he relied on an exception in the statute, which exempted procedures which hasten or increase the risk of death, where the intent is to relieve pain and discomfort. Evidence was given that without Kevorkian's intervention, Hyde would have eventually choked to death on his own saliva. Fieger railed at the jury: 'What kind of people would we be that we would treat Thomas Hyde worse than our pets, worse than a dog or cat, lying there begging for mercy with no hope of survival?'[41] Kevorkian, meanwhile, sat in court studying Japanese verbs and mirror writing.[42]

After nine hours of deliberations, the Detroit jury acquitted Kevorkian, citing as their reasons uncertainties over his motive, the wisdom of the Michigan law, and the place of death.[43] Kevorkian opponents claimed that the verdict 'unleashed the floodgates',[44] a Detroit senator claiming that 'Dr Kevorkian will continue his spree, and that makes me nauseous.'[45] Wayne County prosecutor O'Hair said 'I think he's been absolutely lawless, but I credit him with bringing to the forefront this very profound issue that faces society'.[46]

By late 1994, state appeals over the constitutionality of the (now expired) Michigan statute prohibiting assisted suicide had reached the Michigan Supreme Court. The court held that the statute did not infringe the Constitution, and that in addition, assisted suicide could be prosecuted in the absence of a statute, as a common law felony.[47] Kevorkian responded at a news conference: 'This is a perfect, clear manifestation of the existence of the Inquisition in this state, no different from the medieval one. That may sound melodramatic, but it is true'.[48]

Charges that Kevorkian had committed a common law felony by assisting suicides reached trial in May 1996. It was Kevorkian's third trial. Donning a white wig, tricorner hat, blue britches, gold brocade coat and buckle shoes, Kevorkian declared, 'It's silly to have modern dress when you're dealing with ancient jurisprudence'.[49] He was acquitted of the charges, having assisted in his 28th suicide between sessions in the witness stand.[50]

By late 1998 Kevorkian had admitted to presiding over 130 suicides. He had been acquitted of criminal charges by a jury on three occasions. In another case the jury was discharged after failing to reach a verdict.

Things took a different turn, however, on 22 November 1998, when '60 Minutes' broadcast a videotape of Kevorkian injecting 52-year-old Thomas Youk, a patient with Lou Gehrig's disease, at Youk's home in a suburb of Detroit. Kevorkian had chosen to intensify the debate by video-taping himself administering a lethal injection, in contrast to his usual practice of assisting the patient to suicide in private. 'They must charge me', Kevorkian told '60 Minutes'. 'Because if they do not, that means they don't think it was a crime'.[51]

Three days later, Kevorkian was charged with first degree murder. At the trial in March 1999 he ignored advice and acted as his own lawyer. When cautioned by Judge Jessica Cooper that he could face a prison term for the rest of his life, Kevorkian replied, 'There's not that much of it left, Your Honor'.[52] 'He seems to yearn for martyrdom', commented the *New York Times*,[53] as Kevorkian's legal advisers, stranded at the bar table, tried desperately to attract his attention, and Judge Cooper repeatedly disallowed his questions and arguments.

'Jack Kevorkian murdered Thomas Youk', the prosecutor, John Skrzynski told the jury. He came 'like a medical hit man in the night with his bag of poison'.[54] That was not the way Thomas Youk's brother saw things, commenting, after the trial had ended, that Thomas was 'caught in hell', with spasms of choking on his own saliva.[55]

'Do you see a murderer?' Kevorkian asked the jury, in a theatrical closing argument. 'If you do then you must convict. And then take the harsh judgment of history or the harsher judgment of your children and grandchildren if they ever come to need that precious choice'.[56]

On 26 March 1999 the jury returned a verdict of second degree murder, which carries a recommended minimum sentence of 10 to 25 years in prison.[57] Judge Jessica Cooper's remarks in sentencing Kevorkian were broadcast around the world. 'This trial was not about the political or moral correctness of euthanasia', she said. 'It was about you, sir. It was about lawlessness. You had the audacity to go on national television, show the world what you did and dare the legal system to stop you. Well, sir, consider yourself stopped.'[58]

More than anyone else, Kevorkian has brought medically-assisted suicide into the American public arena. According to his friend, Dr Stanley Levy, 'He is the only one to do it, because the medical profession won't. The profession's response is the hospice system. It says "You can die, but you have to take your time doing it" '.[59]

Kevorkian will be 79 by the time he becomes eligible for parole in May 2007.

Australia: Nitschke, Syme, and the 'Melbourne 7'

Australia, like other western democracies, has its share of media savvy, dissident doctors. One of the 'Melbourne 7', respected urologist Rodney Syme, has detailed a quiet history of euthanasia spanning more than twenty years.[60] Others, such as Melbourne general practitioners Darren Russell and Norm Roth, have advocated euthanasia as an option for people living with AIDS. AIDS GP Jonathan Anderson made front-page news with his admissions of euthanasia, but 'without a body' he remains safe from prosecution.[61] There has been a constant trickle of similar admissions in recent years.

In March 1997 federal legislation introduced by a Catholic Parliamentarian, Kevin Andrews, overturned the Northern Territory's *Rights of the Terminally Ill Act*, which had been in force since 1 July 1996. With euthanasia once again illegal, Australian right to die campaigners have used a variety of tactics to keep euthanasia on the public agenda. Philip Nitschke, the Darwin doctor who presided over all four of the legal euthanasia deaths under the Territory legislation, has achieved the highest media profile. In some ways Nitschke is Australia's answer to Jack Kevorkian. He has risked all for the euthanasia cause: career, reputation and income.

Within days of famously burning the Andrews legislation outside Parliament House in Canberra at 2 a.m., following news of its successful passage through the Senate, Nitschke announced his support for a national register of doctors and nurses prepared to perform euthanasia.[62] Two weeks later, in April 1997, he put palliative care practices to the test by announcing that he had provided coma-inducing drugs to a patient who died after four days of 'pharmacological oblivion'.[63] A month later he announced that he was building a prototype coma machine to assist the terminally ill to achieve terminal sedation. The machine monitors the patient's brain activity to a constant drug infusion of morphine and a sedative (midazolam), in order to keep the patient permanently unconscious.[64] In September 1997 Nitschke announced that he was working on a machine that would assist a patient to die by carbon dioxide narcosis, using a gas mask attached to a plastic bag.[65] Similar devices are also being used by North American activists.[66] 'The Andrews Bill forced us back into the jungle and this is the sort of behaviour you'll see', Nitschke told a reporter.[67]

In 1998 Nitschke moved to Melbourne to stand against his nemesis, Kevin Andrews, in federal elections. While the attempt was always doomed, Nitschke secured 9.3 per cent of the primary vote, forcing the seat to preferences.[68]

In November 1998, as Americans watched Jack Kevorkian inject Thomas Youk on "60 Minutes", Nitschke revealed that he had helped fifteen patients to die in the twenty months since the Territory legislation was overturned.[69] More recently, Nitschke has opened advice clinics in Sydney, Melbourne and other state capitals, flying between cities and offering advice to people referred to him through voluntary euthanasia societies.[70] In May 2000 Nitschke was reported to be seeking legal advice over the possibility of a 'death ship' for carrying out euthanasia in international waters.[71] In November 2000 Nitschke's Voluntary Euthanasia Research Foundation announced the setting up of a laboratory in the Northern Territory, which would provide substance analysis of old prescription drugs and poisonous plants, together with advice about their potency for euthanasia purposes.[72] In January 2001 Nitschke was again in the news when a cancer patient under his care, who had initially tried to starve herself to death, overdosed on sedatives and liquid morphine.[73]

Nitschke faces ongoing opposition from the medical establishment. The Australian Medical Association wants him deregistered, and has lodged complaints to the Victorian Medical Practitioners Board. Nitschke admits that he fears entrapment by a patient. 'I'm careful and I don't want to expose myself to untoward hazards and difficulties', he says, 'but at some stage I have to stand up and be counted'.[74]

It is not every doctor who assists a terminally ill patient to die who achieves notoriety or celebrity status. When doctors kill, they usually do so quietly and discreetly. Euthanasia bubbles away beneath the surface, erupting into the public arena only when doctors (or others) are 'caught' transgressing key legal boundaries,[75] or when they grow tired of the deception, and go public in a blaze of martyr-dom. Euthanasia is not an isolated breakdown in medical self-discipline; it is a worldwide phenomenon, at least in western democracies where technology can prolong both dying and the pain of living, and where the ethic of libertarianism gives moral substance to patient demands for swift release.

3

Voices in the euthanasia debate

I've got the hardest selling job in America.[1]
Derek Humphry, author of *Final Exit* and right to die advocate

I give up the fight: let there be an end,
A privacy, an obscure nook for me,
I want to be forgotten even by God.

Robert Browning

What has happened to the sanctity of life ethic, that it can now be challenged so publicly, in many cases with apparent impunity, and broad community support? There is, after all, something heartwarming in the idea that all human life is equally and intrinsically precious, regardless of its value as perceived by others. The sanctity of human life ethic of the Judeo-Christian tradition, with its prohibition on intentional killing, has been central to the moral foundations of society for many centuries. Although far from secure in the face of religious persecution, ethnic cleansing, capital punishment and war, its presence has nevertheless been profoundly civilising. In the words of one New Zealand judge, the preservation of life is an ideal 'which not only is of inherent merit in commanding respect for the worth and dignity of the individual but [it] also exemplifies all the finer virtues which are the mark of a civilised order'.[2] In affirming the sanctity of all human life, we save the old and the feeble, the disabled and deformed, the ugly and the strange. By affirming life for all, we affirm the value and meaning of our own lives and our common humanity.

But times are changing. Legislatures are beginning to experiment with compassionate killing, and vocal 'celebrity doctors' are leading a passionate public debate. Even so, the process is complex and far from complete. Right to die campaigners have a long way to go. In Australia the Northern Territory's *Rights of the Terminally Ill Act* (1995) was overturned by federal legislation, while in the United States Oregon's assisted suicide statute may face ongoing attack in Congress.

Rather than seeking to provide any overarching review of the social forces behind the assisted death movement,[3] this chapter will focus on some of the most prominent 'voices', and issues, present in the euthanasia debate. It will then consider the impact of AIDS on euthanasia advocacy.

Why now?

Why is the euthanasia debate placing so much pressure on the sanctity of life ethic now, when the Hippocratic injunction against taking life has been a central feature of medical ethics since 400 BC? One contributor to the *Age* argues that

> The debate is about the limits of individual freedoms and the political power of the Baby Boomers, now at the age when they are beginning to contemplate their mortality. It's about an ageing population and a limited health dollar. It's about an increasingly educated population losing its awe of the medical profession. And it provides an intriguing look at religion in a secular society.[4]

Central to the mindset that fuels euthanasia advocacy is the emerging ethic of 'liberal individualism'. According to Professor Margaret Somerville,

> We are now societies based on intense individualism—possibly individualism to the exclusion of any real sense of community, including in situations facing death and bereavement . . . Matters such as euthanasia, that would have been largely the subject of moral or religious

discourse are now explored in our courts and legislatures, particularly through the concepts of individual human rights, civil rights and constitutional rights.[5]

One should also mention the declining influence of the churches in shaping social policy. Those with a tradition of hierarchical authority, as well as the fundamentalist churches, maintain that euthanasia, like suicide, 'represents a rejection of God's absolute sovereignty over life and death'.[6] But regardless of religious belief, many opponents of legalised euthanasia are simply more 'communitarian' in outlook, believing that individual freedoms and interests should be tempered by communal values, social goals, and traditional constraints.[7] Euthanasia, in contrast, is atomistic in its philosophy, an affirmation of individual moral freedom in a world lacking moral absolutes.

The euthanasia debate can also be seen as a reaction against the technological determinism and bureaucratic processes which characterise modern medicine. Drugs and medical machinery have enabled us to procrastinate our death. At the same time, many feel that the life thereby 'saved'—frequently endured without privacy in the goldfish bowl of the hospital ward—violates their dignity and tramples over the values that have characterised their entire lives.

Margaret Battin argues that, increasingly, and for the first time in human history, the majority of people in western societies are dying from diseases which are characterised by an 'extended deteriorative decline'. The predictability of this downhill road is having an important cultural effect, focusing attention on how we die, and the norms that surround the death process.[8] This is particularly true of AIDS, which shares the deteriorative decline, yet is unique among recent illnesses in its capacity to decimate young and healthy populations (in western societies, mostly men) in a way not seen since medicine arrested the typical killers of past centuries: typhoid, tuberculosis and smallpox.

Not everyone, of course, accepts that euthanasia advocacy is a response to declining church influence, an expression of rising individualism, a reaction against the impersonal, biology-driven achievements of modern medicine, nor the epidemiology of death in the twentieth and early twenty-first centuries. Some see the push for euthanasia primarily as a symptom of the failure of doctors to communicate with their patients, their failure to respect patient choice and to discontinue treatment when it is futile, and their failure to practise good palliative care.[9] Others point to the ageing population, and economic pressures to free up hospital beds.[10]

Who's being heard in the euthanasia debate?

The public

Although there are vocal and influential opponents of euthanasia, Australian opinion polls have repeatedly confirmed broad community support for voluntary euthanasia legislation. A 1996 poll showed 75 per cent support for legalised euthanasia, although there was less support for, specifically, lethal injections (63 per cent).[11]

A review of United States polls presents a similar picture. Majority support for legalising medically assisted death has existed since 1973 (53 per cent), rising to 60 per cent in 1977, and 63 per cent in 1991.[12] A 1996 Gallup poll reported 75 per cent in favour of lawful, medically assisted death.[13]

Poll results should, of course, be taken with a grain of salt. Attitudes towards assisted death are complex, and little of this subtlety is captured in opinion polls. Surveys have tended to quantify public attitudes towards assisted dying in an abstract, depersonalised way. As Ho points out, approval levels may vary according to whether respondents have themselves in mind, a significant other, or a hypothetical third person. The nature of the euthanasia (active, passive, voluntary, involuntary), and the nature of the suffering justifying intervention (pain, debilitated body, stress caused to family), are all important variables influencing opinion.[14] It is also possible that significant differences may exist between the opinions of the well public on the one hand and sick patients and their families on the other.[15] Quantifying levels of support for assisted death among sick populations would be an interesting exercise in view of the concerns expressed by opponents of assisted death that legalisation would be used to the detriment of the sick and vulnerable.

The medical profession

While levels of support for legalised euthanasia within the medical profession do not approach those of the general community,[16] Australian studies nevertheless show majority support. For example, Baume and O'Malley's 1994 study of 1268 doctors in New South

Wales and the Australian Capital Territory reported that 46 per cent of respondents had been asked by a patient to hasten his or her death. Twenty-eight per cent (12.3 per cent of all respondents) had complied with the request. Fifty-nine per cent agreed in principle that active euthanasia is sometimes right, and 58 per cent called for legal change.[17] Table 3-1 summarises the major Australian studies quantifying levels of involvement in assisted death.

Table 3-1: Health care workers' attitudes to active voluntary euthanasia: selected Australian studies

Study	In-principle support	Compliance with patient requests	Law reform
Kuhse & Singer: 869 Victorian doctors (1988) Sample: 1893 (46% response rate)	It is sometimes right for a doctor to take active steps to end a patient's life at the patient's request: 62% to 34% in favour	40% of doctors (354) asked by patient to hasten death; 29% (107) of 369 doctors had taken active steps to end a patient's life	60% to 37% in favour of pro-euthanasia law reform
Kuhse & Singer: 951 Victorian nurses (1992) Sample: 1942 (49% response rate)	75% to 25% in favour of Australia adopting the Netherlands situation permitting active voluntary euthanasia in certain circumstances	55% of nurses (502) asked by patient to hasten death, 333 nurses received requests for direct assistance; 5% (of 333) took active steps to hasten death without a doctor's request; 25% (of 502) were requested by a doctor to take active measures to end a patient's life and 85% of this number complied	78% of respondents in favour of pro-euthanasia law reform
Stevens & Hassan: 298 South Australian doctors (1994) Sample: 494 (60% usable returns)	Is it ever right to bring about the death of a patient by active steps? 18% said yes, 26% said yes, but only if requested by the patient	33% of doctors asked by patient to hasten death by taking active steps; 19% (56) had complied with the request	45% in favour of legalisation of active euthanasia (39% opposed)

Table 3-1 (cont'd)

Study	In-principle support	Compliance with patient requests	Law reform
Baume & O'Malley: 1268 New South Wales and ACT doctors (1994) Sample: 1667 (76% response rate)	59% agreement that it is sometimes right for a doctor to take active steps to bring about a patient's death	46.4% of doctors asked by patient to hasten death; of those asked, 28% had complied with the request (12.3% overall); 7% had provided the means for suicide	58% in favour of changing the law to permit active voluntary euthanasia
Steinberg, Najman, Cartwright: 159 Qld general practitioners (1997) Sample: 387 (67% response rate)	52% did not agree that active euthanasia would undermine trust between doctor and patient; 48% agreed	43% of doctors had been asked by patients to administer something to end their life	33% favoured law reform to allow active voluntary euthanasia; 36% favoured a law allowing physician-assisted suicide

These studies illustrate the comprehensive fragmentation of attitudes towards euthanasia within the Australian medical profession.[18] A significant proportion of the medical profession has participated, illegally, in assisted death, and presumably will continue to do so.

Similar, if more modest, themes emerge from studies in the United States. A national survey of 1902 American physicians published in 1998 found that 3.3 per cent had written at least one 'lethal prescription', while 4.7 per cent had provided at least one lethal injection.[19] Eleven per cent of physicians agreed that there were circumstances in which they would be prepared to (illegally) prescribe medication to assist a patient to suicide, and 36 per cent would do so if it were legal. Seven per cent were prepared to (illegally) give a lethal injection, and 24 per cent would do so if it were legal. Table 3-2 summarises the findings from other major American studies.

Levels of involvement may be higher in certain specialties. A 1992 study of San Francisco physicians specialising in AIDS reported that almost a quarter of respondents would be prepared to prescribe a lethal dose of medication to a competent terminally ill

Table 3-2: Physicians' attitudes to assisted suicide and active voluntary euthanasia: selected American studies

Study	Willingness to assist	Compliance with patient requests	Attitudes towards law reform
Meier, Emmons, Wallenstein et al. (1998, national survey: 1902 physicians from 10 specialties) Sample: 3102 (61% response rate)	11% would be prepared to (illegally) prescribe medication to assist a suicide; 36% would do so if it were legal 7% would be prepared to (illegally) give a lethal injection; 24% would do so if it were legal.	18.3% (320) had received requests for medication to assist in suicide; 16% (of 320) had written a 'lethal prescription' (3.3% of sample) 11.1% (196) had received a request for a lethal injection; 4.7% of sample (59) had given at least 1 lethal injection	
Lee, Nelson, Tilden et al (1996: 2761 Oregon physicians). Sample: 3944 (70% response rate)	46% (1257) would be prepared to prescribe a lethal dose of medication to assist a suicide if it were legal; 52% would not be willing	21% (570) had received a request for a prescription for a lethal dose of medication within the past year; 7% (187) had written a 'lethal prescription'	60% believed that physician-assisted suicide should be legal in some cases
Bachman, Alcser, Doukas et al (1996: 1119 Michigan physicians) Sample: 1518 (74% response rate)	If physician-assisted suicide were legal, 35% willing to participate if asked; 22% willing to participate in either PAS or active euthanasia; 13% only in PAS; 52% would participate in neither		40% favoured the legalisation of physician-assisted suicide; 37% preferred no law (no government regulation); 17% favoured prohibition
Doukas, Waterhouse, Gorenflo et al (1995: 154 Michigan oncologists)		38% had been asked to provide assistance in suicide; 18% had provided assistance. 43% had been asked	21% favoured the legalisation of physician-assisted death; 44% were unsure, and 35%

Table 3-2 (cont'd)

Study	Willingness to assist	Compliance with patient requests	Attitudes towards law reform
Sample: 250 (62% response rate)		to administer medication to cause the patient's death; 4% had done so	opposed legalisation
Slome, Mitchell, Charlebois (1997: 118 San Francisco AIDS physicians)	48% would be likely to assist an AIDS patient to suicide, based on a case vignette	53% had assisted a patient to suicide at least once (mean number of times: 4.2)	
Sample: 228 (52% response rate)			

patient with AIDS.[20] In 1997 Slome and colleagues reported that a majority of respondents drawn from a network of San Francisco HIV/AIDS specialists had, *in fact*, assisted a patient to suicide by prescribing a lethal overdose, although the response rate was low (52 per cent).[21] Similarly, in Australia, a 1995 survey of members of the Australasian Society for HIV Medicine (ASHM) reported that nearly one in five doctors had helped an HIV patient to die, responding to 52 per cent of patient requests for assistance.[22]

The fragmentation of medical attitudes towards euthanasia has been obscured by the conservative stance of professional bodies such as the Australian Medical Association, and the American Medical Association, which are perceived to speak for the profession as a whole. Professional bodies are influential in the euthanasia debate, due to their representative status, and the 'sovereignty' or influence they seek to exercise over issues of health policy and ethics.

The 'neutrality' of the Oregon Medical Association, in the lead-up to the 1994 referendum over Oregon's *Death with Dignity Act* split the traditional alliance between the profession and churches against assisted death, and was a key factor in the success of a referendum to legalise physician-assisted suicide in that State.[23] The church/profession alliance, which held strong in earlier referendums in Washington State (1991) and California (1992), provides an impressive defence against law reform efforts, even where polls show high levels of popular support for change. Churches and doctors' groups have access to the media, captive audiences in parishioners and patients, and an 'hierarchial structure from which campaign rhetoric [can] flow freely to potential voters' [and legislators].[24]

Issues in the medical debate

Part of the opposition to pro-euthanasia law reform is the assertion that palliative care can adequately relieve pain and distress, thereby obviating the need for a 'euthanasia escape route'. Baume and O'Malley argue that the levels of participation in assisted death revealed in their 1994 survey suggest 'a substantial level of need among patients for symptom relief which current arrangements do not provide'.[25] Palliative care specialists, on the other hand, are keen to draw attention to the successes achieved by their speciality, and regard much of the impetus for euthanasia reform as based upon lack of information and ignorance of these achievements.[26] The assumptions of the 'palliative care model'—which may require the relentless, round-the-clock ministrations of a multidisciplinary team—have in turn been questioned.[27]

Even if one assumes that doctors *are* seriously ignorant of advances in palliative care, debate nevertheless persists over the ethics and the implications of these same comfort-care techniques. The use of sedation to induce a coma in a distressed and dying patient (a practice sometimes called 'pharmacological oblivion', or 'terminal sedation') has been widely acknowledged in the literature, provoking debate over whether the practice is medically indicated, or ethically justifiable.[28] Any distinction between coma-inducing sedation, and the intentional hastening of death, becomes increasingly blurred when intravenous feeding and hydration are withheld from the comatose patient.[29] Opponents of euthanasia face the challenge that terminal sedation is 'slow euthanasia',[30] and that evidence of its practice illustrates the limitations of 'orthodox' palliative care in responding to suffering. The latter issue was nicely put by Robert, an AIDS physician interviewed in this study, who observed, 'If palliation includes rendering the patient unconscious, *it always works*'.

Pro-euthanasia campaigner Mr Rodney Syme argues that 'for some patients sedation may be an appropriate alternative . . . It certainly protects the conscience of the doctors and provides immunity from the law. But in my view it is a crude exercise in medical futility'.[31] Admittedly, Syme's view ignores the strongly-felt emotional and moral distinction that physicians, and the public, draw between killing people, and letting them die.[32] But while some take comfort in the time lag in 'terminal sedation', Syme sees a procedure marked by 'futility, inefficiency, hypocrisy, and dishonesty'.[33]

While sedation can dull pain, pain is only one of many issues motivating requests for assisted death. Adelaide palliative care specialist Dr Roger Hunt, who has 'broken ranks' with his speciality, argues:

> But what can be done for those patients who have unresolvable pain? And what about common problems such as weakness, loss of independence, incontinence, loss of dignity and a sense of meaninglessness due to a progressively diminishing quality of life? Such problems cannot be eliminated by palliative care teams.[34]

Conceding that palliative care has its limitations, other specialists are concerned that killing patients provides an easy answer to complex clinical challenges, undermines medical skills, retards medical progress, and may encourage the under-funding of palliative care services.[35] The 'easy marriage between respect for autonomy' and 'the need for greater cost-containment' is an alarming prospect.[36] Many would be concerned at comments made by the United States Court of Appeal for the 9th Circuit, which conceded: 'We are reluctant to say that, in a society in which the costs of protracted health care can be so exorbitant, it is improper for competent, terminally ill adults to take the economic welfare of their families and loved ones into consideration'.[37] Nevertheless, the resources to eradicate economic incentives for euthanasia are as remote as ever. The United States, in particular, lacks a comprehensive and publicly funded health insurance system. Where adequate palliative care is unaffordable, should doctors ignore the suffering of their patients, in the vain hope that politicians will listen?

The churches

According to Anderson and Caddell, religious opposition to euthanasia, particularly from conservative churches within the Judeo-Christian tradition, focuses around three ideas: resistance to playing God, 'Thou Shalt Not Kill', and the potential spiritual benefits of suffering.[38] The Northern Territory's *Rights of the Terminally Ill Act*, for example, was condemned both by the Vatican[39] and the Australian Catholic Bishops Conference, the latter reminding parishioners that while 'there is no virtue in suffering for its own sake . . . the experience of death is a profoundly Christian experience when we go to meet God at the moment when God chooses to call us'.[40] Catholic opposition to euthanasia also includes 'secular' arguments about the effect of euthanasia upon the provision of palliative care, and the danger of the 'slippery slope' caused by the weakening of the sanctity of life ethic.

In their 1988 study of Victorian doctors, Kuhse and Singer found that of the 62 per cent of respondents supporting, in principle, active voluntary euthanasia, Roman Catholics were the only group not to give majority support.[41] In their 1995 study, Baume, O'Malley and Bauman also reported that Catholic practitioners were most opposed to active voluntary euthanasia (AVE) and physician-assisted suicide (PAS), agnostic/atheist practitioners were most sympathetic, and Protestant practitioners fell midway in between.[42] Similar themes emerge from studies of American doctors.[43] Interestingly, Baume and colleagues found that 'non-theists' were more than twice as likely to know of other doctors who practised AVE, and were more than three times more likely to think AVE to be sometimes right, compared to 'theist' practitioners'.[44]

American research confirms that individual attitudes towards euthanasia correlate with religious affiliation. Caddell and Newton's 1995 study found conservative Protestants and Catholics least supportive of active euthanasia, with higher levels of support amongst liberal Protestants, Jews and those with no religious affiliation (63 per cent support overall).[45]

Similarly, in a study of attitudes of members of the Hemlock Society, and the California Pro-Life Council (CPLC), Holden confirmed that 'Christian religious training most influenced opposition to euthanasia, whereas death-proximate experiences most influenced approval of euthanasia'.[46] 'The largest proportion of the CPLC members identified themselves as Catholic and as believers in a consequential afterlife, whereas the largest proportion of Hemlock respondents described themselves as atheist/agnostic and as not believing in an afterlife.'[47]

Religion makes sparks fly in the euthanasia debate. The perception that churches are attempting to impose their doctrinal beliefs upon a pluralist society remains a source of criticism.[48] In Australia, Melbourne's Archbishop expressed the Catholic view as follows:

> Does our society want the healing profession to become a killing profession? . . . To kill a dying patient is the ultimate abandonment, an irrevocable statement that you will not share their passion any longer, that you are not compassionate . . . I believe our humanity will be seriously eroded if our response to weakness, suffering and the process of dying is euthanasia, that other name for the crime of homicide.[49]

Mr Rodney Syme, one of the 'Melbourne 7', responds:

> The Catholic Church argues much about intent—the intent of the doctor—but ignores the consent of the patient and the motive of the doctor. The primary intention of a doctor in assisting suicide for terminal suffering is to relieve that pain and suffering, but also recognises that in certain circumstances, this can only finally occur by death. The doctor's motive is pure, based on compassion not, as in homicide, on greed or hate or revenge.[50]

Other critics save their harshest words for the theological underpinnings of religious opposition. Faust quips that '[absolutist] religions don't like euthanasia because it might lead to free will'.[51] Tallis notes that 'only those theologians who believe that there are more important things than human happiness feel that the dying should earn their death the hard way and go the whole distance along the tunnel of barbed wire'. He adds that one cannot feel safe at the hands of those for whom, after all, 'excruciating pains have a deep and inalienable meaning as the "kisses of Christ"'.[52]

Church opposition to euthanasia cannot simply be dismissed on grounds of theology. A recurrent 'secular' concern is the 'slippery slope' argument, or fear that 'if voluntary euthanasia was permitted, it would not stay voluntary for very long'.[53] In its most extreme form, this 'thin end-of-the-wedge' argument is a charge levelled at doctors who would become uncontrollable 'rambo-types', 'prone to a lust for killing that could end in a Nazi-like holocaust'.[54] One of the more measured slippery slope theorists is Robert Manne, who argues:

For anyone who understands social process the expansion of the circle of those who can be killed will come as no surprise. For once we agree to the principle of doctors performing voluntary euthanasia by what effort of societal will, on what rock of ethical principle, can we resist its extension to ever new categories of sufferers? There is no such will: no such fixed and reliable principle . . . The slippery slope . . . involves a subtle transformation of ethical sensibility. Over time we become blind to how we once thought.[55]

Manne neglects to mention that the law has already significantly watered down the sanctity of life ethic (see Chapter 4). He is probably right, however, to argue that legalisation may influence our moral perceptions. Euthanasia is new ethics. Legalising it *will* change norms and values. Euthanasia reflects a shifting of moral weight from the sanctity of life ethic, which protects longevity by prohibiting intentional killing, towards a liberal, individualistic ethic which focuses on individual perceptions of quality of life. Charlesworth argues, however, that 'we are on a slippery slope only when we move away from seeing the decision to end one's life as a moral decision belonging to the individual patient, and as being grounded in the patient's right to moral autonomy'.[56]

The slippery slope argument, as advanced by moral conservatives, serves an important function. It focuses attention upon the bedrock values of society, and upon the subtle changes that have crept up on us over decades. It challenges euthanasia advocates to articulate stable boundaries for the right to die. On the other hand, to assert a slippery slope is not to demonstrate the preconditions for Auschwitz. The social preconditions to communal moral deterioration are worth studying but, as Burgess points out, slippery slope theorists bear the burden of proof and must put forward a detailed case.[57]

Politicians

In Westminster-style democracies whose Constitutions lack substantive rights guarantees, such as Australia, the prospect of euthanasia law reform is remote in the absence of legislative change. This is in contrast to the United States, where law reform has been pursued through private challenges to the constitutionality of legislation criminalising physician-assisted suicide, as well as through citizen-initiated referendums.

Within a parliamentary context, the reform process relies not only on broad public support, and successful advocacy by major players in the political debate, but also on parliamentary facilitators. This creates problems, for pro-euthanasia measures are too divisive to be embraced by the major parties; and for a law reform Bill to succeed on a conscience vote requires advocates to do battle with the consciences and re-election aspirations of every member.

In the Northern Territory the passage of the *Rights of the Terminally Ill Act* was largely due to the hard work and personal commitment of the former Chief Minister, Marshall Perron, whose private member's bill was backed by a considerable degree of personal influence. On the other hand, Australian Prime Minister John Howard and Opposition Leader Kim Beasley were both known to support the federal Andrews Bill which overturned the Territory legislation in 1997. Although the Andrews Bill attracted a conscience vote, federal politicians were savvy enough to know that, come election time, they risked losing more from the vocal minority (the Catholics and moral conservatives who were vehemently opposed to euthanasia) than they did from the majority whose support was, by contrast, muted.[58]

Right to die societies

The right to die movement has become a well organised machine. There are voluntary euthanasia societies in many countries, many of which are also members of the international federation of right to die societies.[59] Although the mostly older-aged volunteers who make up these societies are no match for the churches in terms of membership and financial muscle, individual societies such as the US-based Compassion in Dying,[60] and the Hemlock Society,[61] have achieved good media access, and have funded constitutional challenges to anti-assisted suicide statutes.

More recently, as Ogden points out, 'some proponents within the right-to-die social movement . . . have adopted an entrepreneurial approach, rejecting the notion that physicians need to be involved in assisted death'.[62] This was evident, for example, at a conference held in Seattle in November 1999, where twenty-eight right to die advocates from six countries met behind closed doors to share recent developments in 'deathing' technologies, including the 'Debreather' and 'Exit Bag'.[63] These devices, which have already undergone 'clinical trials', cause death from lack of oxygen. The 'Debreather', for example, is a 'modified piece of sea-diving equipment':[64] the 'client' re-breathes their own air, while the device removes the carbon dioxide in order to make the process more comfortable. In an era of legislative intransigence, these devices may represent the future of the right to die. The 'deathing' process is simple, painless, inexpensive, demedicalised, and impossible to police.

The media

Here, as elsewhere, the power of the media in defining, promoting and influencing the euthanasia debate is unrivalled. As discussed in Chapter 2, the media have nurtured the careers of a class of celebrity law-breakers, dissident doctors who openly flout the law. Somerville notes that 'we are . . . media societies. We are the first age in which our collective story-telling takes place through television. A terminally ill person, begging for euthanasia, makes emotionally gripping television'.[65]

The impact of AIDS on euthanasia advocacy

Since its appearance in the mainstream press in late 1981 AIDS has exercised the public imagination like few other diseases.[66] Twenty years into the epidemic, AIDS remains the disease that most justifies the right to die.

AIDS: the medical impact

HIV, the virus which causes AIDS, weakens the body's immune resistance, causing normally containable illnesses such as tuberculosis to be virtually untreatable. In the late 1980s and early 1990s diseases such as Pneumocystis Carinii Pneumonia (PCP), Kaposi's Sarcoma, and Cytomegalovirus (CMV) entered mainstream vocabulary as major AIDS-defining illnesses. Many of the interviewees in this study began their euthanasia careers in response to these conditions.

In western countries, however, with the arrival of AZT and other first generation (antiretroviral) drugs, these diseases are no longer the primary cause of death in AIDS. The availability of

protease inhibitors from the mid-1990s, and their use in combination with antiretrovirals, has been highly successful in reducing
viral load. This has fuelled tremendous optimism that HIV will ultimately become a chronic, but manageable, infection. Nevertheless,
toxicity issues remain a threat; combination therapy does not always
work for patients who have developed resistance to the earlier drugs;
and some still suffer debilitating side effects, including nausea and
diarrhoea. AIDS continues to manifest itself in chronic wasting
syndromes, lymphatic cancers, AIDS-related dementia, cryptococcal
meningitis and other infections involving the central nervous
system.[67]

As a spectrum of infections which frequently require hospitalis-
ation, yet rarely kill straight away, AIDS produces a fluctuating and
highly uncertain terminal phase. The form that future illness will
take is unknown: AIDS is a lottery.

AIDS: the social impact

While the irrational fear and punitive social responses to it appear to
have diminished in recent years, AIDS remains a highly stigmatised
condition. The psychosocial impact of living with AIDS is enormous, and may result in financial problems, discrimination and loss
of privacy.[68]

Within the gay community, which still bears the burden of HIV
in 'Pattern I' countries including Australia and the United States, the
burden of AIDS and its 20-year legacy of communal grief must be
understood within the context of a culture of body-consciousness
and hedonism, within a community revitalised through the 1970s,
and finding a political voice. The physical stigmata of AIDS were the
antithesis of tolerance and new-found freedom. As Sontag wrote in
a well-known passage:

> . . . to get AIDS is precisely to be revealed, in the majority of cases so
> far, as a member of a certain 'risk group', a community of pariahs.
> The illness flushes out an identity that might have remained hidden
> from neighbors, job-mates, family, friends. It also confirms an identity
> and, among the risk group in the United States most severely affected
> in the beginning, homosexual men, has been a creator of community
> as well as an experience that isolates the ill and exposes them to
> harassment and persecution.[69]

Similarly, as Justice Michael Kirby of the Australian High Court observes, 'the connection with blood, sex and death presents a metaphor which is vividly etched upon the consciousness of society. If cancer is a predicament causing death which has to be whispered, HIV/AIDS is all too often the condition that dares not speak its name'.[70] Patients may conceal their illness from family, friends and even sexual partners. If one factors in the issues of guilt and unresolved sexuality that arise in some cases, one begins to glimpse the immensely problematic context of AIDS-related euthanasia.

The medical realities and the social construction of AIDS, while perhaps enough to distinguish AIDS from other diseases, do not entirely explain the legitimating effect which AIDS has had on the push for euthanasia reform. Seale and Addington-Hall note that pro-euthanasia advocacy has been associated with 'modern, urban cultural conditions'; the AIDS community, in turn, is predominantly urban, young, male and liberal or non-religious.[71] It follows that the philosophical preconditions to pro-euthanasia attitudes are more likely to be present in the HIV/AIDS community. Many of those with HIV, or at higher risk of contracting it, are gay, educated, articulate, and come from an activist community capable of pursuing this aspect of patient self-determination with a zeal similar to that with which other gay and HIV patient issues have been pursued.

Research suggests a high level of support for the option of euthanasia within the HIV community. In a 1993 Sydney study by Tindall and others, 90 per cent of men with AIDS indicated that they would personally wish to have the option of euthanasia if a life-threatening diagnosis were made. Interestingly, 86 per cent of the 105 subjects stated that they were afraid of suffering, but only 19 per cent feared death itself.[72]

Studies also confirm that euthanasia is practised to a significant degree within the HIV/AIDS community. In a 1998 San Francisco study of the involvement of informal care givers in assisted death, 12 per cent of a sample of deaths investigated were found to have been intentionally hastened by the patient or care giver through administration of narcotics or sedatives.[73] Similarly, in a Dutch study of homosexual men with AIDS, 22 per cent were found to have died through assisted suicide or euthanasia, 12 times the national euthanasia rate of 2.1 per cent.[74] In the United States Battin claims that physician-assisted suicide is 'so widely accepted that it is virtually legal . . . among people with AIDS in the gay communities of the US west coast'.[75] This observation is consistent with Ogden's pioneering study of euthanasia within the HIV community in Vancouver, Canada (1994),[76] and my own San Francisco interviews.

It is difficult to predict the future of AIDS-related assisted death. The hope is that demand for assistance will diminish with the success of protease inhibitors. But not everyone is so optimistic. Russell, a hospital physician interviewed in this study, fears that in the 'protease inhibitor world', people will die instead of 'non-traditional' HIV-related illnesses. He tells of a friend with HIV who had 'zero viral load' but who died rapidly, in extreme pain, from a previously-rare fungal infection that expanded through his sinuses into the brain. He had 'tubes running into his brain', infused with antibiotic. It was 'horrendous torture', 'disfiguring', 'demoralising', and the pain was 'over-riding'.

While patients will live longer and more comfortably with protease inhibitors, Russell fears that over the long term they will be continually 'dodging the side effects of medicines', and will die of 'weird presentations'. He believes that this, in turn, will alter the context of assisted death. 'We're going to see people who are used to feeling great and all of a sudden they have a very serious problem, and [they'll be saying] "if you can't get me back to the way I was last month, I'm out of here"'.

If protease inhibitors do fail to live up to their promise over the longer term, there is a significant reservoir of HIV infection that will continue to fuel the demand both for the legalisation of assisted suicide and euthanasia, and in the meantime, for illicit assistance. The trend towards home nursing also facilitates assisted death, since the absence of institutional constraints will mean fewer disincentives to involvement in euthanasia.

Underlying the euthanasia debate is an ideological struggle between competing world views. Opposition to legalisation reflects a perspective which is conservative and communitarian, and which is more likely to be informed by the teachings of an authoritarian and hierarchal church. Advocacy for voluntary euthanasia, on the other hand, reflects a perspective that is liberal, individualistic, and more likely secular.

Society has prohibited euthanasia for at least two thousand years. Support for the legalisation of euthanasia in the community, or in sections of the medical profession, does not automatically translate into law reform. Despite an intense and ongoing debate, euthanasia advocates have only posted modest gains. Euthanasia policy is delicate, and legislators are reluctant to intervene. The following chapter will review recent legislative experiments with assisted death, asking the question: where does the law stand on assisted death, and where is it going?

4

Sanctity of life:
the slow death of an idea?

We are modifying the Christian religion; we are saying that the Sixth Commandment—'Thou Shalt Not Kill'—needs to be modified: Thou Shalt Kill in certain merciful situations. The authoritarian, dogmatic people in religion will not accept this modification.

Derek Humphry[1]

It is no fluke that countries such as Australia, the United States and the Netherlands have begun experimenting with laws permitting assisted death. After all, the law has long since retreated from the position that there is always a duty to preserve life. Legislation giving patients the right to seek assistance in ending their lives is in some ways a logical next step.

This chapter will review some of these legislative experiments, focusing in particular on the Northern Territory's *Rights of the Terminally Ill Act*. To put these initiatives in context, it is important to see how the sanctity of life ethic—understood as a prohibition against intentional killing—has been undermined by a series of developments in the law. These developments have made the law more friendly to the sick and dying. But they have also helped to create the conditions for head-on confrontation with the prohibition against killing.

Retreating from life

Re-defining death

The ability of artificial respiration and life-support systems to sustain the biological functions of the body almost indefinitely, despite the permanent loss of consciousness, has created a sharp conflict between 'those who prize the principle of human life' and 'those who value the capacity for human living'.[2] One way the law has delayed facing up to this conflict is by re-defining the concept of death. Following the work of the Harvard Brain Death Committee,[3] legislatures in the United States, Australia and other countries have recognised 'whole brain death' (the loss of all brain function, including brain-stem function) as a legal criterion of death, in addition to 'heart/lung' death.[4]

The 1990s saw a push towards a further re-definition of death to include 'higher-brain death'. Interest in higher-brain death has accompanied the ability of medicine to preserve life in patients who are in a permanent coma, or a 'persistent vegetative state' (PVS). A PVS can arise following irreversible damage to the cerebrum, which—whether alone or in interrelationship with the brain-stem— is thought to control 'higher-brain' functions including consciousness, thought, feeling and memory.[5] A prognosis of PVS implies the permanent loss of consciousness, cognitive function and sensory capacity, although the patient may breathe without assistance, and may 'live' for many years with artificial feeding and hydration. The plight of patients with PVS was dramatically illustrated in England in the case of 17-year-old Tony Bland, whose lungs were crushed in the fatal crush at the Hillsborough football stadium on 15 April 1989. Through prolonged deprivation of oxygen, Tony's cerebral cortex had 'resolved into a watery mass'.[6] In the United States, well-known PVS cases include Karen Quinlan in the 1970s,[7] and Nancy Cruzan through the 1980s,[8] both of whom sustained irreversible injuries as a result of oxygen deprivation.

Advocates of higher-brain death admit that their preference for labelling such patients as 'dead' is based on the moral judgment that the essence of personhood or 'being human' is the integrated functioning of mind and body. It follows that death might be defined as the 'irreversible cessation of the capacity for consciousness'.[9]

Catholic bioethicists disagree, arguing that 'permanently unconscious patients and new-born babies, including anencephalic infants,
are human subjects with personal dignity whose lives are morally
inviolable'.[10] Australian bioethicist Peter Singer has taken a third
view, arguing that while it is counter-intuitive to refer to a PVS
patient as 'dead', it is nevertheless morally acceptable to harvest
organs for transplantation from people who permanently lack the
capacity for consciousness and feeling.[11]

   'Higher-brain death' has not yet achieved the degree of social
consensus necessary to be adopted as a legal criterion of death. On
the other hand, 'higher-brain' death has been accepted as sufficient
justification for the withdrawal of life-sustaining medical treatment.

'Futile' lives

The question facing Britain's highest court, the House of Lords, in
the Anthony Bland case, was whether there was a duty to continue
providing medical and nursing care to a young man who would
never regain consciousness, thought, or feeling. The law Lords
agreed that doctors owe a duty to act in the best interests of incompetent patients. When a patient is permanently unconscious, however, their Lordships agreed that those 'best interests' do not require
the provision of ongoing medical care. One judge, Lord Mustill,
observed that Anthony Bland had 'no best interests of any kind',[12]
while another, Lord Keith, remarked that 'it must be a matter of
complete indifference whether he lives or dies'.[13] Their Lordships
were unanimous that where a responsible body of medical opinion
decides that further medical treatment will be of no benefit to an
unconscious patient, there can be no duty to provide it, and medical
treatment may be withdrawn.[14]

   Underlying this decision is the recognition that 'higher-brain
death' is a sufficient basis for withdrawing the medical treatment on
which Anthony Bland's life depended. Lord Mustill justified this
conclusion on the basis that continued treatment could 'no longer
serve to maintain that combination of manifold characteristics
which we call a personality'.[15] Further treatment—and it must
follow, Anthony's life, in its current state—was pointless and futile.[16]

   What happens when medical treatment is withdrawn from an
unconscious patient? If antibiotics are withdrawn, the patient may

catch an infection and die of pneumonia, while if intravenous nourishment and water are withdrawn, they will die of kidney failure or starvation. To put *Bland* into practice is to ensure that death comes faster than it might have. Withdrawing such treatment is only compatible with the judgment that PVS patients are better off dying sooner (rather than later). It makes little sense to argue that death was foreseeable, but unintended, when one is intentionally performing actions whose inevitable effect is to hasten death.

In the *Bland* case, although they authorised the withdrawal of Anthony's treatment, their Lordships emphasised that euthanasia remains unlawful,[17] thereby requiring a distinction to be drawn between the two. They did this by arguing that the lawful withdrawal of medical treatment is an 'omission', rather than an active measure (e.g. a lethal injection) which directly causes the patient's death. Thus, their Lordships reasoned, when Anthony dies, it will be his underlying injuries, rather than the withdrawal of treatment that will be regarded as the *cause* of death.[18]

A critique: The 'acts/omissions' distinction is problematic in end-of-life jurisprudence. In *Bland*, their Lordships frankly admitted that it was 'morally and intellectually dubious',[19] 'illogical',[20] and hypocritical.[21] In the United States the Ninth Circuit Court of Appeal saw little difference between a doctor who pulls the plug on a respirator, and a doctor who prescribes a lethal overdose,[22] although the Supreme Court reaffirmed the acts/omissions distinction in its 1997 decision, *Vacco* v *Quill*.[23]

When you have a ventilated patient, it is disingenuous to try to avoid moral responsibility for the inevitable consequences of one's actions by claiming that death was foreseen, but not intended, or that the removal of the ventilator was but an 'omission' which didn't *cause* the death which followed.[24] There is 'nothing psychologically or physically passive about taking someone off a mechanical ventilator who is incapable of breathing on his or her own'.[25] The criminal law would not permit an intruder who sneaked into a critical care ward and turned off a ventilator to argue this, and nor should doctors. Since doctors have the ability to prolong life through the use of medical technology, we must accept that the intentional withdrawal of such treatment will inevitably shorten life, and precipitate an earlier death.[26]

There is, of course, an important distinction between Tony Bland's doctors and the intruder. In clarifying that difference, we are forced to ask ourselves whether there are ever *good enough reasons* for permitting doctors to cause or hasten death.[27] *Bland* suggests that the permanent loss of consciousness may provide one such reason. The same challenge applies in cases where a neonate is so gravely disabled that doctors believe that the provision of further life-support serves only to defer an inevitable death, or to perpetuate a life of cruel suffering. Asking whether there are good enough reasons to hasten a person's death forces us to articulate the moral values we hold about life, and this is a good thing.[28] However, the fact that we may not hold a doctor culpable for the death of a patient, or that due to terminal disease the patient would have died soon anyway, should not blind us to the consequences of what doctors do.[29] It is little wonder that one law Lord recognised that the *Bland* case might well be seen as an example of 'euthanasia in action'.[30]

In the United States, unlike Britain, courts have tended to make medical treatment decisions for incompetent patients through a process of 'substituted judgment' which involves trying to determine what the patient 'would have wanted' in those circumstances. While 'second-guessing' the patient may be artificial, it brings us to a third development which has undermined the sanctity of life ethic.

The right to say 'no more'

British Commonwealth and American law respects the right of competent adults to decide whether or not to accept medical intervention. Provided the patient is competent, the law will respect this right, even if the patient will die as a result.[31] Where the patient is not competent, doctors must continue to act in his or her best interests (Australia, England), or must follow the course the patient 'would have chosen' in the circumstances (substituted judgment, as adopted in some American states). The basis for the right to refuse medical treatment, as the United States Supreme Court pointed out in *Washington* v *Glucksberg*,[32] is the principle that forced medication is an assault. The right to refuse medical treatment is an expression of the right not to be assaulted.

In the United States the right to refuse life-supporting treatment is not just a common law right, but an aspect of the 'liberty' that citizens enjoy under the Fourteenth Amendment to the United States Constitution. In the Nancy Cruzan case, the Supreme Court assumed that 'the United States Constitution would grant a competent person a constitutionally protected right to refuse life-saving hydration and nutrition'.[33]

The right to refuse treatment has also been recognised in legislation, in a variety of ways. In California, and some Australian states, patients can make an advance directive or a 'living will' enabling them to refuse all, or particular, forms of treatment, if they later become incompetent and terminally ill.[34] Legislation also permits a person to confer an enduring medical power of attorney upon an agent, who then has authority to refuse medical treatment on the patient's behalf, if the patient becomes incapacitated.[35]

In two 1997 cases (*Washington* v *Glucksberg*, *Vacco* v *Quill*), the United States Supreme Court refused to accept that the constitutional right to refuse life-supporting medical treatment encompasses any broader 'right to die'. As a result, the Court upheld the lawfulness of statutes in Washington State and New York that prohibited assisted suicide.[36] In *Vacco* v *Quill*, the Court relied on similar reasoning to that adopted by the House of Lords in *Bland*, distinguishing between the withdrawal of treatment (an omission), and assisted suicide or active euthanasia (an act). When life-support is withdrawn, the underlying illness will be treated as the cause of death, not the action of the doctor. On the other hand, a lethal injection *causes* death and is therefore unlawful.

A critique: The distinction between acts and omissions allows a doctor to disassociate himself or herself from the consequences of withdrawing life-preserving treatment. On the other hand, by giving priority to the patient's right to make treatment choices, the law enshrines a right to suicide, at least for patients who depend upon life-support and can therefore choose to die by refusing further treatment.[37] But if doctors can honour a patient's request to assist suicide by withdrawing a patient's treatment, why can't they also assist by drawing up a lethal injection? The law quarantines itself from assisted suicide only by applying an incredulous theory of causation, and by ignoring the intention of the sympathetic doctor who withdraws life-support at a patient's request.

The right to adequate pain relief

A final development which has put pressure on the sanctity of life ethic is the principle of 'double effect'. According to this principle, it is lawful to administer sedating drugs that may have the effect of hastening the patient's death, provided that the doctor's purpose is to provide relief from pain and suffering. Decent, palliative care in hospitals and hospices depends heavily on this principle.[38]

The dividing line between intending to relieve the pain of an exhausted and dying patient, and intending to expedite their inevitable death by sending them permanently to sleep, may at times become difficult to maintain. One Oregon physician comments: 'Dying patients are given larger and larger doses of morphine. We talk about the 'double effect', and know jolly well we are sedating them into oblivion, providing pain relief but also providing permanent relief, and we don't tell them'.[39] Indeed, the *modus operandi* of some of the doctors interviewed in this study was to trade on the 'moral luck of the double effect',[40] intentionally administering ever-increasing doses of sedatives *for as long as it took*.

While the distinction between pain relief and assisted death is the intention of the doctor (if not the size of the dose), health carers may periodically come to a point where they believe that the next injection will precipitate respiratory failure. Perhaps the most honest way to deal with this situation is to accept that providing relief from distress constitutes a *good enough reason* for hastening and causing death.[41] This involves taking moral responsibility for precipitating an earlier death, even if one persists in arguing that—although foreseen—the death was not intended. A recurrent concern in the literature is that because doctors do not see 'terminal sedation', the withdrawal of hydration, and other end of life practices as euthanatic in character, there is seldom any independent review, and few safeguards against abuse.[42] Ironically, by claiming that *doctors do not kill*, the law may leave patients open to abuse.[43]

To summarise: 'higher-brain death' is not a legally-accepted criterion of death; patients can refuse treatment of any sort even if they die as a result, and the principle of double effect excuses doctors who hasten death, provided their intention is to reduce pain and distress. Life-preserving treatment can be withdrawn from incompetent patients if it is 'futile', or so burdensome that it is no longer in their 'best interests', and doctors are not expected to perform medical heroics when a patient is terminally ill and 'actively dying'. Nevertheless, assisted death remains unlawful, despite attempts in the United States to persuade courts that assisted suicide is a constitutionally protected right. As a result, assisted death has passed into the political arena. It has become a question for legislatures.

Experimenting with death

Euthanasia in the Northern Territory

In late February 1995, barely three weeks after first announcing his intention to introduce legislation recognising the right to die, the *Rights of the Terminally Ill Bill* was tabled by Chief Minister Marshall Perron in the Northern Territory Legislative Assembly. In the course of his first reading speech, Perron said:

> Through the laws in place today, society has made an assessment for all of us that our quality of life, no matter how wretched, miserable or painful, is never so bad that any of us will be allowed to put an end to it. I am not prepared to allow society to make that decision for me and for those I love.[44]

Perron's initiative ushered in three months of frantic lobbying in the Territory, as well as a raucous, nationwide debate. Perron observed wryly after the Bill had been safely passed that in his experience there were few 'swingers' in the debate, and that both inside and outside politics almost everyone retained their original support for, or opposition to, voluntary euthanasia, despite the arguments presented on both sides.[45]

The *Rights of the Terminally Ill Act* 1995 was passed in a conscience vote at 3.15 a.m. on 25 May 1995 by a 15 to 10 majority of the Northern Territory Legislative Assembly.[46] The Act legalised both assisted suicide, and active voluntary euthanasia. It was greeted with hostility by the churches, and by the Australian Medical Association,[47] which subsequently mounted a legal challenge with church support.[48] Margaret Tighe, leader of 'Right-to-Life Australia', predicted that the Northern Territory would experience a surge of 'one-way tourism', especially 'AIDS sufferers'.[49] Seventy-year-old Marta

Alfonso-Bowes, a retired poetry lecturer from Monash University, who was suffering severe pain from tumours in her colon and intestines, was one of several patients to arrive in Darwin hoping to use the legislation, only to learn that it had not yet come into effect. Unable to find help, Marta died 'alone, like an old dog', from an overdose of tablets in a Darwin hotel room.[50]

The *Rights of the Terminally Ill Act* contained a variety of safety mechanisms designed to prevent abuse. The Act only applied to adults suffering terminal illnesses, who were experiencing pain, suffering or distress to an extent unacceptable to them, where no treatment (other than palliative care), was available. Two other doctors were required to be involved: a psychiatrist, to certify that the patient was not suffering a treatable clinical depression, and a second doctor (who had special qualifications or experience in the patient's particular illness), to certify the prognosis and terminal nature of the disease.

The first case of legalised euthanasia under the Act took place on 22 September 1996. Sixty-six-year-old Robert Dent, a former carpenter and pilot, who had suffered from prostate cancer for five years, died at home following a lethal infusion supervised by Dr Philip Nitschke.[51] The death came about using Nitschke's computer-controlled, self-administering 'death machine', with software (entitled 'Final Exit') written by collaborator Des Carne. (The machine is now on display in the British Museum.)[52] To die, Dent moved through three interactive computer screens, the last of which said 'If you press *Yes*, you will cause a lethal injection to be given within 30 seconds, and will die. Do you wish to proceed? "YES/NO" '.[53] By tapping the space bar on the laptop computer, Dent initiated an infusion of barbiturates. Early prototypes of the machine had a range of CD music to choose from, and ended with the farewell: 'Good-bye and good luck'.

After the death, Robert Dent's son, Rod, a postman and local Liberal Party official from Bowral, New South Wales, praised his father's courage, and vowed to carry on the fight. Janet Mills, who suffered from a rare and terminal form of skin cancer, became the second to die on 2 January 1997.[54]

Meanwhile, a Catholic federal Parliamentarian and Liberal Party backbencher, Kevin Andrews, was gathering support for a pri-

vate member's bill to overturn the Territory Act, using the Commonwealth Parliament's constitutional power to make laws for the
Territories. Although the leaders of the Labor, Liberal and National
parties supported this Bill, the Parliamentary debate which followed
to some extent cut across party lines. While the issue bubbled away
in the media, a group called 'Euthanasia No', based on Catholic
connections, and originally formed to oppose euthanasia initiatives
in New South Wales,[55] quietly recruited friends and opinion-makers
to lobby federal Parliamentarians.[56] The ultra-low profile 'Euthanasia No' campaign was supported by grassroots activism from
church members and right-to-lifers, who flooded the Senate Committee (which was conducting hearings into the Andrews Bill) with
anti-euthanasia submissions.[57]

The debate was not without its twists and Damascus conver-
sions. In an open letter to Parliamentarians before his death, Robert
Dent had written, 'If you disagree with voluntary euthanasia, then
don't use it, but don't deny me the right to use it if and when I want
to'.[58] Following his father's death, Rod Dent had campaigned for a
national referendum on euthanasia, and brought a much-needed
human face to the debate. In a dramatic twist, however, he switched
sides, publicly declaring his support for the Andrews Bill, in the
belief that toeing the party line would facilitate his career with
the Liberal Party.[59]

The Andrews Bill was passed by a majority of five votes in the
Australian Senate, early in the morning of 25 March 1997. The vote
was welcomed by the Catholic and Anglican churches, but condemned by State Premiers.[60] Despite this, other attempts to introduce euthanasia legislation into other Australian Parliaments have
so far failed. Euthanasia is divisive, and will always be treated as a
harm minimisation exercise by the major parties. Religious affiliations, and personal lobbying, become highly significant when voting
takes place on conscience grounds. Churches and professional medical bodies make an impressive coalition, opposing legalisation with
greater passion than the majority of voters who support it in vaguely-
drafted polls. Marshall Perron has predicted that euthanasia will be
legalised across Australia in the next decade.[61] While the social and
legal developments canvassed above suggest that euthanasia laws
are a logical next step, law reform may stand a better chance in

places where citizens have direct input into the legislative process through citizen initiated referendums.

Assisted suicide in Oregon

In November 1994 the state of Oregon, in a citizen-initiated referendum, narrowly voted in favour of the *Death with Dignity Act* (known as 'Measure 16'), which legalised physician-assisted suicide.[62] Unlike earlier citizen-initiated laws which were voted down in Washington State and California, the Oregon law did not seek to authorise active euthanasia.

Due to constitutional challenges (which failed), the law did not come into effect until 27 October 1997.[63] In the intervening time, Catholic and anti-abortion groups had convinced the Oregon Senate to conduct a referendum on whether to repeal the law.[64] In November 1997 the Act was passed by Oregon voters for a second time, with an increased majority of 60 per cent. 'This is a tragic day for Oregon, the nation and the world', said Bob Castagna, of the Oregon Catholic Conference.[65]

Like its Northern Territory counterpart, the Oregon experiment with assisted death faces resistance at the federal level. In October 1999 the House of Representatives passed the *Pain Relief Promotion Bill*, which made it an offence for a doctor to prescribe federally-controlled drugs, such as barbiturates, specifically for the purposes of assisted suicide. All fifteen patients whose deaths were reported under the Oregon Act in its first full year of operation in 1998 used 'lethal prescriptions' of drugs supervised under federal law.[66] The Bill stalled in the Senate, however, due to concerns that the legislation would have a 'chilling effect' on doctors' willingness to prescribe adequate pain relief. At the time of writing, it is not known whether any fresh attacks on the Oregon law are planned in Congress, or by the Bush administration.[67]

Assisted death in the Netherlands

Contrary to popular belief, it is still illegal under Dutch criminal law to assist in suicide or to terminate life upon request. Since 1973, however, Dutch courts have recognised a defence of 'necessity' which permits a doctor to avoid liability by pointing to his or her duty 'to reduce suffering or to respect the 'personality' [i.e. autonomy] of the patient'.[68] The requirements for the necessity defence have undergone subtle elaboration over the past three decades. In November 2000 the defence was, for the first time, given an explicit statutory basis, following the approval of amendments to the Dutch Penal Code by the Lower House of the Dutch Parliament.[69] These amendments were passed by the Upper House in April 2001. To avoid liability under the Penal Code, doctors will be required to satisfy the 'due care' requirements set out in the *Termination of Life on Request and Assisted Suicide (Review Procedures) Act*.[70] In addition, the doctor must report the death to the municipal coroner as required under Dutch burial legislation.

Under the 'due care' requirements, the assisting doctor must be convinced that the patient's request was voluntary and well-considered, that the patient's suffering was unbearable and that there is no prospect of improvement. Together with the patient, the doctor must reach the conclusion that the patient's condition is hopeless and that there is no other reasonable treatment alternative. The doctor must consult with at least one other, independent, physician who must see the patient and give a written opinion on the requirements above. The death must be reported as assisted suicide or euthanasia, and a regional review committee is required to assess whether the doctor acted with 'due care'. A case is only to be referred to the Public Prosecutor if the committee believes that due care was not taken.

Under the due care requirements, it is not necessary for the patient to be suffering physical pain: unbearable mental anguish is sufficient. Similarly, there is no requirement for the patient to be in the terminal phase of an illness, or indeed to be suffering from any (physical) disease at all. A physical disability, or a condition of 'untreatable misery' (as in the *Chabot* case), will suffice.[71] Where the patient's suffering is non-somatic in origin, the new legislation does not explicitly require the treating doctor to arrange for psychiatric review, although this seems implicit in the requirement that the independent doctor must certify that the patient's condition is hopeless and without prospect of improvement. More generally, however, 'due care' does not require depression, or any psychiatric illness, to be excluded.

The new legislation permits persons aged sixteen years or older to make an advance directive requesting euthanasia if they later become incompetent. The doctor may act on this, provided the due care requirements are otherwise satisfied. In addition, the legislation authorises children aged 16–17 to request assistance, provided parents are 'involved in the decision process'. Parental approval, however, is required for children aged 12–15.

The intention behind the amending legislation was to 'put an end to the hypocrisy of having an officially "tolerated" practice that is technically illegal', and to try to improve the historically high rates of non-reporting, by doctors anxious to avoid investigation.[72] After the law was passed, the Dutch government began distributing booklets through its embassies warning that 'suicide tourism' will not be available to non-residents.[73]

The rate of euthanasia in the Netherlands is a topic of bitter dispute. In 1990 the Remmelink Committee estimated that 1.8 per cent of annual deaths in the Netherlands were due to active voluntary euthanasia, and 0.3 per cent were due to assisted suicide. A further 0.8 per cent of deaths (1000 deaths) were attributed to non-consensual euthanasia.[74] In 1997 Kuhse and colleagues published a study comparing end-of-life decision-making in Australia with the Remmelink study. They concluded that 1.7 per cent of Australian deaths in 1995/96 were the result of active voluntary euthanasia (an additional 0.1 per cent were the result of physician-assisted suicide). More surprisingly, an estimated additional 3.5 per cent of deaths involved non-consensual euthanasia (termination of life without an explicit request).[75]

At the time of writing, Oregon's *Death with Dignity Act* is the only assisted death legislation in the English-speaking world. On 16 August 1995 the New Zealand Parliament rejected by a 61–29 majority a private member's *Death With Dignity Bill*, which would have legalised voluntary euthanasia for the terminally ill.[76] In England a 1994 House of Lords Select Committee report opposed legalising euthanasia,[77] a conclusion shared by the majority of the Canadian Special Senate Committee on Euthanasia and Assisted Suicide, which presented its report to Parliament on 6 June 1995.[78] The Canadian Supreme Court had determined previously in the *Rodriguez* case that the prohibition of assisted suicide does not violate the *Canadian Charter of Rights and Freedoms*,[79] a conclusion the United States Supreme Court also reached in the *Washington* v *Glucksberg* and *Vacco* v *Quill* decisions. The European Commission on Human Rights has held that English legislation criminal-ising assisted suicide does not violate the right to 'respect for private and family life' in Article 8 of the *European Convention on Human Rights*.[80]

Despite some tentative experiments with legalisation, a vigorous debate and open defiance in some quarters, assisted death remains illegal almost everywhere. This does not mean it is not practised. The following chapters return to the 'euthanasia underground'. Chapter 5 begins by locating assisted death within the broader context of the challenges of palliative care.

5

Exploring the meaning of suicide talk

It was like the 2nd or 3rd week . . . it was really hard to watch because . . . he was just gasping all the time . . . I was sitting there at one point and his mother looked at me and said 'You know that when your children are born you just pray—when the doctor holds them up and slaps them—you just pray their hearts and lungs work. Now I just pray that [his heart] would just stop, you know' . . . So at a certain point I said 'You know I think it's time', and I started to turn the morphine up.

Bill, hospice nurse

Where a lethal injection has been legalised, as in the Netherlands, the threshold to unconsented euthanasia is soon crossed. Death becomes an alternative to care and lives are arbitrarily valued on a scale that many have no choice about . . . Let's concentrate on helping the dying, not disposing of them.

Kevin Andrews, Australian Federal Parliamentarian[1]

According to Kevin Andrews, the Australian politician who introduced the federal Act which overturned the Northern Territory's euthanasia legislation, euthanasia is the antithesis of care. It has no place within the caring paradigm.

This is a fundamental claim made by opponents of legalised, voluntary euthanasia. It was also a sentiment echoed by a small minority of the health care workers I interviewed in this study. According to Richard, a doctor with a large HIV/AIDS clientele, the prohibition on killing patients is 'almost a chromosomally deter-mined rule' which has parallels with the incest taboo. To kill a patient as part of the treatment process is an 'extraordinary' and 'monstrous event'.

But not everyone shares this view. Jane, a GP with extensive euthanasia experience, characterised her involvement as 'a non-Medicare rebateable aspect of care'. Martin, a community worker, saw euthanasia as 'a continuation of the health management pro-cess: we've intervened to maintain life, [and] when that life is no longer worth living, we actually intervene to end life'. Chris, a hos-pital nurse, emphasised, 'you don't [give] euthanasia instead of offer-ing palliative care, you offer euthanasia as an option, as part of that whole package'.

The question 'Can euthanasia ever be an act of medical care?' is one that medicine, and society generally, cannot avoid debating. It cannot be answered from the splendid isolation of the university or seminary, but only by drawing near to the challenges of palliative care, through the experiences of those who have logged up hours at the bedside.

This chapter explores some of the challenges of palliative care in order to better understand the context within which 'suicide talk' arises. The experiences of nurses, in particular, provides a powerful lens through which to investigate two issues. Firstly, how do patients raise the issue of medically-assisted death? Secondly, what motiv-ations underlie a patient's desire to die? Following on from this, Chapter 6 will review the different ways that euthanasia requests are actually resolved in health care settings.

Raising the issue

The interviews with nurses, doctors and therapists confirm that patients with HIV frequently raise issues of suicide, euthanasia and death with those they trust. Kerry, a hospital-based consultant nurse, thought that 'there would be very few people that I've spoken to who at some stage didn't raise the issue of death as a theme, and very very frequently within there is the notion of suicide'. Ria, a palliative care nurse, estimated that at least 40 to 50 per cent of her patients had expressed 'a genuine wish to end their life at some period during their illness'. Anne, a counsellor, put the figure as high as 90 per cent.

Estimates vary according to the interviewee's particular professional role. Not surprisingly, those working in hospital or home-care environments face the issue more frequently than doctors and nurses in suburban practices. For example, Tim, a GP in a group practice, thought that only 5 to 10 per cent of his patients wanted to talk about euthanasia, and only a few actually wanted to talk about it seriously.

Stage of disease

Interviewees pointed out that themes of suicide and euthanasia are more likely to be raised by well patients at the time of HIV diagnosis, and again during advanced illness, as patients get sicker and more distressed, with more frequent hospital admissions. Research suggests that the risk of suicide may be particularly high at these times,[2] although conversely, several studies have suggested that there is *less* suicidality in AIDS patients than in those with symptomatic or asymptomatic HIV infection.[3] Gay, an HIV/AIDS community worker, observed that 'as they get sicker they tend not to [talk about euthanasia]: they need to do it while they're well because as they get sicker life gets very precious and they hang on to every bit they've got'. The truth of the matter was probably best summarised by Damian, a medical practitioner, who noted 'a huge individual variation as to when patients want to end their lives'.

AIDS and cancer

The apparent willingness of HIV/AIDS patients to consider assisted death may distinguish them from patients with other life-threatening illnesses. This discrepancy was noted by interviewees who were experienced in both HIV and non-HIV care. Anne, a counsellor who had moved from cancer into AIDS, observed that 'the first thing I noticed was that practically everyone diagnosed with HIV/AIDS talked about suicide and euthanasia'.

Some of the social factors that may explain this have already been explored in Chapter 3. For Ria, the major difference was that if a cancer patient chooses palliation, 'the chemo stops, the radio therapy stops, generally their symptoms are managed'. But this is not the case with AIDS. If a patient has CMV (cytomegalovirus, an AIDS-defining illness), then

> three times a week they have to be hooked up to have a cytotoxic drug pumped into their body just so they don't go blind, they have to continue their thrush medication so they don't end up with thrush from mouth to anus . . . you've got people who are barely conscious and yet you're crushing up tablets, syringing tablets down their throats, just to try and make sure they have a bit of dignity [rather than] an overgrowth of horrible opportunistic infections.

According to Anne, society has become much more educated around cancer, whereas HIV/AIDS is still perceived as a 'plague'. Many gay patients 'feel somehow on the outside of society', and their fear of abandonment contributes to thoughts and talk of suicide. '*I'm going to be left alone to die, alone with my pain and my fear, and my diarrhoea, and everything else.*'

The context of the request

Patients raise the idea of euthanasia in different ways, depending on their physical and mental state, and who they are speaking to. Some raise it bluntly in the context of an acute episode. One hospital nurse spoke of patients '[who have] been in excruciating pain for weeks and they say "just kill me"'. By contrast, Paula, a GP, thought that there were two types of patients: those who have already made up their minds, and who want euthanasia in the near future and want to know whether you will do it, and those who are just a little bit uncertain, yet regard euthanasia as 'one of a number of options'.

For hospital nurses like Kerry, there was a continuum of language and intention ranging from people talking vaguely about euthanasia in the future to people talking about it now. Patients will frequently raise the issue in an oblique way. Ruth, for example, had never been asked explicitly by a patient to assist in death. Instead, patients asked questions like 'Do you think if I took 50 sleeping tablets I'd vomit?', in an effort to glean some information or precipitate discussion.

Within the safety of gay-friendly, community AIDS organisations, requests are more explicit. Martin, a community worker, reported, 'I probably speak to half a dozen people a week, either over
the phone [or] they come in and have a chat with me, about what
their options are around euthanasia'. Frequently, these clients 'want
a recipe or they want a doctor who will assist'.

Several interviewees admitted to *initiating* discussion of euthanasia with patients. Erin, a community nurse, notes that when a
patient is 'running pretty stable, if I get what I call a "window of
opportunity", I try very hard not to miss it'. If a patient drops a
comment about what will happen when the end comes near, 'I try
to work that into the conversation'. Dean, a GP with a history of
involvement, was more circumspect. 'The patient will always raise
it first, and even then I am fairly cautious and non-committal, and
that's a reflection of my dis-ease, of my ignorance of how to do
it well'.

Exploring the meaning

Euthanasia requests usually precipitate a process of assessment by
the doctor, nurse or therapist, in order to clarify the unmet needs of
the patient, to improve patient care, or to determine whether further
action is appropriate. Requests are seldom taken at face value. The
resulting 'assessment process' will sometimes be the first step in a
chain of events leading to active involvement in euthanasia. For the
purposes of this chapter, respondents' discussion of the 'assessment
process' provides a window through which to explore the challenges
of palliative care, and through it the contested role of euthanasia
within the caring paradigm.

Suicide research

Isolating the psychiatric, social and medical factors which underlie
thoughts of suicide is an important area of research. American
studies have suggested that the increased risk of suicide in men with
HIV/AIDS is between 7.4 and 66 times greater than the general
population.[4] This increased risk may largely be due to pre-existing
psychosocial factors (including psychiatric and emotional problems,
poor social support networks) associated with populations at risk of

HIV infection (homosexuals, bisexuals, IV drug users etc), rather than to serostatus itself.[5] Although contested,[6] this view may fuel the assumption that suicide by people with HIV/AIDS is unrelated to illness and is therefore irrational or pathological.[7]

Even assuming that the relative rates of suicide risk do not differ between HIV+ and HIV– groups sharing similar demographic characteristics and lifestyles, HIV/AIDS is nevertheless a daunting challenge that creates the context for suicidal thoughts. In one study Schneider and colleagues examined the AIDS-specific 'stressors' that may encourage suicidal thinking, by comparing groups of infected and non-infected gay and bisexual men. They concluded:

> Whereas among HIV– men, the report of suicide ideation was mainly associated with current depression and hopelessness (as has been found among the general population), among HIV+ subjects, mood disturbance, loneliness, lack of perceived control over AIDS risk, and AIDS-related life events (including news of decreasing CD4 T-cells), were associated with reporting suicidal ideation.[8]

An important finding from Schneider's study, which concerned relatively asymptomatic men, was that suicidal thinking in HIV+ men was a coping mechanism for anticipated pain and distress.[9] This factor was also strongly evident in my interviews, and was related to the fact that many patients had seen lovers and friends suffer and die.

Psychosocial factors

Although interviewees felt that suffering, and fear of future suffering, were important motivations for patient suicide talk, they were also alive to the influence of pre-existing psychosocial factors. Gordon, a GP, remarked that 'so many gay men are just utterly miserable and this is one of the reasons I believe that there's such a high suicide rate'. Gordon added that he asks his patients ' "If you had a pill that could make you straight, would you take it?" And by and large, most people say 'yes', which suggests that they're not accepting who they are'.

Harry, another GP, said, 'I've hardly ever had a [patient with AIDS] who died peacefully with dignity, with loving people around him; it's always drama, there's relatives that won't speak to lovers, or won't have anything to do with their gay friends; it's horrendous'.

Perhaps the saddest account of a family's inability to accept their son's homosexuality came from Erin, a gay community nurse, who was involved in the care of a 23-year-old man dying from liver disease. This 'young kid had been beaten by his father and his older brothers because he was gay', said Erin. 'His brothers sent him to the hospital, they beat the shit out of him—in a good family, [a] good Catholic family'. The young man had attempted suicide by overdosing on Tylanol and now he was dying of liver disease. The young man was about to be intubated, and a priest had been sent for so that he could make his confession while he was still able to talk. The young patient asked Erin to stay in the room while he spoke to the priest because 'he didn't have the guts to tell the priest his sins [alone]'. The priest agreed to this on condition that Erin understood the seal of confession would also apply to him. Erin continues:

> If I can paraphrase what this kid said: '*As a Catholic I was taught that suicide was throwing life back in the face of God*'. And with tears in his eyes he said '*It isn't that I'm throwing my life back at God, it's that I know life with God has got to be better than this hell on earth*'.

'He was actually having a leap of faith', said Erin. 'In any other context that kid would be a saint.'

'His father stood outside of the room telling fag jokes', Erin recalls. 'I'm not a violent person, but I wanted to go out and put my fist in [his] face. [The family] never got the message, and that kid died.'

Why do patients want to die?

While the motivations for suicide talk are complex, the desire to die is certainly mediated through patients' struggle with their disease. Both in conversation and in the subsequent questionnaire, interviewees explored the factors which in their view contributed to patients' desire to die. Table 5-1, based on questionnaire responses from thirty-five interviewees, confirms the wide variety of factors that motivate 'euthanasia talk'.

As reflected in the Table, questionnaire respondents identified these factors with greater or lesser degrees of generality, and there is

Table 5-1: Factors motivating requests for assistance in dying by terminally ill patients with AIDS (as interpreted by interviewees) (n=35)

Factors motivating patients' requests for assistance to die	No. of interviewees who mentioned this factor	No. of interviewees who regarded this as the most important factor
1. Intolerable/unresolved/ chronic pain or physical discomfort	21 (60%)	9 (35.7%)
2. Emotional pain	2 (5.7%)	
3. Spiritual pain	1 (2.9%)	
4. Chronic wasting/diarrhea	5 (14.3%)	
5. Blindness/going blind	1 (2.9%)	
6. Vomiting/nausea	3 (8.6%)	
7. Devastating and unrelieved symptoms	1 (2.9%)	1 (2.9%)
8. Indignity	1 (2.9%)	
9. Severe deterioration in quality of life/lack of quality of life/unable to enjoy life	8 (22.9%)	5 (14.3%)
10. Don't want further illness, pain, suffering	1 (2.9%)	1 (2.9%)
11. Anger at condition	1 (2.9%)	
12. Frustration at loss of independence/loss of control/ need help for everything	6 (17.1%)	1 (2.9%)
13. Sick of being sick/spending more time in hospital than out than out	2 (5.7%)	
14. Not wanting to be a burden	8 (22.9%)	
15. Desire to remain in control	1 (2.9%)	1 (2.9%)
16. Disgust at one's body/ drastically altered body image	4 (11.4%)	
17. Fear of loss of independence/ loss of control	4 (11.4%)	
18. Fear of loss of body image/ fear of how they are going to die ('bag of bones')	3 (8.6%)	

Table 5-1 (cont'd)

Factors motivating patients' requests for assistance to die	No. of interviewees who mentioned this factor	No. of interviewees who regarded this as the most important factor
19. Fear of wasting	1 (2.9%)	
20. Fear of going blind	1 (2.9%)	
21. Fear of dementia	7 (20.0%)	
22. Fear of process of dying/ not wanting to suffer as others have suffered/fear of suffering when dying	13 (37.1%)	4 (11.4%)
23. Fear of lingering on	1 (2.9%)	
24. Fear of seeing carers watch them die/stress on loved ones as they become more dependent	2 (5.7%)	
25. Fear of being abandoned to die alone	1 (2.9%)	
26. Fear of family's reaction to news of the illness	1 (2.9%)	
27. Fear of pain	5 (14.3%)	1 (2.9%)
28. Fear of the future ('how much worse can I get?')	2 (5.7%)	1 (2.9%)
29. Impending dementia, neurological impairment	1 (2.9%)	1 (2.9%)
30. Depression	5 (14.3%)	1 (2.9%)
31. Dementia	1 (2.9%)	
32. Loss of sense of self and identity	1 (2.9%)	1 (2.9%)
33. No hope left/no chance of recovery/death imminent	3 (8.6%)	2 (5.7%)
34. 'Over it'/tired of fighting/ exhaustion and hopelessness	17 (48.6%)	6 (17.1%)
35. Ready to die; feel they have completed their life	2 (5.7%)	

considerable overlap in the factors mentioned. Items 1–9 focus on the patient's current symptoms and medical condition, items 10–16 on interviewees' perceptions of what patients were feeling about their current condition. Items 17–28 relate to perceptions of the patient's fears for the future, and the remaining items are ungrouped.

Respondents were asked to list those factors they regarded as most important in motivating requests for assistance to die. Pain and discomfort (and more generally lack of quality of life), fears for the future, and feelings of exhaustion, hopelessness and being 'over it' are the recurrent themes. These themes encapsulate the challenges faced by those involved in care: responding adequately to symptoms of disease, addressing fears of future deterioration and suffering, and re-creating hope and a sense that the present has meaning.

The interviews provided a flexible environment within which to explore the ambiguity and complexity of euthanasia talk. Three clusters of issues stand out in the interviews, and will be explored below:

* fear, uncertainty and loss of control;
* pain, distress and indignity; and
* depression and dementia.

Fear, uncertainty, and loss of control

When people ask about euthanasia, the sub-text often is: are you willing to look after me if things get bad?

Gordon, GP

Talking scared

A recurrent theme in interviews was that fear motivates suicide talk, but that talking about the issue plays an important role in reducing fear and in achieving a sense of control. Kerry, for example, notes that patients 'commonly talk about suicide in the context of their fears about what the future will bring'. Kerry's response, like that of other respondents, was to encourage patients to verbalise their fears and to validate the normalcy of such feelings, while still recognising *fear* as the motivation.

Responses such as 'that's a really frightened thing [to want] to do' also reflected Kerry's perception that thoughts of suicide were both the result, as well as a source, of fear for the patient: 'people can be very frightened by those sort of thoughts, frightened that if they have those thoughts maybe they'll do it, and they don't really want to do it'.

Frequently, it is not death itself that patients fear, but painful and undignified decline. Some patients are terrified of a particular kind of death: for example, losing their sight (if they have CMV retinitis), or choking for air, vomiting blood and coughing up one's lungs (if they have *pneumocystis carinii* pneumonia, or internal Kaposi's Sarcoma). These fears are all the more real because patients with AIDS are an incredibly educated population, fully aware of the suffering AIDS can cause.

An insight into this process was given by Martin, a community worker who has AIDS, who said in interview:

> Anyone who argues that life is worth hanging on to right till the very end has never witnessed anyone with a bedsore. A bedsore sounds sort of 'oh, is that uncomfortable?' but I've actually seen when they've gone right the way through into the bone. You can actually see people's bones and I'm sorry, that's not a *polite bedsore*, that's a *gaping, pustulating, vile wound that's painful beyond belief and it's impossible to heal*. That, in conjunction with people crapping them-selves, being unable to take water by themselves; no I'm sorry, that's no life, that's not living; anything's better than that.

Kerry, a consultant hospital nurse, comments that sometimes 'the sense of projected experience can be a lot more fearful and anxiety-provoking' than the reality. Sometimes, merely acknowledg-ing a patient's fear will be enough. 'People say they're afraid of the pain, they're not afraid of dying but they're afraid of the pain. And if you can give them some assurance that you will at least attempt to make them as comfortable as possible, then often you can talk people through it . . .'

Ria's strategy in responding to euthanasia talk was to acknowl-edge that 'they've got every right to feel that they want to die, and then try to shift the focus on to "well what can we do to change this?", particularly if there's issues of dementia, pain or suffering'. 'You've got to teach people how to die', said Gordon, 'find out where they're coming from, what their family experience has been, often only basic information is what's needed'. Ruth, a community-based nurse, notes that 'you just have to reassure them that some of their fears can be addressed'. But she added, 'for some people, their fears can't be addressed'.

Building a rapport

A feature of nursing care is the intimacy and trust that must be established before the issue of euthanasia can be properly aired and discussed. Breaking down the professional boundaries between patient and nurse makes such a discussion more likely. According to Terri, nurses 'become family'. 'Patients divulge their innermost secrets and we are entrusted with fantastic details of life, of their lovers ... what they want to achieve before they go, if they are alienated from their family, and how we can bring the family together if that's at all possible.' *'We are the people the patients say to: "Is it going to be a good death? Are you going to be with me? Will you help me with my pain?"'*

Amanda, a community nurse, reflects that when you go into a patient's home 'you lose to a large extent your character as a nurse and you actually become a friend ... quite often you're the first person that they actually mention euthanasia and assisted suicide to, because they've got your trust'.

Doctors, by contrast, were perceived by nurses to be remote from this level of interaction. Terri notes that 'doctors ... are not comfortable talking to patients about assisting their death'. Patients, for their part, 'don't talk to doctors on that one-to-one basis ... doctors are still seen as people in authority—the white coat'. Remarks such as this, repeated in a variety of contexts, suggest a deeper (thinly disguised) antipathy towards doctors. The important theme, however, is that nurses have, and perceive themselves as having, unique knowledge of, and access to, the realities of patient suffering. Talking about suicide and euthanasia is frequently part of the process of building a rapport, a trusting bond, which may last until death intervenes.

Kerry felt that sometimes patients are 'testing you out, wanting to know to what extent I can trust you with how I feel'. Similarly, Amanda referred to the exclusivity of many of these conversations. Often the issue is raised in a very confidential manner: 'I'll tell you because I know you won't tell anybody, don't tell my doctor, don't tell my partner, don't tell anyone, it's just between us'. Discussion of assisted death is an intimate, secret, hushed affair which contrasts sharply with the multidisciplinary approach to patient management in large hospitals.

Suicide as metaphor

The notion of control is inseparable from the fear and apprehension that patients bring to their disease. As Marzuk notes, patients 'speak about powerlessness and dependency, with suicide serving as a metaphor for achieving control over their destiny'.[10] An insight into this process was given by Damian, a medical practitioner whose involvement in euthanasia had included giving advice and writing 'lethal' prescriptions:

> Many patients speak about wanting to end their lives and not infrequently it's a question of maintaining control over their lives. The great problem with [AIDS] is this lack of control. Their lives are controlled by the disease process and they have to hand over control of their lives to doctors, and this loss of control is a major issue for them. Not infrequently patients discuss suicide in the earlier stages of the disease—perhaps [at the time of] the first bout of pneumocystis or the first AIDS-defining illness—at that stage they feel this loss of control and will discuss suicide. [But] when you give them back the control, and discuss [options] with them . . . assuring them that there are ways and means available to them, that nobody is going to be judgmental if they decide to take that road and that in fact there's help available, [then] not infrequently they are quite satisfied . . . and [they] decide not to commit suicide.

Paradoxically, by *not ruling out euthanasia as an option*, doctors and nurses can assist in dispersing patients' fear of the unknown. By recognising assisted death as an option, patients feel a sense of control which may reduce the incidence of 'prophylactic euthanasia'.

A number of interviewees recognised this dynamic. Stephen, for example, was a psychiatric nurse who had shared information about drug combinations, and the identity of 'sympathetic' doctors. For Stephen the decision whether to share information depended on factors including 'whether I thought . . . I could help this person

improve their quality of life so [that] they wouldn't want to do it—
let them know that they had the means to do it so they then had
some control and wouldn't want to do it'.

'My life belongs to me and no one else'

It is possible that issues of control assume a higher profile among
AIDS patients, particularly gay men, than with other patient groups.
Zane, a palliative care physician, refers to the not uncommon practice of patients stockpiling morphine obtained from previous doctors
and specialists, as an insurance policy: 'they want to be in control of
the situation, and it's often part of their personality, *all their life they
wanted control*'.

What is so important about control? Where does the focus on
'control' come from? Martin, a community worker, explains:

> In my experience, most people with HIV/AIDS have had a very pro-
> active role in their treatment strategy. They don't [just] sit in their
> doctor's office and do as they're told. They become aware of the
> options that are available to them, they discuss those options, not
> only with the doctor but with their peers and then come up with a
> strategy that is right for them. In many instances they've been in
> control of their health management for a long period of time and they
> actually see euthanasia as being a continuation of that proactive
> process.

Martin attributes this proactive stance to the skills the gay community developed in response to gay discrimination during the
1980s: 'In a perfect world where we wouldn't have been discrimi-
nated against on the grounds of our sexuality, we probably wouldn't
have the skills in place to challenge the discrimination around the
disease'.

Warren, a psychotherapist who works intensively with a small
group of clients, expanded on this theme:

> Nearly all my clients are gay men and they're romantic secularists.
> They believe in this life, and they believe in romantic relationships,
> including very sexual ones, and a natural outgrowth of that is that
> they want the life that they currently have to have value and meaning
> on its own terms . . . They're used to having enormous control over

their lives and their bodies, and of negotiating relations with professionals where they have a lot of control . . . they don't like surren-
dering themselves to the authority of medical . . . professionals.

One reason why AIDS is fuelling the euthanasia debate is
because of the values and beliefs of those who have most felt its
impact, particularly gay men. AIDS has impacted upon an urban-
ised, hedonistic, largely post-Christian population focused upon
body image, personal identity, and achievement. It is a population
with a high level of knowledge about the disease process. For Gary,
an activist doctor, the implications and contradictions of this were a
source of surprise:

> They've faced up to death; they've accepted it and almost embraced it
> as a release . . . It's the courage that surprises me, I mean, you know—
> queens, faggots, they're weak men, you can bash them, you can do
> anything, sissies—and yet these guys willingly go to death, and trusting
> me that I will do a good job which I find really humbling, that some-
> one would trust me to end their life properly.

The shifting goalposts

The role that euthanasia talk plays in articulating patient fears
about losing control is a crucial issue for nurses and counsellors.
Usually the hunger for control will never translate into suicide or
euthanasia. Patients will die a relatively comfortable, natural death,
without using the drugs they had stockpiled in the fridge. 'What
people actually wanted was a choice', says Martin. 'It's like having a
condom in your pocket', says Stanley, 'you don't always have to use
it, it's just . . . nice . . . to know that you can'.

Michelle, a community nurse with four years experience, comments that when the end comes, patients usually change their mind:
'the basic primitive instinct to survive comes to the fore and they
will fight to the very last'. Ruth, a community nurse, referred to this
phenomenon as 'the shifting goalposts'. The goalposts get shifted
because when the patient reaches the point where they had previously decided life would be intolerable, it has been a gradual
process, 'it's sort of snuck up on them, and it's not as bad as they
thought it was going to be'.

'People . . . draw lines in the sand', says Stanley. They say ' "if
I can't walk then I'm going to kill myself". [But] when they get to the

point where they can't walk, they find another reason for drawing another breath, and then they move on'. To recognise 'the shifting goalposts' is to recognise that remarkably, despite feelings of grief and despair, many patients do adjust to the things that most scare them.

Patients may sometimes feel trapped or 'locked in' by earlier requests for assistance. Kerry recalls one occasion where friends of her patient 'wanted to take him home and kill him, basically', honestly believing that was what he wanted. The patient had become very ambivalent, and kept making excuses about why he wasn't ready to be discharged. He found it very difficult to admit that he had changed his mind.

'Sometimes there is a notion in the HIV area', says Kerry, 'that suicide is the noble way out, that suicide is what really strong people do'. In this case, the patient was not discharged and died naturally a week later.

Tara, a clinical psychologist, picked up on the same theme of 'subtle peer pressure', noting that some of her clients felt 'almost a sense of duty to self-deliver', as if suicide was 'the model way to die'.

It would be self-serving to dismiss all euthanasia talk as peer pressure or as a way of maintaining control. Michelle, Ruth, Helen and other nurses were adamant that there were some patients who made a decision about the quality of life that they wanted, and maintained that decision, without ambivalence, when that quality was no longer available to them. There are some patients who 'never ever ever digressed from that [decision] from the minute they got their first AIDS-defining illness to the minute they breathed their last'.

This poses a dilemma for conservative nurses who—while recognising the rubbery edges of pain relief—feel uncomfortable with euthanasia as part of medical care. Sometimes the goalposts do not shift. Sometimes 'euthanasia talk' is not ambivalent. Sometimes talking about it does not defuse the death-wish.

Pain, distress and indignity

> *Sometimes palliative care works really well, but there's 1 in 20 or 1 in 40 whose pain you'll never get under control who will die in pain.*
>
> Dianne, palliative care nurse

The public's sympathy for euthanasia is greatest when we hear of cases where medicine has failed to control pain. On the other hand, the notion of pain is a complex one. In AIDS, as elsewhere, the emotional, psychological and spiritual components of pain combine with the physical.[11]

Acute pain

Interviewees gave different perspectives on whether the dying process in AIDS is accompanied by acute pain. The fact that AIDS is a spectrum of illnesses may account for this, as well as the differing practice contexts respondents worked within. According to Gary, a GP, 'patient suffering is more important than pain . . . people [with AIDS] die with very minimal pain, they don't get big nasty growths in places that are pressing on to other things, they don't get broken bones'. Another GP noted that rather than pain, the major problem is the 'overwhelming, profound, mind-numbing lethargy'.

The perspective of hospital nurses was somewhat different. AIDS-related tumours and lymphomas can cause acute pain. Dianne, a palliative care nurse, recalls

> I've had some patients where no matter what amount of morphine or narcotics you give them it just doesn't kill the pain. In the case of someone with gross Kaposi's Sarcoma, their whole body is encased in this sort of shell, and they're incapable of doing anything themselves; no amount of morphine will kill the pain.

Ria, another palliative nurse, described the shooting, tingling pain and the sensations of burning in the extremities caused by peripheral neuropathy. Morphine is ineffective against nerve-based pain, and in one case she was involved in, the drugs used for neuralgic pain were neutralised by the patient's continuing narcotic need. Other interviewees spoke of the inability of narcotics to control pain in IV drug users with AIDS who had developed a high tolerance to morphine, pethidine and other drugs. A similar tolerance may arise in patients with intractable diarrhoea, who have received consistently high doses of codeine phosphate.

Pain: not a neutral concept

It was nurses who best articulated the complex nature of pain, and its relationship with social, emotional and spiritual factors. Several spoke of the 'total body pain' some patients experience in the terminal stages of AIDS. By this point, patients may be profoundly anaemic, showing symptoms of muscle wasting and severe weight loss. They may suffer from increasing fatigue, breathlessness, and aching. The pain and discomfort they experience may have a strong psychological component. These processes are illustrated in the following vignette, as told by Terri.

'Dean' was a man with AIDS who had lost his partner four years earlier. He had nursed his partner with love and devotion. He had not told his parents that he was gay, let alone HIV positive, and he certainly hadn't told them that he was in the last phase of his life; he'd always covered it over with some illness or pretext.

We finally convinced him that he must speak to his parents, and this caused him a great deal of guilt and anxiety—he even tried to commit suicide because he couldn't face up to what he had to do. He jumped out of a hospital window, landing on a roof below. He didn't kill himself, he didn't even break a bone but he bruised himself severely and ended up in another ward for a few days. This gave him time to think through the processes and to give himself strength to face his mum and dad.

We finally got the family together. His sister-in-law had been his main support; she knew of his illness and had begged him to tell his mother and father. They were all there together when the mother and father were told. The parents just didn't know how to cope; I mean to have a gay son was one thing, that was difficult enough, to have him dying of AIDS and to find all this out within one day was more than these 70-year-old darlings could cope with. The sister-in-law was then attacked verbally because *she knew*, and *how could she be more important than [the] mother and father*? In the midst of all this stress, Dean became totally overly-anxious and quite psychotic, he would just lie in bed and scream and groan. This was not a pain that you could relieve with oral medication or an injection—there was nothing we could give him to reduce his anxiety.

He ended up living another six weeks. He was frightened to death of dying, he wanted people to be with him: 'don't leave me alone, don't switch off the light'. We gave him a lovely stuffed doll, it sounds crazy, but he had to have something to cuddle. His parents didn't ever really come to terms with him; the father could not look at his son without crying and saying 'where did we go wrong? Where did we go wrong?'

We all gave Dean a commitment that he would not die alone. His sister-in-law said she would be there day or night. Nurses said 'you will not be alone'. And yet when the time came—8.00 a.m. on a Saturday—he asked us to go and get his medication, and when we came back after ten minutes, he had died, and he died alone. Actually, this gives me the idea that he had come to terms with what was going on. Patients are very clever in that they choose the time they are going to leave this earth; it has happened so many times that I don't even question it now. I like to think this man had said 'I am not going to leave this earth crying, gibbering, squealing and asking for everybody, I am going to take control of these last few moments of my life, I am going to send you away, you're going to go and get my medication, and when you come back, I will have died'.

He could have lasted quite a lot longer. But I truly believe he chose the time to die. Maybe in that small moment he regained his own self-control, self-respect.

Although Dean had attempted suicide in order to deal with an unresolved family issue, he later feared death. Even so, his case illustrates the complex nature of pain, and the fact that pain, particularly when used as a justification for euthanasia, is not the monolithic, neutral concept some assume it to be. The argument for euthanasia reaches its highest point when a patient is in screaming agony. But few would approve of euthanasia to blot out the feelings of guilt caused by unresolved sexuality, or the pain of family conflicts. One exception was Michelle, a community nurse—and no stranger to euthanasia—who commented: 'I can see their need to escape all that bullshit, especially the ones who haven't told, for whatever reason, their family'.

We love to call it 'pain relief'.

Donald, palliative care nurse

If palliation includes rendering the patient unconscious, it always works.

Robert, hospital physician

'Pain relief' and 'pharmacological oblivion'

The provision of pain relief to terminal patients is a source of criticism by euthanasia advocates, who see an uneasy hypocrisy at work. Warren, a psychotherapist, tells his patients: 'It's pretty likely that you won't die in pain, and one of the reasons for that is that pain control regimes are so generous that effectively you can have a nice, soft, fuzzy euthanasia death under another name'. Some see this 'pharmacological oblivion' as preferable to euthanasia, while others regard a drug-induced stupor in a patient who has requested release as a cruel denial of patient autonomy at a time when the patient is most vulnerable to abuse.

If the 'pharmacological oblivion' solution to the problem of terminal suffering troubles us, it is perhaps because we are evading the moral issue of actually killing. We might, as Little points out, permanently relieve suffering by rendering a patient decerebrate and permanently unconscious.[12] If this seems an absurd solution, perhaps it is because we associate the value of life (at least partly) with consciousness, and with the patient's ability to derive meaning from their experience of life. Perhaps we also feel troubled by the selfishness of ending our patient's consciousness of life on our terms rather than on theirs.

Hospital and hospice deaths are achieved in all sorts of informal and unspoken ways, with the provision of pain relief and sedation being central to the process. This process is not unique to AIDS, as several interviewees point out. Stephen comments: 'This stuff goes on in general hospitals all the time; you know, "give the little old lady with the 'fracky neck' who's going to die in a week a little bit extra Brompton's cocktail" '.[13]

Dianne and Ria, both palliative care nurses, gave examples of AIDS patients who, at their request, were sedated into unconsciousness through regular injections of drugs through a catheter, or by sustained-release infusion. Since it was standard practice not to give intravenous fluids to an unconscious patient, the patient's death was hastened by dehydration. Zane, an experienced palliative care physician, explained how benzodiazepine derivatives such as midazolam suppress breathing, causing the oxygen level to drop to a point where the patient slips into unconsciousness, while the morphine prevents distress and breathlessness. Sometimes Zane had made the decision to continue heavy medication so as to prevent a patient from waking up, while also withholding fluids. He explained: 'If you gave intravenous fluids, at the same time as giving morphia for breathlessness or pain, *you could keep the patient alive for weeks*'.

Far from being the alternative to euthanasia, physician-induced coma, and the non-provision of water, was one method of choice for precipitating the patient's death. This kind of scenario was recognised by all interviewees with experience in palliative care.

Escalating doses

A recurrent theme in interviews was that once a patient switches from oral morphine to subcutaneous morphine administered via a syringe driver, the dosages are usually increased quite rapidly. At this point, Terri comments, 'it's just a matter of time, and it's generally days'. Patients who have requested assistance in dying draw reassurance from this. Terri tells her patients: 'This is going to keep your pain under control, it's going to ease the way for you, we're already on that path, we're heading down the road you want to go on'.

Break-through doses

A common hospital procedure allows nurses to give 'break-through' doses of morphine or other analgesics when existing dosages, administered every few hours, are not having their intended effect. Dianne explains, 'if you go and move a patient and they grimace, well they must be in pain, so you give them a break-through dose'. As the patient deteriorates, nurses will often reach the point when they realise that the next injection may be the last. Secure in the knowledge that it was the doctor who charted the medication, none of the nurses I interviewed had any problem with 'giving the last dose', even when it was clearly excessive. Michelle commented, 'it's an unspoken thing that happens between health care professionals: you know that the four o'clock dose of morphine is going to be the last dose that anybody's ever going to give that patient . . . *it's just done*'. Sometimes the patient will realise this as well, a fact smoothed over with the linguistic veneer of 'symptom relief'. 'Quite frequently', Terri says, 'they will look at you and they know what's going to happen and you say 'this is just going to ease your breathing', but they generally know just as we know that it's going to be that last injection'.

Residual morphine

In addition to 'break-through' doses, nurses have flexibility in responding to patients' pain by saving the morphine left over after the charted dose has been administered. Chris explains: 'One of the fabulous things about morphine ampoules is that they come in standard strengths, 10, 30 and 120 mls. So if you've got somebody who's on 60 milligrams of morphine and you use a 120 ampoule . . .'. 'Of course', he adds, 'with drugs of addiction, another nurse is supposed to witness the destruction of the other half—but it's not hard to fudge that'. In Chris' opinion, '20 or 40 or 100 milligrams of morphine in the last two days of their life when you think they're in pain or they're moaning or groaning or whatever is completely irrelevant as far as I'm concerned'. Chris worked in a Catholic hospital, and estimated that he had administered 'residual morphine', with the collusion of dozens of nurse colleagues, over the years.

The circumstances in which 'residual morphine' is administered are revealing. Chris spoke of the tension and fatigue of the drawn-out death-bed scene, a scenario familiar to nurses. 'You've got a family who are just flipping out because this is dragging on—you call them in Sunday night and [now] it's Thursday and it's still going on.'

Conversely, Chris noted that on other occasions he had worked incredibly hard to keep a patient alive for an extra twenty-four hours because their sister or relative was expected to arrive the next morning. He adds: 'once the sister's arrived, and they say "hello", it's like, "yeah, let's do it, triple the morphine, you know"'.

Sometimes the provision of 'pain-relief' clearly becomes a form of euthanasia, while in most cases it just inhabits the no-man's land between what is clearly legal and what is clearly not. This uneasy state of affairs is nicely encapsulated by Grimley Evans, professor of geriatric medicine at Oxford University, who is quoted as having said, 'Doctors shrink from active euthanasia because they are trained to kill only by accident'.[14]

Other interviewees were less charitable. One referred to the 'Soviet levels of dishonesty' surrounding practices that 'everybody knows are occurring', but which 'nobody is willing to acknowledge or take responsibility for'. Death by palliative care is 'packed in this sort of soggy cotton wool of evasion so we don't know what other people's motives are'.

Purists in the euthanasia debate may argue that there is no moral difference between administering several semi-lethal infusions, and giving a single lethal dose.[15] The interviews with palliative care nurses, however, suggest an important emotional difference. In hospitals, responsibility is diffused, and a nurse who causes a patient's death by escalating medication levels does not feel the moral responsibility of someone who gives a lethal injection. This, of course, begs the question: Is medicine taking full responsibility for its actions?

> *We can control their pain, and we can do this and do that—yes! Big deal! But wake up! Smell the coffee! They're not always in pain— some of them are just 'over it'. You know—at 32—if I looked like something out of a Godzilla film I'd probably be over it too.*
>
> Michelle, community nurse

Distress and indignity

Euthanasia is not just about pain relief. Research indicates that indignity, dependency and lack of control are more important than pain in motivating the desire to die.[16] In a series of 187 case studies of assisted suicide that were investigated as part of the Dutch Remmelink study, loss of dignity was mentioned as a reason for requesting death in 57 per cent of cases, pain (46 per cent), dependency (33 per cent), and tiredness of life (23 per cent). Pain was the sole reason for requesting death in only ten cases.[17]

Indignity and existential fatigue are especially important in HIV disease. Virtually every interviewee raised the problem of uncontrolled diarrhoea. Dean, a GP explains:

> There's the personal degradation they go through . . . diarrhoea they can't control, the embarrassment of it, these are young people who maybe as little as a few months ago were at the gym, and going out, and looking good, and feeling good about themselves.

Gary, another GP, expands on these themes:

> They're gay men who may have been quite proud of their bodies, they
> can't do anything anymore, they can't control their bladder or their
> bowels, they can hardly walk, everything is an effort, their hair falls
> out, they get Kaposi's Sarcoma purple blotches everywhere, they can
> swell up, they can have shortness of breath, tiredness, their appetite
> goes down, they don't like being seen in public, some of them can't
> have sex anymore which for a gay man is an enormous problem . . .
> They might be bed-bound for weeks at a time, they start getting pain
> because of bedsores and they're just aching and bony. And then there
> [are] the real existential problems . . . but we haven't got six or twelve
> months of therapy to help them come to terms with their altered body
> image.

Cataloguing the suffering caused by AIDS-related illnesses
makes bleak reading, and does little justice to the courage many
patients bring to their disease. Donald, a hospital nurse, spoke of
'nausea that you just can't control, they don't eat, they throw up . . .
We can't get rid of it . . . no escape, no way out'. 'You couldn't have
picked a worse disease to hit [gay men]', says Bill, a hospice nurse,
'it's hard enough to grow old in the gay community', let alone with
a disease that makes 'young men old' and attacks their vanity. Terri
refers to 'the disgusting feeling of being constantly wet or constantly
dirty, or of not being able to eat or being so weak that you can't lift
your hand to hold a cup'. Patients will say ' "This is no quality of
life, I'm a guy who used to ride a Harley-Davidson, I'm a man who
used to abseil or climb mountains, I used to go dancing, I loved
music, I was an artist but now I can't even hold a cup, how can I
hold a paintbrush? This is not for me—I want out" '.

The metaphors used to describe those in the advanced stages of
AIDS are telling: 'totally disintegrated', 'withered people on sticks',
'stick-men', 'emaciated wrecks, riddled with various infections',
'Auschwitz victims', 'something from Belsen'.

'To say that there is no room for euthanasia if you've got good
palliation is a load of crap', said Amanda. 'It's a gross generalisation
to put on everybody who is dying. I think carers want to do things
to make *themselves* feel better; there's no recognition that some

people just cannot tolerate their life the way it is'. This view was passionately expressed as law by the United States Court of Appeal, 9th Circuit, in the *Compassion in Dying* case:

> A competent terminally ill adult, having lived nearly the full measure of his life, has a strong liberty interest in choosing a dignified and humane death rather than being reduced at the end of his existence to a childlike state of helplessness, diapered, sedated, incontinent. How a person dies not only determines the nature of the final period of his existence, but in many cases, the enduring memories held by those who love him.[18]

Depression and dementia

Euthanasia talk can be motivated by depression and dementia. In AIDS, both are important themes. Unlike pain and suffering, which libertarians may regard as justifying a request for euthanasia, depression and dementia were generally seen by interviewees as factors to be excluded before any further action was taken.

Reactive depression

A reactive depression, arising in response to the suffering and uncertainty of living with AIDS, will frequently precipitate suicide and euthanasia talk. According to Kerry, 'it's unusual for people *not* to have a sense of sadness, a sense of loss or regret; I mean, depressing things are happening; if they were euphoric, that would make me feel a bit uncomfortable'.

A caring response to patient suicide talk is to see if something in particular has happened to trigger the suicidal urge. Has the patient just received a CD4 count of three? Have they just come down with an opportunistic illness? Is it the anniversary of a partner's death? Or has depression been triggered by grief, following the death of a friend?

Kerry points out that the danger for nurses who have worked extensively in HIV and have witnessed terrible deaths is to project their own emotions and meanings on to the patient's experience, to agree with the patient's sense of suffering and futility in a way that legitimates and encourages suicidal ideation. 'I often hear nurses saying things like: "I don't know why they're hanging around, I don't know why they don't just give up". The danger is in thinking: "Yes it *is* terrible, I've seen a hundred people die that way; *yes— die!*", instead of listening to what the person is saying which may be about 'I'm frightened of something, I'm scared of suffering" '.[19]

Kerry gave the example of an extremely articulate man in his early thirties, who was simultaneously diagnosed with HIV, AIDS, and early dementia. The man had some insight into his dementia, and became very actively suicidal. He was in the midst of adjusting to a whole range of things: he was a married, bisexual man, and there were lots of disclosure issues. Nevertheless, 'because he was an extremely articulate man, the medical staff really identified with him [and] they allowed his discharge [from hospital in order] to suicide'.

While Kerry does not believe that suicide can never be a rational choice, she felt that on this occasion the patient should have been certified. She suggested a psychiatric review to the patient's physician, who brushed this aside, saying 'we have no reason to hold him'. Kerry sensed, and resented, the collusion between hospital staff in helping the patient to end his life. In the meantime, the patient jumped off a bridge, survived, and was transferred somewhere else.

Is euthanasia ever a reasonable option, even in the presence of a reactive depression? Damian, a medical practitioner, reflected that as patients get progressively sicker the depression they present with is 'often appropriate . . . you or I would probably respond in the same way if we were in their position, so I can't say it's abnormal or pathological—their desire to kill themselves has to be seen as rational'. In view of this, Damian described his 'primary role' as ensuring that the patient was making a decision in a clear state of mind, that they were 'not suffering from a treatable depression'.

Reactive depression presents difficult challenges for carers. While quality of life inevitably declines in the terminal stages of AIDS, palliative care nevertheless 'aims to provide hope: not just hope for a cure but smaller, achievable 'mini-hopes', like getting out in the garden or going for a drive. Hope is never removed'.[20] One question which Warren, a psychotherapist, regularly asks his patients is: 'What in life are you still enjoying?' He notes that some patients who can't see or who can't enjoy food anymore will nevertheless still enjoy talking about the past or having someone stroke their back.

In this model of palliative care, health carers become, in all but extreme circumstances, *advocates for life*, committed to achieving 'mini-hopes' for their patients right until the end. At the very end of her interview, Kerry told the story of a 45-year-old man with AIDS who became very depressed and suicidal after his partner's death. After jumping out of a hospital window, he was sent to a psychiatric hospital. Two weeks later that hospital sent him back with a letter, the import of which, according to Kerry, was 'yes of course he's depressed, he has AIDS and he's going to die, what do you expect?'

The patient was sent to another psychiatric institution which treated his depression, and he recovered from it and lived for another 18 months, including over 12 months of good, active life. Against this background, the unqualified views of nurses like Peter, who stated 'I'm comfortable with people's decisions if they wish to end their life because they're terminal and the prognosis is shit-house', may reflect some of the same burn-out and depression manifested by patients.

The really hard questions, of course, begin when nurses or therapists do reach rock bottom; when it becomes clear over time that there simply is not, on any fair and reasonable view, anything more to squeeze out of life. It is here that moral questions about the meaning and purpose of life are sharpest.

Organic depression

Several interviewees distinguished reactive depression associated with failing health, from a deeper, pre-existing, organic depression. Warren commented that organically depressed people have poor psychological judgment, so that 'if you're going to assist their rational selves, you have to be certain that [it is] their rational self [that] is making the judgment about their life'. Organic depression, in Warren's terms, is like the patient saying 'he's feeling rat-shit today, therefore he's going to be feeling rat-shit forever and probably everyone feels rat-shit forever', whereas 'somebody who is despairing but making good judgment has a very rich view of the world, it's just a world that has turned very dark blue for him'.

Making judgments at this time is, however, 'complicated by the fact that people are passing in and out of comas, quite often they're on pain control drugs which also diminish their judgment', so that often only a very elaborate inference can be drawn about what their 'rational decision' might be.

Remarks like this one, from an experienced psychotherapist, highlight the risks of assessing the mental state of a patient who wishes to die. It is significant, however, that Warren himself did not see these difficulties as insurmountable, pointing to the 'cowardice' of the psychiatric profession, which—having the clinical expertise to exclude organic depression—refused to accept that people *can* make a rational decision to kill themselves. Tara, a clinical psychologist, was less confident, pointing out that there are treatable conditions which, if poorly managed, can 'mimic' the symptoms of organic depression, such as insomnia, poor concentration, anorexia and pain.

AIDS-related dementia

HIV dementia is increasingly common, due to increased longevity and the success of protease inhibitors and combination therapies in combating many AIDS-defining illnesses which were previously lethal. Dementia can begin with subtle memory problems and progress to a full-blown AIDS dementia complex involving severe cognitive changes.

The following vignette, drawn from Ria's experience, gives a taste of the nursing challenges posed by AIDS dementia:

> 'Darren' was a patient who spent five months with us. He died recently. His parents were elderly and quite unwell, and couldn't cope with him at home. Darren was incredibly demented, there was a slight element of aggression with his dementia, and he had no insight into the process at all. The first three months were terrible because he felt imprisoned. He didn't understand why he couldn't go home; I found notes written by him saying 'the police should be informed of what's happening here'.
>
> He absconded twice, we didn't know he'd gone he was that quick. He walked to the pub one night and got a barman to ring him a taxi. Even with full-on dementia he was able to direct the taxi through the eastern suburbs. He knocked on his parents' door and said 'Hi, I'm home'.

He had no concentration span. He basically sat, watched television, and smoked copious amounts of cigarettes. After a period of time, as his dementia progressed, the impulse to abscond left him, and he no longer felt imprisoned.

We had a lot of behavioural problems with him, like with smoking. It got to the point where we could no longer let him have lighters or cigarettes or matches because he was lighting fires in bins in the ward, and there's compressed oxygen canisters in the hospital. In the end we managed it by taking a cigarette up with him to the smoker's room, lighting it, and waiting while he smoked it. I would do 30 trips to the smoker's room in one 8-hour shift, and he became so demented he would only have two puffs, put the cigarette out, then come back to the nurses station, wait for a while, and then he'd get really aggressive: 'I want a cigarette, nurse!' And he'd start yelling, and I'd have to get a cigarette out of the locked draw, walk him up to the smoker's room, sit him down, give him the cigarette, light it . . .

He was 34. He got exceptional care. At one point he was transferred to another ward that couldn't cope with his behaviour and they just sedated him with psych drugs to manage his symptoms. His only pleasures . . . were cigarettes and chocolate. Poor bugger, I'm a smoker, so I could empathise with him. All I could do for him was to make sure he had a pack of cigarettes in one 8 hour shift, and there'd be a smile on his face. Other nurses would try to put him back to bed, but he'd literally lie down, you'd tuck him in and he'd be back up at the nurses station 'I want a cigarette, I want a cigarette', and this went on for months and months and months until he died last week. He died of system failure, he just deteriorated, he was so skeletal, probably only forty kilos, but he didn't require morphine until probably the last three days of his life when he was bedridden and started to develop some body pain.

Research suggests that AIDS dementia may be associated with increased suicide risk,[21] and there may be several reasons for this. Interviewees noted that unlike some dementias, AIDS dementia frequently affects the frontal lobes of the brain which control socially appropriate behaviour, with the result that patients will display increasing disinhibition, impulsiveness and mood swings. Kerry, for example, had heard demented patients ringing up friends to say

'Bring over a gun: I want to shoot myself'. She noted that although —if the patient had the gun at that moment—they might use it, such behaviour did not necessarily signify ongoing suicidal ideation. Even so, such behaviour can be enormously distressing for carers.

Several interviewees also noted that, in its early stages, AIDS dementia may not affect linguistic skills. Dementing patients may also retain significant insight into their dementing process. Along with incontinence and visual deficits caused by CMV retinitis, memory loss, inability to concentrate and patient insight over increasing dementia were recognised over and over as 'the last straw' for many patients. Kerry explained how, superficially, dementing patients may appear quite articulate, while formal testing would reveal significant memory problems, major problems with organising and planning their lives, and impulsive behaviour. The risk is that health carers may underestimate the significance of a patient's cognitive decline in motivating the desire to die.

Interviewees expressed differing views about whether it is appropriate for health carers to euthanise a demented patient. One doctor felt that it was reasonable 'to inform the patient and let them take a decision for themselves before the dementia is [so] advanced that they're not capable of making a rational decision'. Another thought that 'I suppose it depends on the degree of dementia, but if we're talking [about] a matter of days or weeks, [it] hardly seems to matter'.

Where a patient has consistently expressed a desire for euthanasia when a certain point is reached, the doctor may feel justified in assisting the patient, even when dementia intervenes in the meantime. The situation is more complex, however, where the health provider is not privy to any previously-expressed wishes, which must now be mediated through friends and relatives. At this point, intervention takes the form of non-consensual euthanasia. A variety of examples of this emerged from interviews.

In one case, a general practitioner supplied morphine to the teenage children of a patient, who 'helped [their father] on his way'. Recalling the patient's condition, the doctor said 'I knew him, there was no way that this was good for him; mentally he died . . . weeks before . . . he didn't know who he was or where he was in the last few weeks'.

Other issues

The interviews revealed a grab-bag of other issues that may underlie a patient's desire for death. Butch, a hospice physician, explores a series of possibilities with patients who have requested assistance to die: 'Is there any particular treatment that you're finding especially burdensome? Do you feel pressure from the people around you to 'get it over with?' Are you worried you're going to run out of money? Are there any issues of guilt related to having AIDS or the lifestyle that led to AIDS? Can a chaplain do something?' But despite addressing just about everything, there are still a 'few people', who, 'for their own reasons, want to die'.

Ruth points out that patients will sometimes get to the point where they say 'I just don't have any more energy left to fight this disease, I've been doing it now for 12 years, and I've run out, all I want to do is die'. This sentiment was echoed over and over, strengthened by the unpredictability of AIDS, and by recurrent hospitalisations over a period of years.

The role of anger in euthanasia talk deserves special mention. Like sadness and depression, patients frequently experience anger during the course of their illness: anger at diagnosis, anger at being unable to do things, anger at the loss of control, anger towards oneself and other people. Bill, a hospice nurse, tells of a patient who told his mother he was going to kill himself. The mother immediately booked a flight to come and see her son, who didn't want to see her but couldn't tell her that because it might hurt her feelings. 'There's so much ambiguity in that', reflects Bill, adding that anger can serve to 'coalesce' the mind, to assist patients in 'grounding themselves' at a time when their mind may be slipping due to dementia. Some patients have been 'angry all their lives', and death acts 'like a magnifying glass'. It 'enrages' them.

Kerry, a consultant psychiatric nurse, tells the case of a hospital physician with AIDS who spoke freely about his suicide and openly revealed the date. It became clear, however, that this talk was more a context for acting out his anger against his partner than a cemented intention to die: 'the more angry his partner [became], the more open and verbal and specific he was about what he was going to do'. The patient died naturally in hospital some months later.

Sometimes the request for euthanasia reflects the distress of family and loved ones who can no longer bear to see the patient suffering. Peter, a nurse with a long history of euthanasia involvement, spoke of the 'torture' suffered by relatives, 'the death scene business, on and on and on and on'. The administration of morphine, which may depress breathing and lead to 'gurgling noises' can also cause distress to relatives, although as Robert noted, 'ultimately you're treating the patient, not the relatives'.

Euthanasia talk is complex, and there are significant risks in accepting patient requests at face value. The constant theme that emerges from the interviews with those involved in palliative care is the great variety of factors that motivate requests for assistance. The following chapter will explore the options health carers have in responding to these requests.

6

Responding to
euthanasia requests

(with contributions from P. H. Ballis)

I'm not here to cure everybody ... Death is part of the natural cycle of life, and as a physician I have an opportunity to grant people peace and comfort in their death, and it's something that I'm not unwilling or afraid to do.

Joseph, HIV/AIDS specialist

It is not medicine's place to lift from us the burden of that suffering which turns on the meaning we assign to the decay of the body and its eventual death ... Medicine should try to relieve human suffering, but only that suffering which is brought on by illness and dying as biological phenomena, not that suffering which comes from anguish or despair at the human condition.

Daniel Callahan, bioethicist[1]

This chapter will explore the variety of ways in which patients' requests for assistance in dying are resolved by health carers, and the kinds of deaths that result. We begin by grouping the responses of interviewees to patients' requests for euthanasia into three categories: 'traditionalist', 'conservative', and 'revisionist'. Each category represents a cluster of attitudes and practices towards euthanasia.

While the focus of this book is on assisted death, the vast majority of patients who initially request assisted suicide or euthanasia will die naturally. The chapter continues, therefore, by exploring some of the processes that accompany 'natural death'. It then explores a third alternative, that of 'amateur suicide', before concluding with discussion of the impact of caring upon health professionals.

Responding to patient requests

We grouped the interviewees in this study into one of three categories ('traditionalist', 'conservative' or 'revisionist'), based on their responses to requests by AIDS patients for assisted death. The three categories take into account key variables explored in well-known Australian studies of assisted death by Kuhse/Singer, and Baume/O'Malley.[2] These variables, summarised previously in Table 3-1, include 'moral attitudes towards euthanasia', 'level of involvement in physician-assisted suicide or active voluntary euthanasia', and 'attitude towards legalisation'. A fourth variable which differentiates interviewees is their perception of the professional role. Given the entrenched nature of the prohibition on assisted death in nursing and medicine, the euthanasia question involves a re-imagining of collective professional ethos and 'what it means to be a doctor or a nurse'. Reflecting on the professional role was one important way in which interviewees explained and justified their actions. The three categories assist in demonstrating the variety and complexity of the attitudes and actions which make up illicit involvement in euthanasia.

The 'traditionalists'

Defining characteristics

Traditionalist health care workers have limited knowledge of euthanasia. They have not participated in assisted suicide or euthanasia, and either oppose the concept of assisted death on moral grounds, or believe for other reasons that the current prohibition should remain. The view that palliative care obviates the need for euthanasia fits neatly within the traditionalist mould.

In our sample of interviewees, only three genuinely reflect those characteristics we define as traditionalist, and all were doctors (Table 6-1). Richard, a doctor with a large HIV/AIDS clientele, felt a profound sense of unease over euthanasia. During interview he agonised over whether he should report to police the fact that one of his patients had mentioned an act of euthanasia by another (unnamed) doctor. Richard emphasised the protective function of professional standards, and expressed a distrust of doctors acting as loose cannons. 'I don't idealise doctors as special people who have special personalities and gifts', he said. 'They are fairly ordinary people with many of the same frailties which most people have, although hopefully accustomed to operating within a professional framework.'

Table 6-1: Occupational status and categories of response to euthanasia (n=49)

	Revisionst	Conservative	Traditionalist
Doctor	16	2	3
Nurse	5	11	–
Therapist/Counsellor	3	3	–
Community Worker	5	–	–
Funeral Director	1	–	–
Total	**30**	**16**	**3**

Richard was highly critical of the *secret* nature of euthanasia: 'What would one trust a doctor to do unsupervised?' he asked. 'Should killing someone require less supervision than taking their tonsils out?' If euthanasia is to be practised, 'it needs as much recognition as a tonsillectomy; if you're going to medicalise it and give doctors all this power, then it needs to be subject to scrutiny, like a surgical audit', in order to protect patients from mentally disturbed, impaired or alcoholic doctors.

In an ethical sense, Richard felt that the prohibition on killing patients was 'almost a chromosomally determined rule', 'God's law', or 'an unspoken moral law'. Concern over the surreptitious practice of euthanasia, however, supported Richard's seemingly contradictory claim that euthanasia should 'be legalised and regulated'. Despite the demographic characteristics of his practice, Richard noted that his patients did not talk to him about dying or having a bad death. He admitted that he would certify a patient who he genuinely believed would take an overdose using hoarded medication.

In contrast to Richard, Robert, a physician, did not oppose euthanasia for moral reasons, but because he doubted the law was capable of developing an adequate framework for regulating it. Specifically, he doubted whether legislators were capable of designing laws that were sufficiently sensitive to cultural and religious viewpoints, protected patients from exploitation, and took into account all the 'innuendoes' which inform medical decision-making. 'It's a bit like trying to legislate for the treatment of heart attacks', said Robert. 'It's a clinical judgment. At the end of the day I think we're looking at *clinical decisions*, and [that's why I am yet to be convinced that a law can] cover the range of clinical issues that arise out of that decision.'

A similar sentiment was expressed by Harry, a GP, who said: 'The thought of a committee of people, or even a group of people who *know* the patient sitting around and deciding whether the patient really wants to commit suicide and how it is going to be done, and when, and by whom, just fills me with horror'.

The desire to prevent lawyers, bureaucrats and 'do-gooders' from elbowing their way into the process of clinical decision-making is a recurrent, complicating factor in assessing attitudes in the euthanasia debate. If the interviews are any guide, a healthy proportion of health carers who admit to euthanasia have serious reservations about, or blatantly oppose, legalisation. Bill, a hospice nurse with a long career in assisted death, encapsulates the view as follows: 'Legalisation is an encroachment of the legal profession into the medical community. I do not believe that the medical, ethical, spiritual issues involved can ... be legislated'. Ironically, therefore, advocates and opponents of euthanasia may share similar views about legalisation.

A variety of themes, therefore, can underlie 'traditionalist' opposition to euthanasia. Some are concerned with ethical and professional standards, and fear the social consequences, as well as the consequences for the doctor personally, of medical procedures performed 'on the sly'. Another concern is to avoid outside intrusion into clinical discretion. A final argument, which recalls the controversial practice of inducing 'pharmacological oblivion' (see Chapter 3), is that euthanasia is *unnecessary*. Robert explains, 'if someone is suffering I can make them sleep and then they will drift off, whether it be days or weeks, into their death'.

Whatever their precise motivation, therefore, traditionalists do not practise euthanasia, and support the current legal prohibition.

The 'revisionists'

Revisionists are the 'radicals' in the euthanasia debate. We assigned thirty interviewees to this category, sixteen of them doctors (Table 6-1).

Defining characteristics

Revisionists are articulate, vocal, even militant proponents of the right to die. While many have a political agenda for legalised euthanasia, others, paradoxically, vehemently oppose any legal framework which would impinge upon the free exercise of their clinical judgment. Revisionists challenge traditional perceptions of the professional role by arguing that euthanasia should be seen in appropriate cases as an act of care, and as an expression of medical professionalism. Their deeper levels of involvement in assisted death are accompanied in some cases by intense personal anguish, barely concealed burn-out, and cynicism. Revisionists are usually aware of other colleagues who also practise euthanasia, draw support from this, and express less ambivalence over their involvement in illegal euthanasia. Because of their more frequent involvement, revisionists are more experienced in the 'technology' of achieving death (through drug combinations), and in avoiding post-death legal pitfalls.

While revisionists cover a broad spectrum of practices and personal philosophies, their distinguishing characteristic is their advocacy for change, whether it be legal change, or change in the definition of the professional role and the responsibilities of care-giving.

Zane, a palliative care physician, represented a fairly mild form of revisionism, admitting that:

> I believe there comes a time when you acknowledge all your attempts of treatment have failed, and once the patient says they want to go and they want to go quickly, and you are sure that they have fulfilled all their family wishes and have had reconciliation, seen their relatives for the last time, then I feel it is the physician's role to hasten a person's death if they are symptomatic.

In contrast, Jane, a GP with a long history of involvement and pro-euthanasia advocacy, ridiculed the notion of a separation between one's 'professional role' and personal life. Jane freely admitted that her patients were her friends, and that her medical practice, as a lesbian doctor in a large city, was also her life. Jane's involvement in euthanasia reflected her *personal* philosophy: the notion of a professional role, or of wider professional standards, had limited influence.

At one extreme, some revisionists display what we call the 'Rambo' or 'cowboy' factor: an almost reckless individualism which most readers, we believe, would find disturbing. Putting this to one side, revisionists were nevertheless robust in their attitudes. Peter, a nurse, is a typical example.

> I believe in quality of life, not quantity . . . I've seen enough people go to their end with all the revolting things: dementia, incontinence—I see no other answer for some people. We've got to pull our heads out of the sand and accept that euthanasia is occurring. We've got to start talking about it amongst each other, talk about it for support, talk about it to get information about the right drug cocktails to use, and also talk about how to change laws and structure regulations and ethics to get it done the right way.

While all interviewees were aware of the suffering caused by AIDS, revisionists were particularly sensitive to the limitations of medicine, especially where emotional and existential factors are concerned, or where symptoms are unrelated to pain, as with diarrhoea. Close personal contact with patient suffering, and a strong libertarian ethic of respect for patient choice, feature time and again as justifications for re-casting the doctor's role to include 'compassionate killing'. 'I mean, vets do it all the time, for God's sake', said Tony, a GP. 'If it's good enough for the family cat or dog, it should be possible for us to do it to humans.'

Criteria for involvement

A consequence of revising one's perceptions of the professional role is the need to articulate criteria for involvement in euthanasia. In general, revisionists managed to do so with only a low level of finesse. Stephen, a nurse and volunteer carer, stated that 'it's when I know that I won't feel guilty, or I will feel guilty, that counts. It boils down to whether I think that person should be dead, or alive'. Helen, also a nurse, pointed out that she knew the 'personal feelings', 'lifestyle', 'wants and dislikes' of her patients. 'I . . . understand them as a person so therefore it's not such a hard decision for me.' Tony, like most revisionist doctors, had no mental checklist, but emphasised that 'it's really a matter of getting to know [the patient] very well'.

Relying upon one's intuition does not necessarily suggest a naivety on the part of interviewees—who discussed issues of depression, dementia, family conflict and unresolved sexuality. The assessment process of revisionists was, however, ad hoc and informal. Interviewees told of episodes in which they ignored the very criteria they asserted as guiding their involvement. In the absence of a formalised structure for making decisions, this is not surprising.

Harvey, an unassuming general practitioner, admitted to performing euthanasia 'probably a dozen times' over a number of years. He explains that 'on an intellectual level . . . I support people's right to choose . . . to end their own life'. As an individual, however, he said, 'I find it very stressful dealing with it'. Harvey believes that 'having assisted people before . . . there is only a finite [number] of times you can do it', because it is 'very draining' and 'ugly'.

Apart from drawing attention to the emotional costs of involvement, the interview provided Harvey with opportunity to reflect on his professional role, attitudes towards legalisation, and future intentions:

H [I]f it was legalised I think I would choose not to be involved.

M Why is that?

H Because I would . . . choose to be a general practitioner [providing] palliative care to people and [leave euthanasia to] another health professional who for whatever reason had chosen to be involved . . .

M So why *are* you involved, given that it is illegal?

H Because no one else is willing to be involved.

M It sounds to me as if you're very reluctant to be involved . . .

H Yes, well I am . . . but it's the sort of thing [that] if I don't assist . . . no one else would.

M   Do you have any regrets . . .?

H   I don't have any regrets. I have feelings of ambivalence about the whole issue, but I don't regret doing it.

'Clinical discretion' and the doctor's 'turf'

The above exchange hints at a form of medical arrogance which was by no means unique among interviewees. A number of revisionist interviewees were far from supportive of the prospect of legalisation, fearing that this would burden euthanatic procedures with safeguards that would undermine their clinical discretion. Later in interview, Harvey expands on why he would choose not to perform euthanasia except in a one-on-one context and on his own terms: 'I would find it too stressful getting second opinions or . . . bureaucratising the process'.

The underlying assumption shared by several interviewees was that the doctor's values, and experience, are a sufficient protection for patients whose suffering or depression compels them to seek assistance to die. As Tony states:

> Doctors make decisions about people's lives and well-being all the time . . . It's usually a single doctor making all the decisions about someone's birth. So I'm a bit wary about having psychiatrists involved —they aren't involved in decisions about whether a baby should be delivered by caesarean section, so why should they be involved in decisions about whether someone should die? You've got to be accountable, but doctors have to be accountable in so many ways anyway.

Similarly, Gary says: 'I'd be afraid that if [euthanasia] were legalised that there would be some controlling mechanism which might make it extraordinarily difficult for it to occur, or at least time consuming, and difficult for the patient'. Gary adds that if euthanasia were legal, getting it done would involve 'too much bureaucracy' and take it out of the hands of doctors. Merril—another doctor—agrees: 'I want it to be legalised but I'm not asking for regulation; I have to use my common sense and my professional judgment'.

Other interviewees were concerned to keep euthanatic procedures away from 'dithering ethics committees'. 'Keep it the hell out of the courts!', said one. 'Don't let the lawyers make all the decisions', wrote another in the questionnaire.

Jane, a GP, stressed that legalising euthanasia would be 'dangerous for my community' because it would transform euthanasia from 'being a right' to being something the patient must 'convince somebody else about'. The sub-text is that gay decisions should not be subject to scrutiny by 'straight' regulators. Jane also admitted that she didn't like the idea of 'some stranger . . . social workers, psychiatrists' imposing themselves on the final moments of her patients' lives.

The desire to minimise intrusion into clinical discretion does not only motivate the opposition of *doctors* to legalisation. It motivates opposition from members of other health professions as well —those who might be expected to be *denied a role* if euthanasia were ever permitted under a statutory, 'medical model'. Warren, a psychotherapist and non-doctor, warned that euthanasia was a site for the 'expansion of professional power':

> People are going to be allowed to be put to death, but only if it's under the carefully organised control of a specially qualified and highly paid segment of the [medical profession]. My attitude is: fuck that, what we have to be doing here is respecting the ethical integrity of the client, and you don't need a fucking professional to do that! . . . What we have to do as professionals is to get down on our knees and bow to the autonomy of the client.

It is possible that the submerged desire to remain a 'player' in the euthanasia arena may have contributed to the misgivings certain revisionist nurses and therapists had towards legalisation.[3] Bill, a hospice nurse, believed that euthanasia should be 'limited to . . . trained groups of individuals [from] many fields—[doctors], nurses, social workers, spiritual advisers, working with the patient and the family'. But he had 'difficulty with the intrusion of law into ethical and moral areas of such complexity'. Michelle, another nurse, was more blunt. She feared that legalisation would involve too much 'red tape', and asked 'why should doctors be the only ones who can make these decisions?' Stanley, a therapist, asserted that the decision to end one's life should no more be in the hands of an ethics committee than 'a woman's right to choose to abort a foetus'.

In total, eleven interviewees (seven doctors, two nurses and two therapists) expressed reservations about legalising euthanasia, despite long-standing involvement. This was a surprising finding in light of the size of the overall sample.

While some revisionists had reservations about legalisation because of its impact on clinical decision-making, others were concerned that legalisation could encourage 'inappropriate' euthanasia:

> I would worry that legalising it will make it more acceptable and . . . more of an easy way out for doctors and patients when there are other options (Bob, doctor).

> I do have fears about . . . indiscriminate doctors who might abuse that power . . . In principle I would like to see it legalised but I understand the dilemmas of making it happen (Gay, HIV/AIDS community worker).

It is noteworthy that even those who champion the rights of patients to choose, and who in the past have *trusted themselves* to participate in illegal procedures, may still hold fears for patients under a legalised regime. Margaret, another community worker, admitted to niggling concerns that if euthanasia were legalised, there would always be someone who would 'rort the system'.

In a variant of the above attitudes, others were concerned that doctors would be unable to bear the weight of trust that a *widely-drafted* law would thrust upon them. Harvey emphasised the need for 'very strong safeguards' requiring the involvement of 'two or three' health professionals, a model blatantly out of step with his own preference for one-on-one assistance without collaboration or second opinions. Helen, a community nurse, felt that any 'regulations' must protect patients from those who 'might think they're on a mission from God . . . to put people [to] rest'. Russell, a physician, was concerned that the law not give doctors a 'carte blanche', emphasising that assisted death should remain 'a patient choice and not a physician choice'.

Some important messages emerge from these attitudes. Involvement in euthanasia, and belief in the right to choose an assisted death, do not necessarily equate with support for legalisation. Opinion is divided along a number of fault lines, with revisionists expressing ambivalence towards legalisation because of their desire to avoid regulation, and concerns about abuse.

Contempt for law and professional standards

The reality of revisionists' involvement in euthanasia encourages contempt both for the medical establishment, and for law. Tony states:

> I'm not too fussed about the legal ramifications myself, I'm getting too old and cynical for that, it's all a bit of a game, really. I'd be very unlikely to end up in jail as a result of doing something which I really felt was appropriate and in the best interests of the patient.

He adds that if some 'official' or 'bureaucracy' wanted to take him to court,

> then I'm prepared to take that chance, to stand up and say why I did it [although] I can't believe that I would suffer anything more than some sort of bond. You've got to take a chance, haven't you; I mean, if I wanted to be perfectly safe I'd go and work in a bulk-billing clinic and see coughs and colds and earn twice what I'm earning now.

Revisionists challenge both the law and the medical establishment. They have little respect for the standards of bodies such as the Australian Medical Association (to which they don't belong anyway). Many are gay men, whose sense of loyalty to their community easily outstrips any loyalty to abstract, professional norms. As Tony says, 'since I'm gay I just feel I owe it to all those guys with the virus'. It is this notion of kinship that provides the context for the altered ethic of caring many revisionists share. If euthanasia were ever legalised within a statutory framework, it would restrict the role revisionists have carved out for themselves. It would cramp their style.

The 'conservatives'

Between the extremes of traditionalism and revisionism lies a third category of interviewees whom we call the conservatives.

Defining characteristics

Conservative health care workers see their professional role in essentially conservative terms. Many are palliative care nurses who demonstrate an impressive commitment to improving the lives of dying patients. Despite this, many support the legalisation of assisted death. At the same time, they have little invested—in a personal or political sense—in law reform or current debates. Significantly, a conservative ethos does not necessarily preclude involvement in euthanasia outside the work context. Nor is it incompatible with referring patients along the 'euthanasia network' to others who are prepared to explore the issue of hastened death more directly. Some conservatives have been directly involved in active euthanasia in their professional life, although this was an extreme event which weighs heavily on their emotions. Themes of anguish and ambivalence are common for this group of interviewees whose defining characteristic is the sense that they remain 'advocates for life'.

While media coverage generally presents the euthanasia debate in terms of polarised opposites, interview-based research reveals a more complex reality.[4] A significant feature of our study was the high number of interviewees who reflected an essentially conservative ethos (sixteen, or 33 per cent). An advantage of the unstructured interview format was the opportunity to probe this conservatism, to challenge the 'story' interviewees told about themselves, peeling back the layers to reveal attitudes and involvements which would not have been captured through a short answer survey.

The interview with Ruth, a community-based nurse, provides an illustration of this process. Early on in interview, it was clear that Ruth's conservative ethos was tinged with ambivalence. 'There would be lots of people who are working in the health profession who feel that if someone makes a decision that it's time for them to end their life, then they should be assisted to do that', said Ruth. 'But I know that in myself I couldn't give someone an injection when I know that they would die—which is really a double standard. I don't think it's uncommon to have this sort of ambiguity'.

However, this was not the end of the matter. Asked if she would be prepared to take active measures to hasten a patient's death in future, Ruth replied, 'I probably would, but each situation is very individual . . . a lot of it goes on gut feeling, and that's a very individual thing'. Ruth later admitted to giving—in conjunction with a doctor—steadily increased dosages of intravenous morphine to a patient who could have been managed on oral morphine. The patient had decided that it was time to die, and the morphine was given to control 'anxiety'. It was a case of 'pharmacological oblivion': the patient became unconscious and died.

Ruth's interview also illustrates how the professional limits that nurses set for themselves may differ from the limits drawn in a personal context. Further discussion revealed that in conjunction with a doctor, Ruth had administered an extremely high dose of morphine (2000–3000 milligrams) to her own niece, who had an enormous, fungating tumour eating away her abdomen. Chris, a hospital nurse, had limited his professional involvement to playing fast and loose with 'residual morphine' during the last couple of days of a patient's life, albeit 'with the full knowledge that it's illegal'. Yet he was a complicit witness in the morphine and pethidine overdosing of his father, who had motor neurone disease.

Admissions of involvement by those who had internalised a conservative ethos and who remained, overwhelmingly, 'advocates for life', may suggest deeper levels of involvement than survey studies have evidenced, particularly where involvement takes place in a 'private capacity'. A variety of lesser involvements by conservatives, which indirectly facilitate the practice of assisted death, further underscore the fragmentation of attitudes towards euthanasia among those who superficially might be thought to be opposed to it.

Kerry's view of her professional role, for example, ruled out providing direct information about suicide methods, or assisting in euthanasia. Even so, she was sometimes prepared to refer a patient to a doctor whom she knew gave advice on these matters, provided the patient's desire for euthanasia was an enduring theme which was not precipitated by any recent, 'relievable' event, and provided the patient had seen a psychiatrist.

Given the strength of their commitment to improving life here and now, what motivates the involvement of conservatives in assisted death? For some, like Kerry, the decision to refer patients to 'activist doctors' reflected the desire to avoid perpetuating the 'botched' suicide attempts they had previously encountered. 'If somebody is going to do it and if that's their decision and they're going to get advice, then it should at least be done well.'

For others, such as Liz, who crept away from work to be interviewed in the anonymity of a department store coffee shop (see Chapter 11), involvement in euthanasia arose from 'following doctors' orders'. Some conservatives genuinely regretted, or were ambivalent about, their involvement. Gordon, a GP, had emptied his doctor's bag into a patient in the middle of the night in circumstances which must strike the most jaded observer as inappropriate (see Chapter 10). He now asserts that he would not participate in euthanasia so long as it remains illegal.

Amanda's interview provides another example of the contradictions and ambivalence that are characteristic of conservatives. Amanda told of her experience with a middle-aged man, 'John', a patient with lymphoma who had recently developed CMV retinitis, and had been sent home to die. 'John was progressing quite quickly', said Amanda, 'and he decided that he could't go blind. He had dealt with the lymphoma bit, but then to be told "well you might have six months but you're going to go blind": he couldn't deal with it'.

In response to his requests for assistance in dying, Amanda explained, 'I'm not invalidating how you're feeling, but you need to be aware of what our boundaries are as well'. After a long conversation, John said 'I can't stand this anymore, I want to die and I want somebody to help me to do it and if you're not prepared to do that, then there is no point to this conversation going on'. 'He actually dismissed me', Amanda recalled.

Not long after, John committed suicide by jumping off the roof of his flat. His partner found him and called an ambulance, but by the time it arrived, John had died. There was so much blood around and John's partner didn't want anyone to touch it or clean it up. 'It seemed a really savage and primitive way to kill yourself', Amanda reflected,

> I mean, people who are not half as well educated as this man find more comfortable ways of doing it. I just think the whole thing is disgusting, that a human being needs to go to that sort of length to achieve something that is so important to them.

Amanda revealed that every month she came in contact with patients who were seriously talking of suicide. 'I find it really difficult', she said, 'each time it's like "here we go again, what am I going to do this time"?' Although her professional role ruled out direct involvement, Amanda was prepared to refer clients who were seriously talking about euthanasia to general practitioners who she knew were prepared to assist.

Later in the conversation, however, Amanda admitted that she had participated in euthanasia 'not on a professional level but with a friend of mine' ('James'), a 28-year-old man who had Kaposi's

Sarcoma in the lungs, and also externally. A friend who was nursing James asked Amanda to be involved, for support, because 'it's much nicer to do these sort of things together than by yourself'. 'Once I'd said "Yes"', Amanda recalls, 'I thought "no, I don't think I want to do this", it was a case of trying to separate the personal from the professional'.

In the end, Amanda accessed James' vein and injected five 4-mg ampoules of potassium chloride, and 700 mg of morphine. James had his own supply of Valium and Rohypnol, and he had taken a 'great big handful' so that 'by the time we accessed his vein, he was pretty zonked'.

It took James 23 minutes to die. Amanda monitored his breathing every couple of minutes, and they talked as they waited, saying things like 'Do you think he looks comfortable?', and re-assuring each other that things were okay. 'We weren't sure what to expect', said Amanda, 'but he just sort of stopped like he was asleep'.

'We sat there for an extra five minutes after he had no pulse nor heartbeat just to make sure that we weren't wrong, and we got each other to listen to his heartbeat with a stethoscope and all that sort of stuff.' After that, 'we opened a big bottle of whisky and sat down and probably drank the whole bottle within half an hour between us'.

'The biggest problem I have now', Amanda says, reflecting back on her experience, 'is that it sort of sets a precedent for me; I've done it once, how do you decide when you do or don't do it again?'

'Conservative' health care workers embody the impact of nursing and medical practice upon legal, professional and moral abstractions. They are aware of the realities of patient suffering, and the limitations of palliative medicine in responding to that suffering. Many believe in euthanasia in principle, but they are not evangelists for change. Some have been involved in euthanasia, but with mixed feelings.

Some implications

The traditionalist, revisionist, and conservative positions that emerge from the interviews highlight a number of issues relevant to the euthanasia policy debate.[5] First, they confirm the fragmentation of attitudes and practices in the medical profession over euthanasia. This fragmentation of consensus may be more complex than pre-viously recognised. Part of this complexity arises from the involvement of conservative health care workers in euthanasia in seeming contradiction to their understanding of the professional role. Levels of involvement in euthanasia by health professionals may be deeper than survey studies suggest. Another dimension of this complexity arises from the different levels of involvement by health carers. Lesser actions include referring patients to doctors who are known to be involved, hoarding medication, and giving out 'recipes'.

Secondly, much of the research quantifying levels of involvement in assisted death has focused on doctors, while the involvement of nurses, and other health professionals, has been largely ignored. Nursing is a key variable in the debate. Asch's 1996 survey of American critical care nurses, for example, found that 17 per cent had received requests for assisted suicide or euthanasia, 16 per cent had engaged in such practices, and an additional 4 per cent had hastened patients' deaths by only pretending to provide physician-ordered life support.[6] The interviews confirm that nurses are deeply involved in assisted death, in collaboration with, and independently of, doctors. While doctors represented a majority of revisionist interviewees, Table 6-1 illustrates the involvement of nurses, therapists and community workers in AIDS-related assisted death. One is tempted to ask: do those doctors who oppose legalisation, yet feel comfortable with members of the medical profession exercising their clinical judgment in difficult cases, approve of similar actions by nurses, therapists and community workers?

Thirdly, revisionist health carers present a head-on challenge to the legal and professional prohibition on killing. Legalisation, however, invites the regulation of clinical practice, an area jealously guarded by the medical profession. Medical opposition towards legalisation, by participants in euthanasia, cannot be attributed to respect for the sanctity of life ethic. It reflects, at least partly, a desire for independence from bureaucratic controls. The issue is one of medical monopoly, and not only patient well-being.[7] This has important implications for euthanasia law reform. Such reform faces opposition not only from traditionalists who aren't involved, but from revisionists who do not wish to be monitored.

Preserving clinical independence is not a theme unique to doctors. For revisionist nurses and therapists, the 'professionalisation of euthanasia' would probably deny them a role at all, by granting exclusive control over the euthanasia event to doctors.

These and other policy issues will emerge again in later chapters. Assisted death is only a small part of the caring role of interviewees, even those who were most heavily involved. For all health carers, the challenges of palliative care remain.

Caring to the very end

A constant challenge faced by those working in HIV terminal care is to assist patients to find a sense of meaning and completion in their last days of life. The dying process in modern societies has become regimented and 'bureaucratised' within hospitals and hospices, and the role of nurses in ministering and negotiating meaning at the end of life has grown accordingly. Medicine has ousted the church as 'comforter at the deathbed'.[8] Confessional practices within the modern hospital or hospice now centre upon the nurse or counsellor, who must display the virtues of caring talk and 'emotional accompaniment' with patients who know that they are dying, and whose needs during this time impose unprecedented emotional and professional demands upon carers.[9]

'Caring talk' and 'emotional accompaniment'

These challenges were well illustrated in the interviews with nurses and counsellors. Anne, for example, is a counsellor who uses the symbology of Jungian psychology as a framework for exploring the grief and loss felt by clients. Like many interviewees, she had stepped well beyond the boundary which separates a professional relationship from a personal friendship with her clients. The account below illustrates not only the tradition of caring that AIDS has fostered, but also the burdens of care, and the raw emotion of death which in our society is largely hidden from view.

> 'Bevan' was an architect with AIDS in his early thirties. He talked frequently about suiciding when he became too debilitated. He had one last task he wanted to complete: he wanted to build a round house. In Jungian psychology, we refer to the 'Mandala', which is the potential for wholeness. So he was telling me, in Jungian terms, that he was searching for a wholeness in himself before he died.
>
> He never got to build that round house. Instead, he tore out the guts of his own house and re-arranged it instead. A lot of men, I find,

will work at something, a building project, and when they're doing it they're actually working on their own psyches. Bevan got incredibly ill, then rallied, he got ill again and rallied. He and his partner went overseas, but he was hospitalised in England with a neurological disorder, and a nurse from England accompanied him back here.

By this time Bevan was reporting amazing meditations, dreams . . . he was always in an old town in Europe, there was always a well, and a market square, and in Jungian psychology the square is also the potential for wholeness, and the well can symbolise cleansing or baptism, so I felt that he was getting ready to die.

One day Bevan left a message on my answering machine asking me would I please go down and discuss with him in a logical, rational way, how we could arrange for him to suicide. I shot down there—I was furious—I said, 'Right, we're going to talk logically about this. I don't have the pill, the magic tablet. Can you get the pill?' He said something about knowing someone in another city who could provide the pill. So then I turned to his partner: 'Are you going to sit with him while he actually swallows the pill, or will you go for a walk? Bevan hasn't said goodbye to his mother. She is in England. Doesn't she need the opportunity to say goodbye? Do we just phone her and say "Sorry old girl, Bevan's dead, pity you couldn't say goodbye"!'

Bevan never took the pill, but there were times when he went to try to cut his wrists. But still I felt he wasn't quite ready to die. On one occasion I had six men with AIDS home to lunch, they could hardly walk, one man was just shaking all the time—it was extremely difficult to arrange a meal with such sick people. Bevan came to the lunch. He said to me, 'I've had an amazing experience', and he explained how he kept having the vision about the well. He said, 'But today a Christ-like figure—I don't know who it was but some higher being—got into the well with me and we washed one another'. And I thought, I think he's probably ready to die, and so I told his partner that maybe his mother should come out from England now because he was coming fairly close to death.

Bevan would frequently throw all his psychiatric drugs down the lavatory because—as he said—'I'm not myself when I take them'. He could have easily overdosed on those drugs, and yet he wanted to be himself, he somehow wanted to be part of some natural process that was taking place, and he knew the dreams were all part of that process.

It was a very moving experience to hear him talking; I mean, gay men don't easily talk about dreams, Christ-like figures, and I certainly don't engage in talk about Christ-like figures, I don't work from a religious perspective. But to see his absolute joy, whatever way we want to look at that Christ-like figure, it was something to do with coming together, finding a sense of completion.

Around the same time I, too, had a dream. In the dream I was lying on the bed with Bevan, and the church bells rang and he said, 'You must get me to the church, you've got to get me to that service'. I said, 'I can't get you up and dressed in time for that service, I will take you to the next service'. That dream showed me that he was very ready to die. If his mother could have arrived then, and if euthanasia were legal, I would have had no hesitation in assisting at that point.

He still had tremendous mood swings. One time his partner asked me to look after him while he was away. So I went to Bevan's home, and he said to me, 'Anne, you once told me that if I slashed my wrists, you would sit with me while the blood drained out of me'. I said, 'Yes, I did say that, but now I don't think I've got the guts for it'. And Bevan said, 'Well I'm going to the kitchen and I'm getting a knife and I'm going to slit my wrists now'. He went to the kitchen, and we grappled, he was still very strong, it was a horrendous struggle. I got the knife away from him; later I found out it was far too blunt, but I didn't know that at the time.

After all that he said, 'I'm going for a walk around the block'. I followed him, fearing what he might do, dodging behind the bushes, feeling an absolute fool. That night he asked to be put into hospital for his own safety, and his mother arrived out from England. I think I had some sort of a breakdown myself that night.

Later, when I went to visit him in hospital, he said, 'Anne, I can't bear seeing you, you keep reminding me of death', which I thought was a bit rich. He said, 'You haven't been any help at all, you haven't done anything I've asked you to do [laughing]; the one thing you can do is organise for the euthanasia people to come and see me'.

So I organised for someone from the Voluntary Euthanasia Society to come and speak to him. But they don't perform euthanasia, and Bevan died naturally.

Bevan was a very complex person. I had a close relationship with him and with all my other clients. We went out for coffee and dinner, I went to their homes and they came to mine. I think it was partly that freedom, and partly my own dedication which actually burnt me out.

If nothing else, Anne's story illustrates the massive expenditure of emotional energy by those involved in end-of-life care. Another theme is the benefits of resolving the frayed components of life, and finding a sense of wholeness before death. On one view, euthanasia arbitrarily terminates this process: it is an easy exit from a process which can be emotionally painful, yet richly rewarding for the patient and those left behind.

Ria, a palliative care nurse, told the story of 'Dana', a 32-year-old woman with AIDS who weighed a mere 34 kilograms. Ria overheard that Dana had organised for a drug overdose to be smuggled into the ward, and that Dana intended to slip out into the garden and inject an overdose. Ria explained that nursing staff were unable to support her in this. 'She was a person who had taken little responsibility for her life', explained Ria, 'she was a bit of a nomad, by choosing to overdose, she chose to avoid her last responsibility of going through the dying process'.

As it turned out, there was no drug deal, and Ria was struck by how 'incredibly beautiful' Dana's dying process actually was. Dana had a narcotic need, as well as significant pain caused by microbacterial avium complex (MAC) in the gut. This caused some 'ethical dilemmas', although Ria stated that Dana probably did receive adequate morphine for her pain in the last weeks of life. Towards the end Dana reported seeing visions of her grandparents, visions where the women she played cards with every week walked into her room to say goodbye. Ria explained how Dana bounced back: she found her sitting up in bed, eating lollies and coolfruit, and hiding them under her bedclothes. Ria explains: 'She had amazing conversations with guides who I believe—from my spiritual base—were sent to help her with her transition, and she was saying things like "So we've been here before", and "They give me injections but they don't tell me what they are"'.

'Some people would class that as rambling', Ria added, noting that in the end visitors were restricted to family because each time she had contact with people, Dana would 'do a Lazarus' and bounce back from a semi-conscious state. 'It was almost like she was drawing energy from them.'

When Dana finally died, 'she looked like an angel, she was peaceful, it was beautiful'. Ria concludes: 'I felt that she had the right to overdose, but being with her through her dying process made me think that there is a reason why you go through this time . . . the hard option is to go through that dying process'.

Superficially heart-warming, Ria's account has a bitter edge. Those who do not share Ria's 'spiritual base'—and who do not believe in reincarnation—might well regard Dana's demise into a state of incoherent rambling as far from beautiful or inspiring. Even so, the denouement of life provides unique opportunities for reaching out, and for healing. Gordon, a GP, comments:

> We live in a death-denying society, [but] death is a natural part of life and it can be gentle and it can actually be a good experience; it can be painless; people can reach some sense of fulfilment before they die; the family's loss can be comforted and people can learn to treasure the person.

The fractured family relationships of many gay patients was a recurrent theme in some interviews. Robert, an AIDS physician, noted that palliation and symptom control for patients who continue to live in the community is more difficult with AIDS than other diseases because patients frequently have no network. They may be alienated from their family, or living apart from a partner. There may be no one to care for them.

Happily, family tensions are sometimes, unexpectedly, resolved. Anne felt that 'parents were under-rated' in terms of their ability to cope, and 'quite often a gay man, an IV drug user who had felt enormously rejected by the family, found himself, herself, back in the family fold'. For his part, Robert regretted how patients and their families often fail to exploit the intense emotional opportunities of this time. Relatives 'play charades', pretending that the patient isn't really dying, because they are afraid of dying themselves, and afraid of confronting the death of a loved one. He observes how families that have used this time as a 'closing experience' in their relationship with the patient, suffer less after the death.[10] The role of rituals and pre-death 'wakes' in preparing the patient, and loved ones, for the death, is explored in Chapter 7. But suffering occurs in regret: the things that aren't finished, the things that weren't said, the things the patient would like to have done but didn't.

Choosing the time of death

A feature of the interviews with nurses and doctors was the recognition that, in some sense, patients *choose* their time of death.

> You'll get people that won't die until the sun comes up; you'll get people that won't die until the sun goes down (Paula).

> There are people who will live until [after] Christmas because it's not convenient to die at Christmas, it's so messy to die at Christmas, but they'll die on the 28th of December because that's convenient, and that happens time and time again (Terri).

At one edge of the spectrum are the patients who are still in fighting mode, who continue to insist on invasive treatment 'when they might only have a week to live'. According to Donald, 'there is a huge focus on people living with AIDS, but they're dying with AIDS as well. We need to talk about death more freely so people will accept it more'.

Other patients are not ready to die because something is unresolved in their lives. Mark, a clinical psychologist, tells of a patient who died in his office. For the last three or four months the patient was carried up the stairs by an attendant with a portable IV pump and oxygen, and 'he would go into Cheyn-Stokes breathing . . . while I was talking to him'. Nevertheless, 'it seemed very important to [the patient] to come here . . . I think it was important because I was the one person in his life where he experienced an ability to be himself, and not be ashamed'.

Mark points out that those who have 'felt some satisfaction in their lives, some sense of accomplishment . . . let go much more easily'. But here was a man who at death's door was still grasping at life *'because he hadn't loved it, and he hadn't lived it, and he knew that'.*

Patients may feel they will be letting their partner or family down if they die. A number of interviewees recalled death-bed scenes where the bedside vigil had gone on for days, the family was exhausted, and there was a sense of agitation and anxiety. In these situations Anne would ask the extended family, 'Who isn't ready for [the patient] to die?' She would then explore the unconscious messages that were being sent to the patient: 'Don't die on me now, not yet'. Paula, a GP, would sometimes say directly to a patient, 'You know, it's okay if you die', noting that all some of them needed was 'permission to die'.

For other patients, death follows quickly and naturally from their decision not to fight any longer. Recalling such a case, Tony, a GP, reflects that it 'brought home to me the old stories about the Aboriginal pointing the bone, and how powerful that is, so powerful'.

The reality of 'amateur' suicide

While the focus of this book is on assisted death, the incidence of unassisted suicide cannot be left out of the policy equation. It is virtually impossible to quantify the extent to which the inaccessibility of euthanasia affects the incidence of suicide and suicide attempts. The incidence of suicide in the terminally ill is a poor argument for legalisation where suicide is motivated by depression or psychiatric disturbance. On the other hand, anecdotal evidence from interviewees does confirm that some terminally ill patients suicide because they do not know how else to avoid suffering. Unfortunately, lack of information about effective drug dosages, desperation and psychiatric factors have resulted in suicide attempts that are violent and primitive.

Suicide in patients with HIV/AIDS is well documented in the literature, with jumping from buildings, or under trains, featuring in reports as heavily selected methods.[11] In the present study, 16.8 per cent of the detailed accounts given in interview related to suicide (see Table 7-2). These thirty-four accounts included examples of patients jumping from bridges, flats and other buildings. Interviewees gave examples of suicide within hospital wards,[12] including jumping from hospital windows, crashing through a hospital window and severing the jugular vein, and overdosing on insulin, morphine and other drugs smuggled into the ward and injected into a patient's intravenous line. Outside hospital, suicide methods included hanging in a hotel, slashing one's wrists, and overdosing with sleeping pills while a friend monitored a garbage bag which was placed over the patient's head.

On the few occasions when interviewees broke down and wept during interview, it was as they reflected on 'botched' suicide attempts. The distress caused by unsuccessful suicide attempts was an important factor motivating health care workers to participate in euthanasia. Gary, a GP, began his euthanasia career after a conversation in which the patient baulked at jumping off a building or in front of a train because 'someone is going to find me', and 'it will mar my good looks'.

Nevertheless, participation in 'pre-emptive' euthanasia, in order to avoid messy suicides, carries significant risks. Firstly, suicidal ideation is frequently ill-considered. Recalling one client who had killed himself, Warren, a psychotherapist, said,

> I worried about it because this client killed himself the day after the Madonna concert. The last thing he wanted in life was to go to the Madonna concert. Sometimes I'm willing to go along with that, but there's a certain frivolousness about it which made me wonder whether the patient's judgment was good in this case.

Secondly, as discussed in Chapter 5, many who say they will commit suicide never do so. At the last moment, the 'life reflex' kicks in, the goalposts are moved back again, the patient winds down slowly and dies naturally.

Thirdly, some patients survive suicide and live to regret the attempt. Kerry tells of a patient with AIDS in his mid-forties who took an overdose of sedatives and lay unconscious on the floor for 24 hours. The prolonged unconsciousness caused rhabdomyolysis, a condition caused by the disintegration of skeletal muscle, causing painful contractions, blood disturbances, and requiring lots of rehabilitation. The patient had been very depressed following a drawn-out relationship breakdown, and had made a number of suicide attempts. After this particular episode, however, he decided he wanted to live. His retro-viral drug began to take effect, he put on weight, became physically fit, and actually lived another six months. Kerry had been involved with the patient both before and after the suicide attempt, and her reaction to the episode encapsulates one of the most important themes in the interviews: 'it just raises my ambivalence and my concern', she says.

Coping with caring

HIV, the virus which causes AIDS, is only 1 ten thousandth of a milli-
metre in diameter, yet it casts a long shadow not only over the lives
of those who test positive, but also those who care for them. 'How
do you cope with the emotional demands of HIV/AIDS care?' was a
question Magnusson explored frequently in interview. The responses
below illustrate some of the stresses that accompany caring.

> I see a therapist three times a week and he works his arse off . . . It's
> true you see a lot of suffering and distress in AIDS, and sometimes you
> have to struggle to hang on not so much to your own humanity but to
> your own sense of subtlety and shades. At the same time, you almost
> never have any sense of being bored. In that sense [working in HIV] is
> wonderfully valuable (Warren, psychotherapist).

> I won't go to the funerals anymore. I won't because they're too dis-
> tressing . . . The core of people that work here are people that have
> learned to care for people, [and] be involved, [but] then walk away.
> You've got to be able to walk away (Donald, hospital nurse).

> Until you've faced your own death . . . I don't think you can do it for
> anyone else (Sam, hospital nurse).

> I have a little procedure that I go through when I leave the unit. I
> shake the dust from my shoes, I wipe over the top of my head, and the
> day's activities are left behind me, I don't take them home. You also
> tend to have a very highly developed sense of the ridiculous, a very
> ridiculous sense of fun. We also have very strong support systems
> within our unit; you have people that you know you can go to, if you
> have to unburden yourself (Terri, palliative care nurse).

> Sometimes I just go into a really deep depression. I am lucky I have
> friends who will allow me to talk through issues, and who will say,
> 'listen, you need a break; just go away for the week-end, leave the
> phones to somebody else, and go and hug a tree and roll on the
> ground and do those sorts of things' (John, funeral director).

Some important themes emerge from these responses. Firstly,
there is a need for support, whether from friends, a partner, or other
professionals: someone who is willing to be 'unloaded upon'. Both
conservative and revisionist health carers point out, however, that

the illegality of euthanasia inhibits their ability to talk freely about difficult challenges in patient care. 'I'm afraid of sharing my views', said Tim, a GP. 'It's a real stressor', says Amanda. 'Conversations are often vaguer than you'd like them to be.' Even when a patient is discharged from hospital and health carers know or suspect that friends are going to assist the patient to die at home, 'it's very secret, it's whispered conversation'.

Amanda points to the 'breach between those who will and those who won't', adding that legal constraints create a barrier to dialogue which effectively polarises those who are surreptitiously involved in euthanasia, from those who disapprove. 'It just makes any reflection or examination of processes exceedingly difficult', she said.

This is an important factor. Opponents of euthanasia *are the very ones likely to be kept in the dark* when it is going on around them. But fear and distrust also breed a sense of isolation for those who *are* involved. One interviewee admitted that a collegial conversation that followed a seminar given by Magnusson (part of the recruitment strategy for this study) was in his experience the first time euthanasia had openly been discussed amongst a group of professionals who were 'probably supportive of it'.

Secondly, a complicating factor for many in HIV care, particularly those who are gay or gay friendly, is the relative absence of any dividing line between professional relationships and personal friendships. For some, HIV medicine is a lifestyle as well as a job, and there is no escape.

How involved should a health carer become? Terri, an experienced nurse, tells the story of her intense involvement with a gay patient over a three-month period. 'He became not only my patient, but a very dear friend . . . he grew to trust me and we expressed an amount of love for each other'. Four months after his death Terri reflected on their relationship during interview:

> If you ask me why I made a bond with a gay man who was dying, I couldn't answer you. I think there comes a time when someone comes to each of us [who] was meant to come at [that] particular time. It was the most wonderful, moving experience. It was exceptionally painful . . . There's not a day that I don't think of this person, but I don't think I'll allow myself to let it happen again; you have to protect yourself.

A third issue is the need for carers to come to terms with death itself. Miles suggests, in this context, that the taboo on physician-assisted suicide may 'prevent suicides that are improperly based on a physician's own fear of dying'.[13] To support a patient who is dying, you must not be afraid to go where the patient is going. This has particular implications for professionals and volunteer carers who are HIV infected, and who preview their own demise through their patients.

Fourthly, some health carers are not coping. AIDS care is characterised by uncertainties regarding prognosis and treatment, and by a longer time scale usually involving frequent hospital admissions and thus enhanced opportunities for developing deeper relationships with patients. Earlier in the epidemic, carers faced issues of homophobia and fear of contagion.[14] Although the assumption that AIDS is more demanding than, say, oncology or paediatrics has been questioned, the psychosocial stresses of caring are nonetheless significant.[15] The constant exposure to suffering and death, and over-involvement with patients, can lead to emotional exhaustion, depersonalisation and symptomatic disorders similar to post-traumatic stress disorder.[16] As one doctor wrote in the *Washington Post Weekly Journal of Medicine*, 'Although I have tested negative for HIV and my physical health is good, AIDS consumes me 24 hours a day'.[17] At least one interviewee had had a breakdown precipitated by the stresses of caring, and those stresses were clearly visible in others.

A final factor to bear in mind is the rewards of caring. Although challenging, HIV/AIDS care brings enormous satisfaction. Two Australian nurses expressed this in the following way: 'HIV/AIDS nursing has proved highly rewarding for us, though fraught with difficult challenges, much sadness and emotional strain. The intensity and depth of our relationships with our patients and their loved ones are certainly the highlight of our jobs'.[18] Warren, a psychotherapist, summed it up in the following way: 'the opportunity to live for others in a constructive way is a fantastic opportunity for me and it's one of the best things that ever happened to me'.

The experience of caring for patients with AIDS during the terminal stages of disease was described by one nurse as 'an incredible roller-coaster ride'. For carers who identify with the HIV/AIDS community even more closely, through sexual orientation or HIV status, there is also a sense that they are making history: a sense of mission.

The emergence of combination therapies in the mid-1990s has fuelled the hope that HIV will one day be a manageable infection. One interviewee, who has AIDS, expressed his 'utmost admiration' for those who are 'still hanging in there', showing that 'we can break those boundaries' and 'live longer with HIV and AIDS . . . than we thought possible 5 years ago'.

But despite the tremendous focus on living with AIDS, there are others who are still dying with AIDS. Interviewees reflected on the challenges they face as they accompany patients towards death. Some may argue that euthanasia is an easy option for those un-willing to make the really hard commitments of relating to a dying person, but there was little evidence of this in the interviews with nurses. Those interviews reflect a deep and genuine culture of caring, at considerable personal cost. This was illustrated through inter-viewees' appreciation of 'suicide talk', and through specific accounts of 'emotional accompaniment'.

Nevertheless, as reflected in the 'traditionalist', 'revisionist' and 'conservative' categories, there is a fragmentation of opinion within the health professions over assisted death. The contested place of suicide within the caring paradigm is beginning to be explored in the literature.[19] The euthanasia debate is challenging traditional medical ethics, and substituting new understandings of the ethical precepts of beneficence and nonmaleficence.[20]

7

People, practices and potions

*A huge weight is lifted—they know that their suffering is going to
be finished soon.*

Gary, general practitioner

Who is involved in illegal euthanasia? How is death actually
achieved? And what social practices have grown up around the
euthanasia event? This chapter presents some of the major themes
and findings of my study into AIDS-related euthanasia in Australia
and San Francisco.

I conducted forty-nine detailed interviews with doctors, nurses,
therapists, community workers, and one funeral director. After each
interview I invited interviewees to fill in a substantial questionnaire
to verify issues discussed in interview, and to collect demographic
data. The return rate for the questionnaire was 80 per cent.

As shown in Table 7-1, interviewees were predominantly in mid
career, reporting an average of 14 years professional experience. The
least experienced, a counsellor, had been in the job for 7 months.
The most experienced, a general practitioner, had been in practice
for 39 years. A variety of religious affiliations were reported. Thirty-
eight per cent of respondents identified as either atheist or agnostic.
Two interviewees, highly experienced in assisted death, were former
priests. Some chose unique descriptors, such as 'enlightened RC',

'RC with Buddhist leanings', or 'eastern spiritualist'. While information about sexual orientation was not sought, several interviewees volunteered that they were gay or lesbian. With the exception of one African-American, all interviewees were white. Many were prominent within the gay, and HIV care, communities in their city. Some had national and international reputations, and media profiles.

Table 7-1: Demographic characteristics of interviewees

	Doctors	Nurses	Therapists	Community Workers	Total
Age					
20–29	–	3	1	–	4
30–39	8	6	–	2	16
40–49	6	6	2	1	15
50–59	–	1	2	–	3
60+	1	–	–	–	1
					(39)
Years of experience					
0–4	–	–	1	no data	1
5–9	2	2	1		5
10–14	6	7	1		14
15–19	4	3	2		9
20–24	2	3	–		5
25–29	–	1	–		1
30+	1	–	–		1
					(36)
Religion					
Atheist	2	5	2	–	9
Agnostic	5	1	–	1	6
RC	1	4	–	2	7
Anglican	–	–	1	–	1
Uniting church	1	–	–	–	1
Jewish	2	1	–	–	3
Bhuddist	2	2	–	–	4
Other	2	3	2	1	8
					(39)

The recruitment strategy adopted for the study is outlined in the Appendix. Interviewees were not 'screened' on the basis of any prior knowledge about their participation in assisted death. Nevertheless, 37 of the 49 interviewees (76 per cent) reported participating in specific episodes of suicide and euthanasia. The 'active participants' included general practitioners, hospital, hospice and palliative care physicians, psychiatrists, both hospital and community-based nurses, clinical psychologists and counsellors, community workers, and one funeral director.

In the course of discussing specific accounts of involvement, a variety of third parties were also implicated. They included, predictably, other health professionals, lovers and friends of the patient. Two interviewees in different cities described the actions of Roman Catholic nuns who were present and assisted in euthanatic procedures. Another gave a detailed account of a judge who presided over one euthanasia episode, giving a moving tribute to the deceased, and making it 'clear to everyone that this was actually murder and that anyone that was involved was actually an accessory' (see Chapter 9).

People: admissions of involvement in euthanasia

Involvement in assisted death may take a wide variety of forms. The interviewees in this study covered the full spectrum from 'minimal' to 'maximum' involvement: from exploring 'suicide talk' within the counselling context, to referring patients on to a doctor or carer who was known to be sympathetic towards assisted death, to providing patients with information about lethal drug combinations, to prescribing or supplying drugs and injecting equipment, administering lethal cocktails, and 'finishing the patient off' when an attempt failed. The semi-structured interview format was well suited to verifying and further exploring details of involvement.

The detailed accounts, or case illustrations, which featured in all but two of the interviews, were a particularly important source of information. Interviewees reflected on assisted death through the lens of their own experiences. While general discussion, and the questionnaire, provided opportunities to verify each respondent's 'highest level of involvement' in assisted death, and the frequency of their involvement, the major strategy for verifying *the fact of involvement* was to invite respondents to describe specific incidents.

Specific reports of involvement

As illustrated by Table 7-2, interviewees reported a total of 203 anecdotes, each of which was categorised as relating to nursing and palliative care, suicide, or physician-assisted suicide (PAS) and active euthanasia (AVE).

Table 7-2: Summary of the kinds of anecdote told in interview (n=203)

Category of anecdote	Sub-totals	Totals	Percentage of total
Anecdotes relating to PAS/AVE		105	51.71%
HIV/AIDS related	**91**		(44.8%)
Interviewee directly involved	(75)		
'Hearsay' accounts	(16)		
Non HIV/AIDS related	**14**		(6.9%)
Interviewee directly involved	(13)		
'Hearsay' accounts	(1)		
Anecdotes relating to suicide		34	16.8%
Suicide threats	2		(1.0%)
Successful suicides	21		(10.4%)
'Botched' suicides	11		(5.4%)
Anecdotes relating to patient care		56	27.6%
Other anecdotes		8	3.9%

The 'nursing and palliative care' accounts frequently focused on discussion of a patient's feelings around suicide or euthanasia, in a context where nothing concrete was done to further this aim. The suicide accounts were further divided into 'threatened', 'botched', or 'successful' suicides. Of the 105 accounts of PAS/AVE, a small proportion (17) were 'hearsay' accounts, in the sense that the interviewee was re-telling an account of assisted death that they had *heard*, but were not personally involved in. Placing these hearsay accounts to one side, interviewees gave 88 detailed accounts of PAS/AVE in which they were direct participants. Seventy-five of these episodes related to HIV/AIDS care, while in the remaining cases the patient had some other terminal or progressively debilitating disease.

Specific reports of involvement, whether hearsay or not, were clearly distinguished from the more general rumours and speculation that occasionally featured in interview. One interviewee, for example, had heard a story 'that I have no substantiation for', although the source was a well known and credible AIDS physician. According to the interviewee, there were two physicians in San Francisco who 'you can call on a certain number and they'll come over and kill you'. 'Sometimes they go together and sometimes they go one at a time; they wear disguises ... Groucho Marx masks'. Rumours like this, however, are a world away from the 'first-hand accounts of involvement' which provided verification of each participant's role in assisted death.

Table 7-3: Summary of the nature of interviewees' involvement in 88 first-hand accounts of involvement in PAS/AVE

Nature of involvement	HIV/AIDS anecdotes (n=75)	Non-HIV/AIDS anecdotes (n=13)	Percentage of total anecdotes (n=88)
Hands on	43	7	56.8% (50)
Active at scene	4	2	6.8% (6)
Indirect facilitation	21	2	26.1% (23)
Referral	3	1	4.6% (4)
Discussion	4	0	4.6% (4)
(failed to comply with doctor's direction)	–	1	1.1% (1)

The conversational style of the interview enabled the exact nature of the interviewee's involvement on each occasion to be explored. As summarised in Table 7-3, the precise nature of involvement within each of the 88 'first-hand accounts was categorised into only one of five categories: 'hands on', 'active at the scene', 'indirect facilitation', 'referral' and 'active discussion'.

'Hands on' involvement refers to direct physical actions performed on the body of the patient in order to hasten death. Examples include setting up an IV line and, in cases of active euthanasia, injecting drug overdoses, or suffocating a comatose patient. No attempt was made to rigidly distinguish between assisted suicide and active euthanasia since both could, albeit in different ways, be carried through with the assistance of an intervener who was providing 'hands on' help, who was 'active at the scene', or who 'indirectly facilitated' the death in other ways.

'Hands on' administration of drug overdoses took several forms. In the community setting, the drug overdose was frequently both massive and explicit, taking the form of a 'death infusion', or 'lethal injection'. Hospital and hospice based interviewees, by contrast, were forced to rely on more surreptitious strategies to avoid detection. Drug dosages were typically elevated over a period of days, and were either not charted, or the chart itself was fudged to reflect increasing pain or a deterioration in the patient's condition (see Chapter 9).

Whatever method was used, the interview process enabled the intention of the health care worker to be explored. The distinction between 'hands on' involvement and established palliative care techniques was carefully investigated. For example, interviewees did not confuse pain control (in circumstances where morphine was medically indicated, yet had the concurrent effect of hastening death), with intentionally lethal drug overdoses. References to 'hands on' intervention cannot, therefore, be misconstrued as palliative care. In 50 of the 88 first-hand accounts of involvement, the interviewee was involved 'hands on'.

'Active at scene' involvement refers to direct actions intended to hasten death, but not involving physical contact with the patient's body. One typical example involved instructing the patient, other health care workers, lovers or friends, how to prepare and administer a lethal drug overdose. More generally, it included the provision of assistance and moral support at the scene, to the 'hands on' interveners. It also encompassed acting as an accomplice in the sense of being complicit, supportive, and giving the consent without which the process would not have gone ahead. Bill, a hospice nurse, noted that on occasions where the patient did not require assistance to take a lethal cocktail, the nursing role is 'to co-ordinate all these people and keep everybody in a pattern where they're not freaking out about the whole thing'.

In a typical example of 'present at scene' involvement, Stephen, a psychiatric nurse, was called in to do an 'assessment' of 'Frank', a patient with AIDS dementia who had suffered an acute episode. Frank had previously hoarded several ampoules of morphine which were prescribed for pain, apparently intending to take a lethal dose. After Frank's release from hospital, Stephen 'borrowed' a syringe from his place of employment and supervised as the patient's lover gave Frank a fatal dose. Even when they did not administer drugs personally, interviewees did see themselves as participants in assisted suicide or euthanasia when they took on the role of advising and mentoring the 'hands on' interveners.

'Active at scene' involvement also encompasses situations where a doctor gave directions to nursing staff to administer an overdose that was intended to hasten the patient's death. In a hospital or hospice this is the usual way that medications will be administered.

'Indirect facilitation' refers to a range of actions including prescribing, donating or stealing drugs, providing the syringes subsequently used in the euthanatic procedure, giving specific advice on how to perform euthanasia (although not at the bedside), being 'on call' while others are attempting to perform euthanasia, and knowingly assisting in covering up evidence of an assisted death, whether by signing the death certificate or providing a discreet burial service.

In contrast to the three categories above, the final two categories refer to relatively modest forms of intervention. 'Referral' relates to episodes where the interviewee actively tried to procure assistance on behalf of the patient from someone else. The lowest level of involvement, 'active discussion', refers to episodes where the interviewee discussed the euthanasia option in detail with a patient, usually over a period of time, and with a view to assisting in future. It was this sense of willingness or activism, conveyed during the recounting of the episode, that explains why these episodes were categorised as examples of 'direct accounts of involvement', rather than as 'care anecdotes'. Typically, the anticipated involvement had not occurred by the date of interview, or the patient had died naturally in the meantime.

The specific reports of involvement provided first-hand examples which verified each interviewee's participation in assisted death. But these reports do not even begin to quantify the number of times interviewees had been involved in illicit, euthanatic procedures. Merril, for example—one of two interviewees who told no anecdotes in interview—estimated that he had facilitated suicide by providing large quantities of drugs, or had injected drugs directly, on forty occasions over the preceding decade.

Interviewees' 'highest level' of involvement in assisted death

I adopted a three-point strategy for clarifying the 'highest level' at which each interviewee had participated in assisted suicide or euthanasia. Firstly, the anecdotes or case illustrations provided concrete examples of involvement. Secondly, the face-to-face interview format provided the opportunity to question respondents directly, and to probe for information. Thirdly, the questionnaire provided opportunities for verification and additional disclosures. Together, these methods give a high degree of insight into the extent of each interviewee's involvement.

Table 7-4 categorises each of the 49 interviewees according to their highest level of involvement in assisted death, using the five categories of involvement described above. Respondents were categorised conservatively; in a couple of cases, ambiguity led to an interviewee being assigned a lower level of involvement than may well have been the case. Kyle, for example, had provided lethal overdoses in a 'hands on' capacity during the Vietnam war (see Chapter 1). Nevertheless, I categorised him according to his more recent actions, which were limited to 'indirectly facilitating' the suicides of AIDS patients.

Table 7-4 only accounts for interviewees' *highest level of involvement*, and this represents only one aspect of overall involvement. For example, a doctor who had been involved 'hands on' (for example, by administering a lethal injection), would frequently have also 'indirectly facilitated' either that or another death, perhaps by advising, supplying the drugs, or lying on the death certificate. Similarly, 'hands on' interveners would frequently have been 'active at the scene' on other occasions. The relative absence of interviewees in the 'referral' and 'discussion' categories suggests that those who were prepared to refer patients on, or to actively counsel them about strategies for achieving death, were also prepared to go further and assist more directly. Overall, 76 per cent of the cohort of interviewees had assisted in specific episodes of suicide and euthanasia in a way that went beyond mere referral or discussion. Fifty-three per

Angels of Death

Table 7-4: A summary of interviewees' 'highest level' of involvement in assisted death (n=49)

Nature of involvement	Doctors	Nurses	Therapists	Comm. workers	Funeral director	Total
'Hands on'	11	9	2	3	1	26 (53%)
'Active at scene'	3	–	–	1	–	4 (8.2%)
'Indirect facilitation'	3	2	2	–	–	7 (14.3%)
'Referral'	–	1	–	–	–	1 (2.0%)
'Discussion'	–	–	–	–	–	0
No involvement	4	5	2	–	–	11 (22.5%)

cent of interviewees had been involved in a 'hands on' capacity. While eleven interviewees had had no involvement in assisted death, their testimony was nevertheless notable for the rich and complex picture it painted of palliative care and end-of-life challenges.

Frequency of involvement

In contrast to the high level of accuracy in clarifying each interviewee's 'highest level' of involvement in episodes of assisted suicide or euthanasia, numerical estimates of the number of times an interviewee had been involved are less satisfactory. There are at least three reasons for this. Interviewees who had been involved on many occasions over a period of years found it genuinely difficult to give a fixed estimate. Some chose expressions like 'immemorable', and 'too many to remember' to describe the frequency of their involvement.

Secondly, in contrast to the specific accounts of involvement explored in interview, overall estimates do not account for the varying nature of involvement on different occasions. Finally, there were substantial discrepancies in some cases between the estimates given in interview, and subsequently in the questionnaire, perhaps for the very reasons given above.

Despite these qualifications, the impressive euthanasia credentials of many of the interviewees are clearly evident. Table 7-5 gives

Table 7-5: Frequency of involvement in episodes of assisted death, as estimated by the 'top dozen' interviewees

Name & occupation	Dominant form of assistance	Total number of times involved (estimated in interview)	Total number of times involved (estimated in questionnaire)	Number of anecdotes told in interview illustrating direct involvement
Jane, GP	'Hands on'—lethal injection at patient's home	50–60 with AIDS patients	50–100	5
Merril, GP	'Indirect facilitation'—prescribes drugs, oversees drug overdose (has given lethal injection)	perhaps twice a year for 20 years	N/A	0
Kyle, GP	'Indirect facilitation'—prescribe drugs for overdose	15 times	N/A	1
Russell, hosp physician	'Indirect facilitation'—prescribe drugs for stockpiling, provide syringes for euthanasia	30–40 times	~10 times	3
Harvey, GP	'Hands on'—lethal injection at patient's home	dozen times	7 times	2
Tony, GP	'Hands on'—steady escalation of morphine, or sudden withdrawal of cortisone drugs	N/A	10–12	3
Peter, comm. Nurse	Hands on'—frequently lethal injection	5–6 lethal injections at patient's home	AIDS patients (20–25 times); terminally ill non AIDS (4 times); able-bodied HIV (3 times)	4
Bill, hospice nurse	Mixed—act as intermediary between patient and doctor; obtained drugs for overdose; educating patient; assisting at scene; lethal overdose (once)	'immemorable'	'greater than 50, certainly'	2
Erin, comm. Nurse	Mixed—procuring drugs, counselling the process, administering drugs	4 times in past year	20–40 (AIDS patients), and that number again with terminally ill non-AIDS	3
Michelle, comm. Nurse	Mixed—liaison role, obtaining drugs, active at scene, lethal injections	6–8 times in 4 years	6 times	3
Stanley, therapist	'Active at scene'—coaching, create rituals; assist drug ingestion	'a couple of dozen, probably'	a dozen (AIDS patients); 5–6 (terminally ill non-AIDS)	1
Mark, therapist	Mixed—active at scene, lethal injection	5–6	5	4

a thumbnail sketch of the frequency of involvement of those who appeared to be most 'active'. Even if one assumes that these numbers are inflated, it is significant that a cohort of less than 50 interviewees, recruited in a variety of ways, should have resulted in so many interviewees who estimated that they had participated in assisted death on a dozen occasions or more. General practitioners like Gary (see Chapter 1), who gave six separate accounts of involvement in interview, don't even make it into the table!

An equally important implication from the table is that euthanasia activism is not limited to doctors, even though community-based doctors (GPs) feature prominently in terms of frequency. A significant finding of the study overall, worth repeating, is that many of the most seasoned operators are not doctors, but community and hospice nurses, and therapists, many of whom have no training or experience in palliative care.

Practices: achieving euthanasia death

Where patients die

Euthanasia death encompasses a wide variety of social practices. There was significant evidence of euthanasia in hospitals, including Catholic hospitals (see Chapter 9). More frequently, patients died at home, in hospice settings, or were discharged from hospital or hospice in order to die at home. Some died alone, overdosing on medications previously supplied or prescribed by interviewees. A recurrent theme in interviews was that patients were concerned not to implicate those assisting them. The self-administration of stockpiled medications was one way of ensuring this. On some occasions, interviewees, friends or family were asked to leave, returning to find the patient dead.

Some patients died in the presence of the interviewee, with no one else present. Interview accounts suggest that this was particularly distressing and exhausting for the interviewee, although it carried the advantage that there were no witnesses to the procedure. Others died with a partner or small circle of friends present: sometimes the death was preceded by a party of friends and family who had gathered to celebrate the patient's life in a 'pre-death wake'. Interviewees were occasionally dismayed by these gatherings. For example, one psychiatrist who arrived to assist in a death promptly turned on his heel when he saw that a 'cast of thousands' was involved.

Several interviewees described death scenes where only some of those present were aware that euthanasia was, in fact, occurring. In a memorable passage, Michelle, a community nurse, describes a failed overdose that took place in the bedroom of a 'very very small house', crowded full with relatives. None of the family realised what was happening, 'except for [the patient's] sister and her husband [who] had cottoned on'. The atmosphere was emotional, and then all of a sudden the patient's niece 'rocked up', a 'registered nurse, [but] fortunately only college trained and only experienced in geriatrics'. On that occasion, Michelle made frantic contact with a doctor who was 'on call', and who came over to administer a subsequent, and successful, injection. As this report illustrates, deception is a constant feature of illicit euthanasia.

How patients die

There is no typical procedure for achieving euthanasia death, but rather a spectrum of practices which reflects the drugs available to the health care worker, their preferred modus operandi, ethical framework, assessment of the risks of detection, as well as the patient's clinical condition. A variety of pharmacological strategies was reported. Some wanted to cause death as quickly as possible. Others were content to escalate the administration of drugs over a period of days. This made good sense in hospital contexts, where doctors administer drugs vicariously through nurses, and where an abrupt death might have looked suspicious without a preceding, documented decline (real or fabricated).

Drug overdoses were the most common strategy for achieving death, whether through a series of injections, infusions or, in one instance, by unlocking the lock on a syringe driver administering morphine. Non-drug strategies were occasionally mentioned. One community nurse performed euthanasia by carbon dioxide narcosis, by interrupting the flow of oxygen through a breathing apparatus, and placing the cardiac monitor on standby. On another occasion, an interviewee dialled down the settings of a ventilator.

Assisted suicide and euthanasia attempts frequently fail. One interviewee spoke of a patient who failed to take an anti-emetic and vomited a lethal concoction of Seconal and yoghurt. He died on the second attempt, after re-ingesting his vomit. Consistent with Ogden's findings in Vancouver,[1] and Jamison's San Francisco study,[2] interviewees gave detailed examples of episodes where they had strangled comatose patients, suffocated them with pillows, or injected air into their veins. 'Botched attempts' are a troubling feature of illicit euthanasia, discussed further in Chapter 10.

Differences between Australian cities and San Francisco

In contrast to Australia, the debate about assisted death in the United States has focused rather narrowly on assisted suicide. Australian interviewees were more likely to see their role as extending to the direct administration of drug overdoses, whereas the focus for American health carers was more towards facilitating either the patient's own suicide, or a euthanasia procedure performed by the patient's partner or informal care giver. In their study of the role of informal care givers in hastening AIDS deaths in San Francisco, Cooke, Gourlay, Collette and colleagues point out that partners and care givers played the central role, with physicians giving input 'from a distance'.[3] Despite this, San Francisco interviewees gave many examples of 'hands on' euthanasia.

Several other themes were unique to, or accentuated within, the Californian interviews. These included allegations of a 'drugs courier service' run by air hostesses between San Francisco and Mexico. San Francisco interviewees focused more on the use of illegal street drugs in euthanasia. The theme of an 'underground pharmacy' for the redistribution of both AIDS medications and euthanasia drugs, while evident in Australian interviews, was more pronounced in the American interviews. The same was true of respondents' discussion of 'underground language', and the role of particular words and expressions in communicating requests for euthanasia, or in conveying advice on lethal dosages.

A final discrepancy related to interviewees' concerns about the risks of making euthanasia legally available to patients who lacked access to appropriate health care. Due to the existence of the national health insurance system in Australia (Medicare), this issue was raised by Australian interviewees *only* within the context of inadequate funding and development of, specifically, palliative care. Several Californian interviewees had more general concerns, pointing to the lack of 'universal healthcare' in America, and the potential consequences for those who were unable to 'mobilise resources for themselves from the health and social service[s] system'.

Overall, the San Francisco interviewees conveyed the impression of a euthanasia underground that was more deeply entrenched, with a longer and richer history, despite the more limited focus on assisted suicide in the Californian arm of the study.

Pre-death rituals

Ritual plays an important part in euthanasia deaths. The pre-death 'wake' is particularly important. It may take the form of a lavish meal with music, farewells, and rituals of blessing, giving and receiving, in the presence of the patient's closest friends or family. The meal itself may be the final phase of a planning process which involves the costing of coffins and funerals, finalising a will, giving farewells and parting messages, as well as planning the death event itself. Patients plan the menu, the music and the guest list.

There is a sense of pathos in hearing interviewees describe these occasions. Stephen, a nurse and volunteer carer, spoke of 'smoked oysters and a couple of bottles of wine or champagne'. Michelle, a community nurse, recalls 'we all had Kentucky Fried together and . . . he did some really stupid funny things'. 'It was a very twisted night, a very twisted night', said Jane, recalling the jokes thrown around at one such party.

Pre-death rituals are deliberate, symbolic acts which provide a context for celebrating the patient's life and finding meaning in the death. One doctor explained how patients with a traditional religious upbringing frequently felt alienated because church standards conflicted with their sexual lifestyle. Because of this, patients 'don't want ministers of religion hanging over the end of their bed when they're dying'. The rituals that occur before death, and at the subsequent funeral, therefore, tend to be both unique to each patient and not overtly religious. They may be fashioned with the assistance of friends, and others who have stepped in to perform a ministerial role at the end of life.

Stanley, an ex-priest and therapist, provides a candid illustration of how the 'ministerial' role can be combined with that of 'euthanasia consultant'. Periodically, Stanley was requested to perform 'assessments' on patients wishing to die, to preside over the death, or to perform the burial service. Stanley described his role in the following terms:

> Most of it's a coach[ing] kind of thing . . . helping people relax . . . creating . . . a peaceful life-affirming environment, trying to keep the chaos that often surrounds death to a minimum. I've tried to help educate people who will survive and attend the dying person on the etiquette of being present at such a pivotal moment, *and there is etiquette*, it seems to me . . . Oftentimes it's helping the dying create a ritual to celebrate this um transitional phase in their life—some people believe . . . in reincarnation or life after death and so it's truly a transition . . .—giving gifts and receiving them, giving blessings and receiving them, saying thank you, saying goodbye, that kind of stuff; all of those things [that] make for a peaceful, wise and good death.

Later in the conversation, I asked:

> M   How does religion fit in with all of this?
> S   You've got me [laughing], I haven't a clue! . . . Nothing in seminary prepared me [for this].

Stanley gave a poignant example of the role of ritual in creating a sense of completion and peace at the bedside. He had been asked to 'evaluate' a patient who was lingering on beyond the time his loved ones had expected him to die. On arriving at the patient's home, Stanley recalls:

> Here was this little stick-man lying in bed. I just took one look at him and I said, 'What in the world are you still doing here? You look like shit!' . . . He had a smile and he goes, 'I don't know what I'm still doing here either . . . I thought I'd be dead by now'. I said, 'Well . . . I feel blockage, something's blocking here' . . . This guy owned a restaurant here in town, he was quite a recognised chef . . . So I asked him, 'Did you sell the restaurant?' And he goes, 'yeah', and I said, 'All the paperwork done?', and he said, 'yeah'. And I said, '[Any] family [stuff] outstanding?' [And he said,] 'No, they're all here' . . . I don't know how this came to me but . . . I said, 'you know we all have a need for immortality . . . do you have such a desire?' He thought for a moment and his eyes welled up with tears . . . He said, 'I've been a

"foodie" all of my life, I've cooked with the best and the best have cooked with me . . . I've been all over the world . . . Now that I'm dying, *no one has asked me for my recipes*'. That struck a chord with me and I immediately called his lover and the other people who were around and we created a little ritual, we lit some candles and some incense and put some soft music on . . . He was working on a cook-book at the time and so all of this stuff was on computer disks, and so we made this ritual where he gave the disks to his friends and he said, 'make me live'. And within an hour he was dead [Stanley weeps].

While some pre-death wakes and rituals were described as 'parties', others were more modest and intimate. Joseph, a physician who had written a 'lethal prescription' to assist a suicide, tells how the deceased man's partner described their final meal together: 'It was Valentine's Day and they had a lovely meal with champagne . . . they held each other, and then . . . his partner took his pills and was released'. Terri, a hospital nurse, described a patient who 'made gifts of his lovely trinkets and his special items . . . [and] told people what he wanted them to have from his flat'. John, a funeral director, described the death of a close friend in these terms:

She woke up [and] was in pain, she asked for something and I said, 'What do you want? I gave you an injection an hour ago, we really can't give you anything more'. And she said, 'I want *it* done, *I do not want to see morning*'. She asked for a cup of tea, so I made her a cup of tea and we settled and we discussed [it] . . . When she'd had her cup of tea she asked for the injection. She had no bloody skin [left], she was just skin and bone, she had no muscle left by that time. I found a reasonable spot on her upper thigh and injected her . . . I said, 'This wasn't in the contract when I met you . . . this wasn't part of the deal' . . . Her final words were 'Well next time you'll read the small print you little bastard!' She was always one for a smart line. [Those] were her last words . . . She just lapsed into unconsciousness, and [I] cradled her.

Fatal moments

Being present during the process of assisted death is an intense experience. Interviewees described how they supported each other during the final moments, checking the patient's pulse, observing 'the difference between looking at somebody [who is] nearly dead and looking at somebody [who] *is* dead'.

Some described a sense of relief, elation and even celebration after death had been achieved. One nurse reports, 'we all just sat there and kissed each other and cried, and laughed and had a drink and all that sort of stuff'. Another says, '[We] opened a big bottle of whisky and sat down and probably drank the whole bottle within half an hour between the four of us and felt much better after that [laugh]'. A third described his embarrassment as members of the patient's family 'thanked me profusely again and again'.

Other interviewees reported feelings of closeness and bonding which resulted from shared participation in both successful and unsuccessful episodes. These bonds—forged in the highly charged death-bed environment—may persist in the future, to be re-awakened each time participants see each other. 'We had a lunch [to] de-brief around how we felt', said one community worker.

> That was really quite a powerful thing . . . [the] bond is still there, three years later. It may sound strange to say, but it was quite a special thing to be involved in, *to know that you're taking . . . someone's life*, [although] the overriding factor for all of us was that he wasn't going to suffer anymore.

But it would be misleading to suggest that all participants feel invigorated or satisfied by their involvement in these procedures. Bill, a hospice nurse, reports that overdosing a patient was 'the hardest thing . . . I was really wrecked for days after that, you know, I really was'. Another doctor admits, 'I obviously needed to [have] some degree of control, but it really . . . blew us both away'. John, a funeral director, reflects,

> it took me weeks [long silence] to re-adjust [to] the fact that I had done the right thing . . . I was fine right up until the day of the funeral and then I just went through sheer hell from the day of the funeral— had I done the right thing? I ended up having to go and see a therapist about it.

In retrospect, John is glad he went through this period of 'doubt and questioning' because it caused him to reassess his beliefs. He reports: 'I am probably more firmly committed to [voluntary eutha- nasia] now than I ever was'. Even so, it is clear that participants in euthanasia do not see their involvement in shallow or simplistic terms. They describe feelings of sadness and ambivalence. Burn-out and emotional exhaustion are very real hazards for those involved on multiple occasions (see Chapter 11). For health carers who performed euthanasia without the support of others, death brings a sense of loneliness, and sadness, as well as a cadaver and the responsibilities of completing paperwork, concealing suspicious evidence and reporting the death.

There were occasional reports of participants going to pieces after a death. Stanley describes the hysteria of a man who felt driven to suffocate his lover with a pillow, as the hours dragged on and a morphine infusion failed to work. 'He called me two days later', recalls Stanley, saying, ' "I killed my lover, I killed my lover!" and I said "well good thing you're having this response . . . because you had to suspend everything that you hold sacred about life . . . to do this heroic act for the man that you loved" '. 'We talked about it a bit', says Stanley, and eventually the man was 'at peace' because he knew that what he had done was 'not a malicious act, but a heroic act'.

Potions and death recipes

Euthanasia is forbidden medicine. Because it is practised in secret, there is no manual on how to 'get it right'.[4] Interviewees earned their expertise through trial and error and, not surprisingly, the interviews revealed an odd assortment of overdose recipes. Many of these had featured in 'botched attempts'. There was little consensus over which recipes were thought to be more effective in practice. The ever-present challenge was to access drug combinations that would cause a quick and gentle death, while minimising the risk of detection.

The most frequent recipes mentioned in interview were overdoses of therapeutic drugs that were medically indicated or could plausibly be prescribed for a terminally ill patient with AIDS. Morphine was readily accessible to general practitioners and physicians and was typically administered intravenously (sometimes in combination with pethidine) together with oral or intravenous overdoses of a variety of other classes of drug. These included antidepressants such as Tryptanol (amitriptyline), and Prothiaden (dothiepin), sedating agents such as Valium (diazepam), Rohypnol (flunitrazepam), and Hypnovel (midazolam), antipsychotics such as Largactil (chlorpromazine), and other drugs including Lanoxin (digoxin, a cardiac drug), aminophylline (a bronchodilator), and Tegretol (carbamazepine, an anti-epileptic). Intravenous potassium chloride, which in high doses can paralyse the heart muscle, was a frequent chaser following one of the above combinations.

The advantages of anti-depressants include their initial value as sedating agents, and their ability to offset the nausea and other unpleasant effects of high-dose intravenous morphine. Zane, a palliative care physician, had carefully thought through the 'combination recipe' he favoured:

> We used an anaesthetic control drug, a hospital drug, midazolam to suppress muscle spasms but also knowing that it will suppress breathing [and] allow waste gases to build up in the body and the oxygen level gradually to drop; the morphia relieves any pain, and also stops the brain being affected by the low oxygen level.

Nevertheless, there are several reasons why morphine and sedatives were frequently unsuccessful in precipitating death. Young patients with unaffected hearts can show extraordinary tolerance to narcotics, particularly morphine, if they have previously received morphine as pain relief, or have a history of IV drug use. Bob, a GP, described a case which had ended only 36 hours earlier, which bears this out. The patient's morphine infusion had been rapidly increased from 15 mg per 24 hours to 360 mg in order to hasten death. Significant doses of Serenace (haloperidol), and Maxolon (metodopramide)—initially used for nausea and sedation—and midazolam, were also administered. But it still took from Sunday to Thursday for the patient to die. Over the last two days Bob administered a further bolus dose of 360 mg morphine, as well as all the midazolam in his doctor's bag.[5] Bob remains unsure whether it was the drugs, or the patient's dehydration and pneumonia, which precipitated death. The limitations of analgesics become apparent when one appreciates that patients with AIDS will not infrequently be on morphine infusions of 400 mg to 700 mg a day, sometimes more.

Further problems may arise where drugs are taken orally. Overdoses of anti-depressants can slow down stomach motility. 'The anti-depressants will actually sit in the stomach and not move', says Damian, a psychiatrist, cautioning that patients can be rushed to hospital hours after ingesting the drug, 'have their stomach pumped and actually survive the episode'.

Patients may also vomit the drugs, or be too debilitated to ingest them in the first place. Many of the successful recipes reported by interviewees, therefore, included anti-nausea drugs or anti-emetics, such as Maxolon or Serenace. Tony, a general practitioner, noted that 'direct tubes straight into the stomach' are 'very handy for administering . . . liquid morphine and Largactil and most other drugs . . . you can just keep on pumping it into the stomach until they die'.

Overdoses of commonly prescribed, therapeutic drugs—such as Valium or morphine—have the advantage of minimising the risk of detection. Michelle, a community nurse, was enthusiastic about the benefits of overdoses of 'insulin for diabetics', and 'KCl [that] can't be traced in the dead body'. John, a funeral director, recalled a death where a mixture of pethidine, morphine and insulin was used for a patient allergic to pethidine.

Zane, a palliative physician, had developed the technique of giving his patients 'quite large doses' of cortisone, before their admission to hospital, conscious of the fact that cortisone suppresses adrenal function and creates a dependency. 'My experience has been that if you suddenly withdraw the cortisone and only gradually increase the morphine then the patient will die within 24 to 48 hours'. Tony, a general practitioner, had also used this strategy with success.

In contrast to analgesics, sedatives and anti-depressants, Australian interviewees noted that barbiturates were controlled substances and more difficult to prescribe without drawing attention to oneself. Even so, both Australian and American interviewees disclosed recipes involving barbiturates such as secobarbital (Seconal). Paula, a GP, told of one (successful) incident where she prescribed a box of pentobarbitone which was ground up by the pharmacist and mixed with alcohol and sugar to make it palatable. Joseph, an HIV/AIDS specialist used a recipe borrowed from a friend, consisting of five grams of secobarbital, and Compazine (prochloperazine, an anti-psychotic). The drugs were mixed into yoghurt, and the patient took them the night before, and an hour before, the event. Joseph adds: 'It's nice to finish it down with a nice glass of port'. Similarly, Merril advocated massive combinations of Seconal and Demoral (secobarbital) with alcohol ('fine wine probably') and anti-emetics.

Barbiturates were also implicated in the 'botched attempts' interviewees reported in this study. Mark, a clinical psychologist, received a phone call from a distressed patient whose partner had taken between 7 and 8 grams of Seconal, together with anti-emetics and a third of a bottle of vodka. The drama only ended when Mark's patient asphyxiated his (comatose) partner using a plastic bag.

Josh, a young GP, told how he had successfully used a drug called Lethabarb (pentobarbitone), sourced from a friendly vet, in two successful episodes. 'I have a joke with the vet that it's "1 ml per kill", meaning 1 ml per kilogram [of the patient's weight]', says Josh. 'Actually it's half a ml per kilogram so it's about 25–30 mls; [the vet] says that's enough to kill a great Dane and most patients in this state are fairly lean'. Josh described death from Lethabarb in the following way:

> It actually causes . . . cardiac arrest pretty quickly, and certainly causes complete neurological desensitisation and death within about a second . . . it's an incredible experience because this person . . . he was alive and talking, and wanting it to happen and within a second or two was ashen and very much dead and not breathing and looked like a dead person.

Josh felt that Lethabarb was 'incredibly humane' and a 'real delivery' because 'you don't have the agonal respirations . . . all that awful stuff'.

Harvey, an unassuming suburban practitioner who had performed euthanasia a dozen times, favoured injections of intramuscular morphine (several hundred milligrams), combined with massive oral dosages of Betaloc (metoprolol), an anti-hypertensive. 'If you've got 5 minutes you can actually swallow hundreds of tablets if you do it calmly', says Harvey, adding that he sits with patients while they swallow 5000 mg of Betaloc, together with sedatives such as Rohypnol and Valium, preceded by 'three or four nips of alcohol to potentiate the action of the drugs'. Harvey, who felt that 'psychologically, I don't think I could cope with giving intravenous injections', points to the absence of 'good quality literature on the subject', but adds that his combination had always been successful within three or four hours.

Apart from analgesics, sedatives, anti-psychotics, anti-depressants, barbiturates and betablockers, some interviewees mentioned the use of illegal 'street drugs' to hasten death. According to one therapist:

> We are a drug culture here, particularly in the west coast and particularly in San Francisco. [People] know a whole lot more about street drugs than they do about pharmaceuticals and they know how to overdose on street drugs: cocaine, heroin . . . they're much easier to get than Seconal . . . There's another way for people to be very proactive by just, you know, going to their local dealers and getting the wherewithal.

The same interviewee admitted to being involved in a number of deaths involving heroin, and 'speedball' (a combination of cocaine and heroin).

The 'death recipes' that emerged from the interviews varied not only in terms of the drugs used, but also in the underlying pharmacological strategy. Participants such as Josh, who had used and supplied other doctors with veterinary drugs, sought to produce an instantaneous death. Similarly, Gary claimed that he had 'refined the techniques', using a (fairly conventional) cocktail of valium, morphine and potassium chloride so that 'I can do it in three or four minutes now'.

By contrast, Tony, another GP, didn't see 'any great advance in having a sharp clinical death . . . Having that last cup of tea—I think that's a bit dramatic'. Like Harvey, Bob, Zane and others, his strategy involved the continual escalation of drugs over hours or days, with a commitment to monitor the process until the end. Martin, a community worker, chose morphine over potassium chloride to assist his lover to die because they had previously discussed the spiritual aspects of dying, and the possible value of *declining*, rather than dying suddenly.

As discussed in Chapter 10, some of the most pathetic and degrading stories came from interviewees who had miscalculated the doses required to achieve death and who, hours or days later, were now desperate to 'finish the patient off', to flee the scene, and avoid detection. Said one community nurse: 'The following day we just gave him every drug we had to try and stop the heartbeat, and that means huge doses of digoxin, and aminophylline—any drugs open in the doctor's box'.

Why do they do it?

This is perhaps the most difficult question of all. An understanding of each respondent's personal philosophy emerged through the interview, and specific motivations were evident from detailed accounts of involvement. Nonetheless, while *ex post facto* reasons for participating in assisted death give important clues, they may also be coloured by self-justification. The strongest theme which emerges for me, having lived and breathed the interviews over several years now, is that health carers participate in euthanasia for all sorts of laudatory, idiosyncratic and reprehensible reasons. Motivations are complex and multi-faceted. A similar theme emerges from research into the reasons underlying the withdrawal of life-support from terminally ill patients.[6]

Belief in the patient's right to choose, a desire to halt the patient's suffering, and a sense of compassion or 'emotional accompaniment' with the patient feature in many accounts. These are conventional, respectable reasons for participating in euthanasia, which readers will encounter throughout this book. But they are not the only ones.

Some interviewees admitted that they were involved in euthanasia in order to ensure that 'it was done properly'. Harvey, a general practitioner, volunteered that 'aesthetically', euthanasia is 'very dehumanising', and that an 'aesthetic death would be good quality palliative care and dying peacefully at home, or in a good quality hospice'. He adds, however, 'I can't necessarily project my value system on . . . everyone else', and that 'I suppose many professional people may do things they're ambivalent about'. Harvey surmises that one reason why he is inolved is because if patients are going to do it, 'it's important that it's done properly'.

Mark, a therapist, raised a similar point. Asked whether he would continue to be involved in assisted death in future, he replied

'I'd rather not, you know . . . I feel like it's not my role'. He then explained that his involvement was an act of 'kindness and decency' which arose 'by default, because physicians are not doing it'.

Some of the reasons interviewees gave for their involvement in euthasasia provide ready ammunition for those who oppose assisted death. In a case explored in detail in Chapter 11, one nurse followed a physician's orders and participated in an episode of what she perceived as involuntary euthanasia because she was 'frightened' and didn't want to 'open up a hornet's nest' by defying her superiors. For another, the sheer excitement and drama of it all appears to have been a major contributing factor. One young doctor was influenced by requests from the patient's family, even though he had no opportunity to independently assess what the patient wanted (the patient was unable to communicate). Another admitted that part of the reason why he emptied the contents of his doctor's bag into a comatose patient was because he had a severe flu, 'felt dreadful and . . . just wanted to get out of there'.

Some readers may be tempted to demonise those interviewees who detailed their experiences of participation in assisted suicide and euthanasia. In my view, this is just a little *too easy*. For all their failings, and in all their complexity, the interviewees were nevertheless hard-working health carers who were deeply committed to their work, who engendered trust, who held positions of leadership and represented their respective professions to the wider community.

The conversational interview format, the detailed accounts of involvement, and the follow-up questionnaire, provided different ways of investigating the 'euthanasia profile' of each interviewee. Inevitably, what we know is limited to what interviewees were willing to divulge. No attempt was made to independently verify individual accounts, as this would have compromised the confidentiality which was central to the study. The limits of any methodology must be acknowledged, and methodology is an easy target for studies which present 'uncomfortable findings'. The following chapter, therefore, aims to make the interview event as transparent as possible, and to give readers a sense of what it was like to listen as interviewees described their involvement in assisted death.

8

Doing fieldwork in the euthanasia underground

(with P. H. Ballis)

We have ... become a singularly confessing society. The confession has spread its effects far and wide. It plays a part in justice, medicine, education, family relationships, and love relations, in the most ordinary affairs of everyday life and in the most solemn rites; one confesses one's crimes, one's sins, one's thoughts and desires, one's illnesses and troubles; one goes about telling, with the greatest precision, whatever is most difficult to tell.

Michel Foucault[1]

The interviews in this study generated both confessional tales of personal involvement in euthanasia, as well as an understanding of a culture of illegal euthanasia. The focus of other chapters in this book is on what the interviewees *did*, in terms of participation in euthanasia. This chapter, by contrast, reflects on the *interview event*: what interviewees *said* about what they did, how they said it, and what they achieved by saying it. Our aim is to make the interview process itself *transparent*, and to illustrate some features of what we believe remains a successful model for conducting fieldwork into concealed and 'underground' phenomena.

For the health care worker, the interview was the occasion for reflection, impression management, self-gratification, and self-justification within a supportive environment. In many cases, the interview performed a therapeutic function, while also providing a context for articulating and refining a personal philosophy. For the interviewer, the interviews provided a window into the hidden underbelly of health care work.

Negotiating intimacy

With few exceptions, interviews began in a meandering fashion, with interviewees invited to speak about the nature of their health care work and involvement with patients with AIDS. The interviews were, on average, a little over an hour in length, and the first third to a half of that time was spent creating an environment of trust and acceptance. The majority of interviewees began to share their self-incriminating stories of involvement deeper into the interview, following an extended period of 'courtship', and only after gentle probing. Eye contact, body language, tone of voice, personal warmth and empathy, appropriate surroundings and careful questioning were central to achieving this state of intimacy, as were the pre-recording discussions about confidentiality and use of pseudonyms. A re-reading of interview transcripts confirms that the interview 'proper' began as the culmination of these initial 'courting rituals', which in some instances lasted up to forty minutes. Sometimes, as in the interview with Tara, a psychologist, the tape was stopped mid-interview, at the interviewee's request, while assurances were given. As Tara's interview illustrates, however, there was little correlation between 'reluctance to talk', and 'depth of involvement'. Tara was a 'conservative' (see Chapter 6) with no involvement in assisted death. By contrast, other interviewees with long careers in euthanasia chatted away quite happily.

A minority of respondents took either an inordinate length of time to be coached into discussing their own involvement, or alternatively launched into a detailed description with little or no prompting. The interviews with Gordon and Peter illustrate these extremes. Peter ('P'), an experienced HIV/AIDS nurse, admitted immediately to numerous acts of euthanasia in an interview notable for its directness and absence of metaphor.

> P   What do you want to know? [very quiet] . . . okay I'm willing to talk I presume you're absolutely confidential; yes I've done euthanasia yes I've killed people ah . . .

M   Do you mind just talking into the [microphone]—

P   Sorry, yes I've done euthanasia. Yes I've killed people; I've ah been involved with when they've done it themselves and I assisted them . . . brought their life to an end . . . by giving them . . . straight-into-the-vein morphine or drugs to kill them . . .

M   How many times would you have—?

P   [pause] five, six. There's other times when I've been a nurse on wards . . . and I've given [the patient] higher-than-you-need-to doses of morphine to kill the person—

M   Higher than is needed for pain relief? And how many times would that have happened?

P   A few hundred.

By contrast, the interview with Gordon reveals an understand-able reluctance to reveal details of an episode of non-consensual euthanasia in the middle of the night, while he was suffering from severe flu. The post-interview field notes record:

> Gordon liked to talk about the 'issues'; pinning him down on his own actions was harder, and there was a subtle evasiveness in the way he kept getting sidetracked, or 'kept on about' general issues. I noticed that he rarely closed his sentences; he kept the process of unburdening himself going by putting "and um" at the end of each sentence. I felt that this also enabled him to control the conversation. It required me to be more aggressive when interrupting him.

Sometimes, despite lengthy discussion of general issues, the interviewer gained the impression that there was something more waiting to be said which would not be volunteered without direct request. This was particularly the case with 'conservative' inter-viewees who reported minimal or low-level involvement in their pro-fessional capacity. Partly by hunch, and partly wondering why they had initially volunteered or agreed to be interviewed, the interviewer probed whether they had been involved in a personal capacity, out-side of work. Amanda, a community nurse, responded with a de-tailed account of euthanasia, performed with a nurse-friend, on a 28-year-old-man with Kaposi's Sarcoma. Ruth, also a nurse, reported having attempted twice to euthanise her 7-year-old niece who was dying of cancer. Chris, a hospital nurse, reported assisting a general practitioner to euthanise his father.

As these examples illustrate, although the interview was 'free-flowing' and conversational in style, it was nevertheless necessary—despite a long period of 'courtship'—to specifically interrogate some interviewees with particular questions that became the trigger for reports of personal involvement. The inability to 'follow up leads', and to tailor the investigation to the particular circumstances of each respondent illustrate the limitations of survey-type studies in researching euthanasia practice. More generally, the 'courting rituals' and the need for a period of 'negotiated intimacy' illustrate the challenges involved in researching 'underground' phenomena, the need to establish a relationship with the research subject, and the advantages of a flexible, conversational format.

Language and emotion

How do euthanisers talk about death? At times colourful, enigmatic, brazen, or infused with emotion, the language interviewees used to describe their role in euthanasia practice never fails to surprise us, despite the long periods of time we have spent with each transcript.

The 'credentialling' of the euthanised

A recurrent feature of the detailed reports was the way in which they were prefaced by remarks about the intelligence, humanity and autonomy of the person who was 'euthanised'. We refer to this feature—which simultaneously permitted the interviewee to pay tribute to the deceased, while indirectly legitimating or justifying their own involvement—as the 'credentialling' of the euthanised. The following are typical examples:

> He was a very intelligent man . . . very gentle, kind, loving man . . . [who] knew more about the virus than we did . . . We learnt a lot from him. (Helen)

> He was intelligent . . . and wasn't depressed . . . [He] convinced me that it was the right thing to do. (Josh)

> He was young, strong and healthy . . . He wasn't wasted . . . this was a patient [who] was able to make decisions. (Liz)

He was a very intelligent [and] articulate man who was very educated. (Amanda)

[He was] late thirties, you know, intelligent and insightful, but angry . . . (Harvey).

This man is actually very special, very clever, very clever (Nola).

Describing death

There is a disarming frankness in descriptions of what the interviewees did, even when the language does not present 'doers' in a positive light. At times, descriptions of the euthanatic process, and of death itself, correspond with stereotypical images of euthanasia as 'happy death': 'they just float out and they stop', or 'he just stopped really quietly, which was nice'. Interviewees spoke of death as 'moving on', 'crossing the river', 'kick[ing] off from the wharf', a 'journey' and 'a release'. Other innocuous metaphors included 'self deliver', 'exit this life', 'leave this earth', 'a transition', or 'finish'.

Some descriptors of death or being dead, however, had a harsher edge; for example, 'knock off', 'put down', 'help them off the hook', 'bumping them off', 'check out early', 'dead as a door nail', and 'off to the big gay bar in the sky'. Jane, a general practitioner, remarked that 'I see it as a termination . . . [but] we always call them 'take-outs' . . . a term we can use in front of other people'.

Like descriptors for death, descriptions of the euthanasia process encompass both positive and negative connotations. 'It's not an unpleasant experience if it's done well', said one interviewee. 'It's quick, they just float out of it, and they stop'. Patients 'quietly [go] to sleep', 'quietly slip away', or they 'spring the mortal coil'. Successful euthanasia episodes are described as 'quite quick and pleasant', a 'celebration', 'really good', 'terrific success', 'an honour', an 'honourable and . . . courageous step', a 'heroic act' and a 'mitzvah'. 'We felt that . . . we had done something really positive', said one, 'that we really helped the person achieve something that was really really important for him'.

One nurse admitted to feeling 'really good about it, if you can say that you feel really good about something like that'. She added, 'I don't go home and have sleepless nights; I have a very clear conscience about it'. Mark, a clinical psychologist, reflected that 'killing someone who is suffering in this way is [an act of] decency and respect'. 'I look at it as being a release', said Peter, a nurse, 'but deep in your subconscious it stays with you'. Gary, a GP, rationalised his involvement as 'hastening things up only a little in the scheme of things', while Stanley, a therapist, described his actions as 'cheating the hangman by a matter of a day or two'.

Interviewees didn't only use metaphor in interview, but reported using metaphor at the bedside. In one anecdote, Bob, a general practitioner, stressed how family members were told, 'tonight [the patient] will go to sleep, he'll be resting, he'll go on his journey'. Between themselves, however, Bob, another physician and a nurse spoke bluntly about the patient wanting 'to be dead' and the fact that the family 'wanted him dead as well'.

Like Bob, many interviewees avoided using 'woolly' metaphors, preferring simple and direct colloquialisms such as 'finishing the job', 'just put a line into a vein, tape it down and then just inject away', or 'I gave him one under the arm and it killed him . . . instantly, two seconds, one second'. Peter referred to doing some 'manual work' (suffocation) and to 'killing patients'. Another spoke of helping patients 'top themselves'.

There were few niceties in the way interviewees report failed euthanasia attempts. 'It was bloody revolting', 'it was hideous', said Gary, a general practitioner. 'It was like Rasputin; we just couldn't finish him off.' Other descriptors included, 'awful', 'dreadful', 'I just thought that was the most horrible thing I had ever done to anybody'. Chris, a hospital nurse, told of a euthanasia attempt upon his father and of ringing his mother to confirm the death. 'I'm on the phone down there', he said. 'Half way through dialling they stick their heads out [of the room] and say, "oh, he started breathing again"', to which Chris responded in interview, 'Fuck, when is this man going to die?!'

These descriptors of death and the euthanatic process may shock some readers. They are less likely, however, to shock seasoned health care workers, who have lost their naivety, and are less sensitised to the fact of death. Importantly, the language interviewees used to describe death and euthanasia reinforces the overall impression of authenticity that emerges from the interviews. While the interview afforded opportunities to self-justify, the experiences were too real and too raw to be camouflaged with posturing or elegant theorising, and the language reflects this.

Emotions during interview

The interviews were rich and emotional occasions. Interpolations made during the transcription process include frequent and some-times lengthy pauses, sighs, nervous laughter, whispering, murmur-ing, faltering voice, and flat monotonic speech. Interviewees cleared their throats, and coughed, while six (Joseph, Martin, Stanley, John, Warren, Anne), broke down and wept during recording. Some inter-viewees were very nervous as they spoke and kept a physical dis-tance. One was palpably ill at ease during interview, moving uncomfortably in the chair and avoiding eye contact with the inter-viewer. Occasionally, some used expletives to emphasise meaning.

The causes of emotionality in interview are complex. Inter-viewees were reporting on past experiences to which they responded emotionally at the time. The process of revisiting the past both generated and re-awakened emotions. Discussion during interview of the current state of euthanasia policy also provoked a range of emotions. These sources of emotion are hopelessly mixed and little is gained in seeking to distinguish between them. While there are many examples that illustrate the intensity and range of emotions expressed in interview, the following are typical.

Anger: During the interview with Martin, an HIV/AIDS com-munity worker with AIDS, emotions overflowed when he reflected on the role of 'right-to-lifers' in opposing legalisation:

> I wonder how many right-to-lifers have witnessed people in the prime of their lives with [a] terminal condition that's as insidious as AIDS actually dying, watching them crap themselves . . . seeing sores that go through to the bone . . . Its interesting that . . . every right-to-lifer that I have spoke[n] to is . . . pro-death penalty and I find that really bizarre. They're control freaks and how DARE they have the right to [tell] someone they have no control over the way which they live [or] . . . die. I would actually like to take all these right-to-lifers into an AIDS ward so they can actually witness young men and women dying in the prime of their lives in the most undignified way I can imagine.

This edited extract conceals the fact that Martin was so angry that it compromised his ability to speak grammatically and blunted the impact of his criticism.

It is worth noting that interviewee anger, frequently re-orienting itself in interview as passionate pro-euthanasia advocacy, came from witnessing 'primitive' and 'barbaric' killings, with or without medical assistance. Tony, a medical practitioner, states:

> I think the ultimate obscenity . . . was one of my patient[s] . . . who helped a friend of his to die at home by helping him take a large quantity of sleeping pills and then holding a garbage bag over his head until he died, and I think that is absolutely . . . appalling and barbaric and primitive . . . The physicality of a garbage bag and someone suffocating inside it, I mean that, to my mind is just appalling, and it makes me very angry about the whole issue . . .

Guilt: Liz, a hospital nurse, gave a detailed account of non-consensual euthanasia in which she had been involved (see Chapter 11). She noted that the relatives had no idea that her patient had died from a lethal infusion. It is not difficult to sense her guilt in the following:

> The worst thing for me is that I'd been close to [the patient's] sister and I see her at school—her kids go to the same school as my kids. She comes up and she gives me a kiss and a cuddle, 'You looked after my brother so well' . . . and its just shitty. They've got no idea, absolutely no idea . . .

In contrast, Margaret, an HIV/AIDS community worker, who participated in a 'botched' euthanasia attempt upon her brother, experienced guilt not because she had participated in the planning of the attempt, but because the attempt failed. 'The only guilt I hold now', she adds,

> is that my mother and step-father were in the house at the time and I didn't feel confident enough to discuss it with them [due to their] extremely strong Christian point of view . . . It wasn't until a couple of days later I overheard a conversation between my mother and my step-father [revealing] . . . an agreement between themselves that they would do it for one another, and then I felt even more guilty because I misjudged them.

Warren, a psychotherapist, felt similarly. He had tried to assist the suicide of select clients by stockpiling anti-depressants. The attempts failed. 'I still find it enormously distressing', he admitted, 'at a psychological level I had failed those people, I'd caused them and their nurses and their families tremendous distress and I still feel that years later'.

Weeping: The interview with Warren took place over cappuccinos in one corner of a busy, and extremely noisy, coffee shop. Warren broke down and wept when discussing the lack of legal avenues for obtaining euthanasia and the acts of desperation some feel driven to as a result:

> I've had . . . patients whose lovers . . . have felt so helpless to aid their lover that they've tried to throttle them . . . Well, I'm certainly having trouble restraining my feelings here [voice faltering, eyes brimming with tears]. To love somebody [who] feels that he wants to die, and to want to help him to die and to have to resort to trying to choke him to death, is a horrible thing for our society to do to somebody [crying].

Six interviewees cried when recalling personal experiences, the memories of incidents involving friends and lovers re-awakening emotions usually kept under control. Warren's reaction was unique in that it was a response not to his own but to his *patient's* dilemma. However, none appeared to weep out of guilt or from regret. Indeed, with the exception of Anne, all were 'revisionists' or strong advocates of euthanasia (see Chapter 6).

Angst: The existential anguish of death was an unmistakable theme in some interviews, combining elements of a great many emotions including rage, grief, fatigue, and even displaced anger towards the writer (who is a lawyer). Peter's interview provides a good example of this complexity:

> It's not easy because they're not patients, they're friends, and you can be all very intellectual and you can do 14,000 PhDs and become a famous lawyer and do your famous research grants, but when you're in that bedroom . . . and it's late at night, and the person lying there is your friend, and the needle you're putting into them is going to kill them—you're going to kill your friend—. . . You're intelligent and they're intelligent and you know what the future holds and you know

that there's no hope at all for them, you just know that when you push the stuff down their veins that they're going to die, it's very, very, very, very hard, very hard.

Peter returned to the same theme several minutes later:

It's sad and it's tragic . . . [and] when they die it brings back all the thoughts and memories and feelings that this disease forebodes, it is terminal and . . . lovely people die from it, you can't deny it when there's a cadaver laying in front of you; you can't just sit around de-briefing or [attend] a lawyer's lecture or a team meeting . . . and go 'waffle waffle'.

Passion and advocacy: For some, the interview provided a con-text for expressing personal and political philosophies. In an inter-view characterised by its passion and energy, Stanley, a therapist, said:

I do lots of memorial services in my business and people say . . . strange things at this time, but one of the things [they say is] 'if only the dead could speak', you know, 'what would Uncle Bob say to me? Or what would my mum say to me now?' And I [say] 'Well the dead can't speak *but the dying can*(!), and that's the next best thing, why can't we listen to them?' [And they say] 'Oh!, we can't listen to them because, you know, they're almost dead!' We *discount* them; I mean if we *listened* to them . . . they'd tell us about the dignity that is incum-bent in being a human being, and what it is to lose dignity . . . It's DIGNITY, not continence that we're talking about, DIGNITY, not sight, DIGNITY, not [being] ambulatory . . . but we don't listen to them, and so we have no wisdom about this.

Others, such as Peter, assuming the interviewer to be in favour of the legalisation of euthanasia, saw in the study an opportunity for pro-euthanasia advocacy: 'I admire you for what you're doing . . . I'm not an idiot, I don't expect that there'll be major miracles . . . but out of little sparks come fires . . . We'll get somewhere, maybe in a decade or two'. By contrast, Liz, a hospital nurse, wanted her experiences included in this study to warn people that non-consensual euthanasia is already occurring.

The interview as therapy: For some interviewees, the interview was an exhausting process. Amanda, for example, a community nurse, exclaimed that she felt 'totally stuffed' as the dictaphone was switched off. Nevertheless, as several others pointed out after recording had finished, the process did assist in clarifying their feelings and beliefs. A number of interviewees had not spoken about their involvement(s) to anyone besides their partner. The interview was a valuable opportunity, therefore, to reveal burning secrets. For Anne, it was the opportunity to recount her years of work as a grief counsellor: 'It's been quite therapeutic for me. I haven't . . . ever talked about these issues at such a deep level'.

Humour: Laughter and humour were the most frequent emotions expressed by interviewees. They provided a mechanism for coping with the intensity and the emotional demands of the interview. Kyle, a GP, when asked how many times he had knowingly prescribed drugs for use in a euthanasia procedure, replied that it was probably 'around 15 now', but then protested with a laugh, 'I don't have a little black book somewhere' to 'record each occasion'. Chris, a nurse in a Catholic hospital, pointed out that little would change if euthanasia were legalised: 'I mean the sisters just wouldn't go for it at all [laugh] . . . forget it!' Gary, recalling an incident presented in Chapter 1, said "I did one a couple of weeks ago with a nurse; I picked her up at her house' [and drove with her to the patient's home]. A couple of minutes later, picking up the same story after a slight diversion, he joked: 'I shouldn't say I *picked up* [the] nurse', agreeing that a better expression would be that he offered her a lift. He then proceeded to tell how he gave the patient a lethal injection, while the patient's family and a priest remained in the next room, oblivious to what was occurring.

John, a funeral director, made jokes during the interview. In the context of emphasising the importance of cremating the body as soon as possible following euthanasia, John adds 'as quickly as [possible, but] never on a Saturday, for God's sake, it's too expensive!' [laughing]. Another illustration came in Butch's interview, when this hospice physician admitted that he wrote 'AIDS' as the cause of death on the death certificate, following a patient's suicide. 'Metaphorically, this is a death related to the underlying disease', he said, before adding, '[although] whether the [Coroner] would see it that way or not, I don't know. He doesn't tend to think metaphorically!'

As frivolous as these illustrations are, they demonstrate the recurrent role of double entendres, absurdities and so forth in lightening the mood and enabling the frank discussion of highly charged events. On some occasions, laughter was prompted by retelling an amusing anecdote the interviewee had witnessed at the bedside. Gary's patient (see Chapter 1), had promised that when he got to Heaven he would speak to the 'big guy' about Tattslotto numbers on behalf of a nurse. Michelle, herself a nurse, joked with a patient that when *she* got to heaven she intended to 'brain' the patient all over again for making her participate in his death in the first place. On other occasions, the presence of humour illustrates what one interviewee called a 'highly developed sense of the ridiculous', which she emphasised was essential for survival in the stressful business of AIDS nursing.

The language and emotions expressed during interview, together with the self-incriminating nature of the disclosures, reinforce the raw authenticity of what was said. Talking was not easy: in view of emotional and legal factors, participating in interview was a bold, generous and, ultimately, a civic act. However one judges the interviewees for what they did, we believe that they were being truthful and honest in their reporting. Their responses are a wake-up call for those who prefer to ignore the euthanasia underground.

Accounts of involvement

As discussed in Chapter 7, the narratives that health care workers gave of their involvement in euthanasia were a salient feature of most interviews in this study. Gee contends that story-telling is 'probably the principal way' that human beings make sense of their experience.[2] Accessing the subjective and specific accounts of participation in euthanasia was therefore an important avenue for understanding 'the world as it is lived and understood by' those who perform illegal euthanasia.[3] As summarised in Table 7-2, interviewees recounted a total of 203 anecdotes in this study, including 88 anecdotes of first-hand participation in assisted suicide or active voluntary euthanasia. The majority of these stories contained information that was highly incriminating, and which did not always cast the interviewee in a favourable light. The term 'confession', defined more generally as self-disclosure, or as the unburdening of one's private self, provides an apt description of many of these accounts.

Below, we present three highly abbreviated versions of 'confessional stories' told by interviewees. These stories were not chosen in order to shock, but to illustrate the different role of anecdotes in interview, and what interviewees gained by telling them. In editing these accounts, we have taken care not to lose the chronology of events as reported, nor the actual language of the health care workers.

Non-consensual euthanasia by a rookie doctor

Tim, a GP, recalled how he first became involved with assisting in someone else's death by repeating a story which, he says, he 'only ever told . . . to one other person'. The anecdote, which is approximately 3000 words long and begins about a quarter of the way through the interview, unfolds in a meandering fashion, with the specific details of what occurred emerging only through persistent questioning.

The patient, who had a 'viral infection in the brain', was discharged from hospital and taken home by his parents to die. Tim says that the patient, whom he had not previously met, 'was not able to communicate . . . had difficulty breathing and . . . seemed to be in pain'. 'Unable to really do much' to help him, family members became distressed and looked to the doctor for assistance. They pleaded with Tim to 'put him out of his misery'. Tim had recently arrived in the area and was not confident 'to approach someone else' for advice. He also admits that at this stage he "hadn't . . . thought much about the issue [of euthanasia]'. An additional difficulty was the fact that the request for euthanasia was 'initiated' by the family. Tim believed the patient was 'brain dead': 'he was awake, his eyes were open, but he couldn't speak', nod or write. All the same, Tim 'was reluctant' to act; he wanted to be sure that family members were clear in their minds about what they were asking him to do. He spent a good part of a day discussing the issue with the ten or twelve family members who gathered at the house. The patient's mother appealed to Tim's sense of compassion, assuring Tim that she had discussed the subject of euthanasia with the son while 'he was able to talk'. Finally Tim was convinced he had 'one hundred per cent support' from the family. The discussions took place in the same room where the patient lay and Tim is 'sure [that] he knew what was happening; I don't think it affected his cerebral hemispheres that much'.

Tim explains that he could have done 'nothing and walked away from it' but he chose to act. 'I guess it was really the unrelenting nature of his distress', says Tim (and, we suspect, the presence of a room full of family members exerting their combined pressure). Tim injected the patient in two stages; firstly, 210 milligrams of morphine and then 'just a box of pethidine'. It took 'a couple of hours' for the patient to die. The family members were in the room the whole time, and even though 'there were a lot of tears . . . and emotion', and the fact that the 'sister was . . . shocked [at] how quickly it happened', Tim reflects that 'overall it was a fairly positive experience' and he 'felt good about it'.

This anecdote is a case of non-consensual euthanasia performed by a 'rookie' doctor upon a patient whom he had not previously met. The doctor lacked the confidence to seek advice from medical colleagues. There are inconsistencies in the telling, including the question of whether the patient was 'brain dead', on the one hand, or conscious, aware, and yet immobile, on the other. The overwhelming impression which emerges from this anecdote was of an inexperienced doctor, ill-equipped to deal with the situation he was thrust into, unsure of where to draw the boundaries, succumbing to pressure from relatives who felt they were acting in the patient's best interests. The experience appears to have been a turning point for Tim, cementing his pro-euthanasia views. The 'telling' had 'confessional' overtones: details were disclosed reluctantly, in a barely audible voice, and in an apparent attempt to self-justify. The whole episode remains, to this day, a closely guarded secret.

A nurse suffocates his lover's 'best friend'

Peter, a nurse, spoke in a serious tone throughout the interview, pausing frequently, and in a voice that at times was barely audible. Peter says that he 'rang around' before being interviewed to seek assurance from colleagues that it was safe to talk. The interview began abruptly with Peter asking, "What do you want to know?'

When told about the study and assured of confidentiality, Peter launched abruptly into describing his involvement in euthanasia (as mentioned above in the context of 'negotiating intimacy'):

> Yes, I've done euthanasia. Yes, I've killed people. I've been involved . . . when they've done it themselves and I assisted them . . . [With others] I brought their life to an end by giving them IVs . . . straight-into-the-vein, morphine or [other] drugs to kill them . . .

Peter's involvement was so frequent that (like a number of others), he had lost count of the number of times he had helped a patient to die. But unlike Tim, whose story was *the context and vehicle* though which to clarify his thoughts and feelings on euthanasia, Peter's anecdotes were short and compressed, and given in order to illustrate very specific issues. The following anecdote was the third of four accounts Peter gave during the hour-long interview. Peter's first two anecdotes were given to illustrate the problem of 'botched attempts', and the difficulties of achieving death using available drugs. His fourth anecdote was told in order to illustrate 'the last one I did', and Peter's general modus operandi. Peter's third anecdote, however, was used to illustrate the point that although he had never assisted a depressed patient to die, he had performed euthanasia on patients who were relatively asymptomatic and not in the final stages of their illness.

Peter told of his lover's 'best friend', Jack, who was in his late twenties. Jack 'had AIDS and a couple of Kaposi's' lesions but was still independent, not 'incontinent' and was able to walk around the house. Peter estimates that Jack 'probably still had a few years [of life] left [but] decided not to go that far'. According to Peter, Jack 'had weighed up all the pros and cons and . . . talked [with] the medicos [about pain management]', but 'decided that the future held nothing for him and that he . . . wanted to die'. Jack 'obtained the medication—pills and potions' and to avoid incriminating his friends (including Peter), he 'said he would do it'.

Peter was present when Jack 'took his overdose'. Having already discussed the anguish caused by botched attempts, Peter then added that 'we just assisted [Jack] at the end by giving him some IV drugs and . . . [by] doing some manual work on [him]'.

When asked to explain what he meant by 'manual work', Peter replied, 'suffocation'.

This is the report of a seasoned participant performing euthanasia in a 'personal' as distinct from 'professional' capacity (see Chapter 11). Peter does not reject palliation as an option for the terminally ill, but there were overtones of contempt for patients who chose to eke out the final moments of their struggle with AIDS. Later in the interview, while discussing the problems associated with burial, Peter refers back to this incident, noting that Jack 'didn't want a funeral, so he could be done ASAP, and that was good, because then we could burn the evidence'.

Two accounts of "botched" euthanasia

The two accounts of involvement reported by HIV/AIDS community workers, Margaret and Gay, are versions of the same event. The patient was Margaret's brother. 'John' had contracted HIV while living in the United States, but with the onset of symptoms, he decided to return to Australia. John was reunited with his family, but at the same time he lost a network of friends who had previously agreed that 'they would actively participate in euthanasia' and 'assist one another when the time came'. In Australia John looked to his immediate family for this support.

Margaret and Gay explain that John, who 'was fairly medically oriented', had decided to end his own life several weeks before his death by 'giving up all active treatment'. Margaret suspects that John thought that by not taking medication he would be 'dead within twenty four hours', but instead he lingered on in frustration. According to Gay, John 'had asked on numerous occasions for some assistance', although Margaret reports that John merely 'hinted' that 'he wanted some assistance' and it was not until the final days that the subject of euthanasia was discussed openly with him. By this stage John 'was totally blind' and the visit of a close friend from the United States was the occasion that brought things to a head. Margaret says, 'I think it became . . . frustrating for him to be alive . . . and blind'.

As John's 'power of attorney', friends looked to Margaret to arrange for her brother's death, insisting 'that is what he wants done'. Margaret wanted to be clear in her own mind that she was acting in accordance with her brother's wishes, to the extent that, she explains, her 'brother was probably getting pissed off' as a result of her constant questioning. The following is Margaret's description of what transpired:

> It was agreed that, yes, this was what we would do. It was discussed between my partner and the palliative care [nurse] as to the amount ... [and] what type of drug would be administered. I felt that I couldn't actually administer the drug, one of the people in the group felt quite comfortable [with] doing that. [When] that was done [we] estimated [that it would take] 15 to 20 minutes. A friend did the bed-side bit. The friend from [the US] was actually taking the pulse ... [which] started to disappear. Then all of a sudden there was a look of panic on [the friend's face] ... because the pulse started coming back. There were all sorts of other emotions that started to take place. It hadn't worked. About two and a half hours [later] the GP visited ... [and he] administered more of the drug and left. He said he'd come back with a death certificate. When he came back my brother sat up in bed and asked for a bowl of ice-cream.

Margaret believes that they failed to take account of the fact that her brother had been an intravenous drug user. The remainder of Margaret's and Gay's account is devoted to discussing the emotions they experienced at the time, and the impact the botched attempt had on each of them.

Margaret says that the euthanasia attempt 'certainly wasn't unpleasant' for her brother, who had 'a wow of a time with all the morphine'—he 'experienced incredible dreams' and 'was quite euphoric'. Margaret says that she 'had never been involved in anything like this before', but while she feels remorse because 'it hadn't worked' and because she had to keep the attempted euthanasia a secret from her 'mother and father [who] were in the house at the time', she does not regret involvement.

After the initial failure, Margaret 'talked [with John] about another attempt'. He declined the offer, because, she says, 'he didn't want to put us in [another] awkward situation'. The attempt to facilitate the death of her brother signalled Margaret's commitment to euthanasia and a willingness to participate further should the opportunity arise.

The same experience left Gay with opposite feelings; the failed attempt has forced her to review her attitudes to euthanasia even though she found it 'hideous to watch' John die, three days later, from dehydration. Gay explains: 'It obviously wasn't right; for some reason he had to live another three days. Whether it was to teach us a lesson or to teach him a lesson or what, I don't know . . . but it's certainly [brought home to] us that we don't have as much control [over our lives] as we'd like to think we have'.

Gay does not regret her involvement, but adds, 'I'd question it for a long time [before] I would ever do anything . . . [like] that again'.

The nature of anecdotes

As noted above, anecdotes of involvement in assisted death were seldom volunteered at the beginning of the interview, but emerged following a 'courting period' of more abstract discussion. Frequently, anecdotes were given as illustrations of particular issues that were being explored in interview. Failing that, they emerged in response to questions from the interviewer, who typically asked the respondent at an appropriate juncture whether there were any *particular* cases in which issues of assisted suicide or euthanasia had arisen in the context of the respondent's practice.

Once committed to the telling, respondents spoke without hesitation, drawing on experiences anchored in memory. The interviewer's role during this time was to focus on the anecdote, trying to facilitate the giving of an ordered chronology, trying to ensure that the teller completed the story before becoming sidetracked by some other issue encountered during the telling, and trying to elicit as much information as possible without spoiling the spontaneity of the exchange. Eye contact, non-threatening comments, and signals of empathy were crucial in conveying understanding and continuing interest, and in maintaining the intimacy and momentum of the exchange. On occasions when this process worked most successfully, anecdotes were detailed and took the form of extended soliloquies.

Interviewees reported their involvements in autobiographical fashion, using the first person singular. This does not mean, however, that specific episodes were reported as an ordered sequence of events linked to form a chronological narrative. Instead, one finds descriptions of events and introspective musings about what happened, and

why, intertwined in the retelling. Interviewees gravitate to presenting highly abbreviated accounts which focus on the most emotionally charged segments of the experiences and work outward from
there only with prompting during interview.

Anecdotes are told for a reason: they generally highlight some
lesson the interviewee took with them as a result of their experience:
its impact on them, retrospective emotions, or subsequent attitudes
towards euthanasia. This is true both of anecdotes focusing on the
challenges of nursing and care, and accounts of assisted death.

Erin tells of negotiating with a doctor so that a dying patient
could spend Christmas (and could die), at home. He summarises:
'I think my role is the same in all those cases. I was trying to be an
advocate'. Martin, like several others, told stories to highlight the
horror of 'botched' suicide and euthanasia attempts, emphasising
that euthanasia is a pretty 'inexact science'. Gary rationalises one
botched attempt anecdote with the words: '[since then we've] refined
the techniques and we seem to have a good combination [and] I can
do it in three or four minutes now'. Others point to positive experiences of euthanasia as (implicit) justification for current attitudes.
Helen tells of one case involving 'four or five of us who had a little
team meeting'. The patient's lover, although 'not happy', was 'at
peace about the outcome', because the process wasn't 'prolonged' or
'painful'. The impact of this experience upon Helen's own attitudes
is evident from what follows: 'I didn't go home and have terrible
sleepless nights, I have a very clear conscience about it and I know
that professionally it's wrong, but I felt really right about it for [this]
person'.

Anecdotes vary in length, from a few lines to lengthy exchanges
that dominate the entire interview. The importance of anecdotes to
the interview was also variable: not all interviews were anecdote
driven. For interviewees like Harvey, Jane, Peter, Merril and John,
the interview consisted of personal reflections which drew upon the
respondent's rich accumulated experience, but which had become
abstracted from specific case episodes. It is ironic that the narratives
reported by some of the most experienced euthanasia participants
were *less* rich in specifics, because the details do not feature in their
consciousness, given their long histories and confirmed identities as
euthanisers.

For most interviewees, however, anecdotes comprise a major portion of each interview. For some, such as Liz, Tim and Bob, the interview was consumed by *one* anecdote: the anecdote *was* the interview, providing a rich environment for the exploration of feelings and attitudes. It is probably fair to say, in retrospect, that these interviewees agreed to talk simply in order to share this one crucial and momentous experience.

More frequently, interviewees told several anecdotes in interview. For 'revisionists', in particular, the anecdote was the focus of emotion, insight and opinion into assisted death. For this reason there is a crudity or 'rawness' to the anecdotes. They are not polished artefacts or 'artfully accomplished constructions'[4] which have undergone modification and refinement through repetition. Indeed, in some instances the interview was the first time the respondents had shared their experiences with someone else. First-hand reports of involvement were, therefore, the seismic epicentre of the interview: everything leading up to them, and everything afterwards, was of secondary importance, because the anecdote was the context through which respondents told of their involvement, made sense of what they had done, and made connections with the wider ethical and regulatory issues that were also implicated.

Lasting impressions

The manner in which respondents spoke, the language they used, the anecdotes they told, and the levels of self-disclosure that these entailed, together with the general atmosphere that pervaded the telling, combine to create a lasting impression on the listener and interviewer. These lasting impressions are not tidy packages that contain everything that the respondents said about their involvement. Rather, they are abbreviations and mental pictures that capture the salient, and possibly most memorable, aspects of what was reported.

For some interviewees the lasting impressions revolve around professional boundaries: the psychiatrist who, in principle, is supportive of euthanasia and has prescribed drugs, but remains professionally distanced (Damian); the rookie doctor who was out of his depth (Tim); the experienced doctor and educator whose one-off involvement was an act of desperation in response to social pressure following a botched attempt (Gordon).

Some are remembered for their inability to maintain personal and professional boundaries: Anne, the emotionally fragile therapist and grief counselor who embodies the burdens of long-time care for dying patients; Terri, the committed carer who fell in love with a gay patient and paid the price emotionally; and Jane, the uncompromising patient advocate and experienced euthanasia participant who scoffed at the distinction between personal and professional relationships with her patients.

The emotional cost of involvement was the lingering theme from some interviews: the guilt-ridden nurse who saw the interview as a way of 'blowing the whistle' on what she perceived to be an execution, without jeopardising her own career (Liz); Peter, the world-weary nurse, who had seen many friends die, and helped them to die, and who feels the anguish of all those years; Merril, the straight-talking, hard-working and religious doctor, who felt driven to assist, but whose involvement sits ambiguously with his Christian faith; Amanda, the community nurse who participated in euthanasia following the bloody suicide of a former patient, who now feels confused by the precedent of involvement; and Erin, the former Catholic brother and 'angel of death', who strained in interview to reconcile his lingering Catholic heritage, his sexuality, and practice of compassionate euthanasia.

The respondent's technical expertise, and professionalisation of the euthanatic role was the dominant theme from some interviews: Gary, the media-savvy advocate, who has perfected the technology of lethal overdoses; Stanley, the therapist/ex-priest, and seasoned administrator of euthanasia ritual; Zane, the palliative care physician and quiet achiever; Mark, the clinical psychologist who has taken on the doctor's persona and now does what doctors do.

Several interviewees stood out in their refusal to become involved in assisted death: Richard, the psychiatrist repulsed by the thought of euthanasia, who saw the ethical prohibition as 'almost a chromosomally imposed rule'; Harry, the GP who lacked the stomach for euthanasia, seeing it as too technical and emotionally troublesome to warrant involvement; Dianne, the nurse who kept a professional distance from patients and chose not to get involved because of the stress.

At the other end of the spectrum stands Bob, the GP who was interviewed with 'blood still wet on his hands', having facilitated the death of a patient thirty-six hours earlier, depleting his doctor's bag of syringes and analgesics in the process; Michelle, the tough-talking nurse caught up in the excitement and drama of it all; Tony, the laid-back cynic of the medical bureaucracy, law, and politics, who feels safe in the knowledge that no one is enforcing the law; Josh, the self-assured GP who obtains lethal drugs from a veterinary friend to 'put down' patients who have requested euthanasia; and John, funeral director of choice to the 'euthanasia underground' in one city.

Secure within the pseudonymous and conversational interview format, interviewees gradually warmed up, and with gentle probing shared secrets that were emotionally upsetting and at times shocking. Interviewees were 'talking on their feet' in interview, and while not every one was able to encapsulate their feelings and philosophies in emblematic quotes, ultimately what one is struck by is how articulate interviewees were in communicating what was important to them.

In the end, anecdotes were the central feature of most interviews, and the most powerful source of information for this study. This chapter has highlighted how these reports of involvement came to be told, and how they were simultaneously the context for describing and justifying conduct, as well as articulating attitudes and personal philosophies. While each interview focused on the involvement of the interviewee personally, evidence of collaborative practices inevitably emerged from the discussion.

9

The underground community

You can never get over the feeling of being executioner—you're turning up at an appointed time; you know that when you leave the room, the person is going to be dead.

Philip Nitschke[1]

Euthanasia is a social process, the product of collaboration between health care providers themselves, between carers and patients, and between patients, family and friends. In Sydney, Melbourne and San Francisco (the major cities where interviews were conducted), euthanasia was facilitated by the network of friendships and professional connections that had grown up around involvement in the gay community and in HIV medicine respectively. This chapter investigates these processes in detail, exploring the extent to which these relationships and connections can be said to constitute an 'underground' or a 'network' for the delivery of euthanasia services. How extensive is the euthanasia underground? How do the connections between participants which go to make it up actually work? What are the implications of this underground for the euthanasia debate?

What is the 'euthanasia underground'?

By 'underground' or 'network' I refer to the informal chain of associations between health carers who tacitly approve of, facilitate, or directly participate in assisted death. The clinical focus which has grown up around HIV medicine, and its partial overlap with the gay community, brings together strong professional and personal associations within the context of a disease which causes great suffering and frequently precipitates 'euthanasia talk' (see Chapter 5). Gay health professionals, and those specialising in HIV care, form the backbone of the AIDS euthanasia underground. Friendships, professional affiliations and shared values cement alliances and facilitate action in a way that perhaps distinguishes AIDS-related assisted death from cancer and other diseases.

The terms 'underground' and 'network' do not imply that each participant in assisted death is necessarily well informed about the activities of other participants. Each person's knowledge of the network is partial, as euthanasia remains illegal and participants are highly selective about whom they confide in. In one city, for example, interviews were conducted with several doctors from the same inner city practice, which was a focus for gay and HIV clients.[2] Three interviewees gave detailed accounts of euthanasia involvement, while a fourth, an advocate of palliative care, had not performed euthanasia, and said nothing to suggest that he knew his colleagues were involved. Nor was it true to say that the three who had been involved knew of each other's involvement. One doctor's only involvement consisted of an episode of non-consensual euthanasia which he had previously revealed only to his lover.

Even those who play a key role within a network of 'co-operative associations' may hide their involvement from close colleagues. Although he was the undertaker of choice for doctors performing euthanasia in one city, and was frequently 'booked' in advance of the death, John, a funeral director and occasional euthanasia participant, shielded this knowledge from his employees. John's involvement is discussed further below.

The limited perspective of some participants in the euthanasia network raised doubts as to its existence at all. According to Damian, a medical practitioner: 'There's no informal network, it's . . . just one or two people . . . that I'm friendly with . . . it's . . . table conversation . . . you know that everybody at the dinner table is of like mind on the subject'. Despite these comments, Damian was aware of a number of colleagues who were involved, and sometimes his advice was sought over whether euthanasia would be appropriate in the circumstances.

By contrast, Gary, another GP, was very clear about the existence of a network encompassing district nurses, several GPs, and a funeral director. Gary's connections also extended to hospital-employed cancer specialists. While confidentiality precluded any attempt to verify (for example) whether Gary and Damian knew of each other's involvement, it is interesting to note that they mixed in similar circles and had mutual friends who were definite participants.

Other interviewees were typically self-effacing. Kyle, a GP, observed that those of us who 'might be looked at as an underground network' were really 'just a very tightly knit group . . . dedicated to making life more meaningful and . . . death less painful'.

How can collaboration be verified?

While survey studies suggest that a substantial proportion of doctors have intentionally assisted a patient to die (see Chapter 3), there has been little or no research into the co-operative nature of such illegal assistance. The claim that the interviews reveal a network of 'co-operative associations' facilitating the organisation and delivery of euthanasia services is therefore novel and requires justification.

Substantiating claims about the communal and collaborative dimensions of euthanasia practice can occur at several levels. One approach was to explore the extent to which interviewees were aware of colleagues who had participated in assisted death, or would be prepared to do so. Interviewees' knowledge of the wider 'euthanasia community' is the result of at least three processes. It arises, firstly, from participants' own experiences in collaborating with colleagues, and, secondly, from reciprocal disclosures made between interviewees and other colleagues, often in a social context, for purposes of mutual support and de-briefing. Thirdly, interviewees may also be informed by their own patients about the involvement of colleagues in euthanasia. While 'hearsay' evidence of involvement must be carefully evaluated, it may sometimes be credible.[3]

In view of the commitment of confidentiality I gave each interviewee, no attempt was made to verify or to particularise membership of that segment of the 'euthanasia community' each interviewee was aware of. I did not ask interviewees whether they were aware of the involvement of other specific interviewees, or third parties. For their part, interviewees kept the identities of their colleagues and associates confidential.

Even so, the recruitment process itself served to confirm inter-viewees' knowledge of the wider 'euthanasia community' within cities, between cities, and internationally. Most interviewees were recruited into the study by volunteering to be interviewed after hearing seminar papers I gave, or following referral by previous interviewees or third parties. Early interviewees played a central role in 'checking out' the study and recommending it to selected col-leagues (see Appendix). In all, 25 interviews came about following referrals given by previous interviewees, or by non-interviewees (see Table A-1). This process enabled assumptions to be drawn about the personal and professional linkages between players. The referral process illustrated, certainly in retrospect, the 'connectedness' of interviewees. It permitted interviewees to disclose their knowledge (or suspicion) of others' involvement, and this knowledge was 'vin-dicated' through subsequent interviews.

Another way of substantiating the collaborative dimensions of euthanasia was to explore the nature and extent of collaboration during the specific episodes of involvement interviewees revealed in interview. Once again, however, confidentiality precluded asking interviewees to specifically identify their associates, even though the identity of associates was occasionally an implicitly shared assumption.

Nevertheless, it was sometimes possible to link specific inter-viewees because of the context in which they were first recruited, together with specific details of the episodes they described. On a couple of occasions the same episode of assisted death was recounted from the perspective of two different participants. On others, the involvement of third parties (who were never interviewed) was corroborated.

It would no doubt have been easier to trace the connections between participants in euthanasia if undertakings of confidentiality had not been given to each interviewee. On the other hand, confi-dentiality was also *the crucial factor* that encouraged interviewees to speak freely. Ultimately, a great deal hangs on the testimony of inter-viewees, their description of specific collaborations, as well as their knowledge of a wider community of like-minded individuals. Both of these aspects are crucially important to understanding the communal dimensions of euthanasia, as detailed further below.

Specific reports of 'collaborative euthanasia'

Table 9-1 describes the extent of collaboration in 88 first-hand accounts of physician-assisted suicide or active euthanasia. The extent to which the interviewee collaborated with others in the euthanatic process on each occasion was explored in interview and quantified. Care should be taken in interpreting the table since certain forms of collaboration were not mutually exclusive (as when an interviewee collaborated both with another health care worker, and a partner or friend of the patient.

As Table 9-1 reports, the interviewee acted alone in nearly 22 per cent of cases. In 53 per cent (47 episodes), the interviewee was assisted by another health care worker. This is a significant finding. If the particular episodes interviewees chose to share in interview are reasonably representative of assisted deaths generally, then this suggests that a collaborative approach to assisted death is not uncommon, certainly in HIV/AIDS.

Evidence of collaboration between *health care workers* in a specific episode of euthanasia is of particular interest, since it may lead to co-operation in future cases. By contrast, one would expect that collaboration between a health carer and a partner, friend or relative of the patient would be a 'once off'. Table 9-1 shows that in 11 per cent of cases (10 episodes), the interviewee was 'actively assisted' by a partner, friend or relative, while in another 13 per cent there was evidence that a partner, friend or relative of the patient was aware of the procedure, and approved of it, but without taking any direct steps to assist. Since the focus of conversation was on the health care worker's own involvement, and any links with professional colleagues, I believe these numbers are a significant under-estimate.

As described in Chapter 7, the exact nature of the interviewee's involvement in each account of assisted death was explored in interview. The interviewee's 'level of involvement' in each case was categorised in descending order of importance, as either 'hands on', 'active at the scene', 'indirect facilitation', 'referral', or 'active dis-

Table 9-1: Evidence of collaboration in 88 first-hand accounts of assisted suicide or euthanasia

Nature of collaboration	HIV/AIDS (n=75)	Non HIV/AIDS (n=13)	Total (n=88)
Interviewee acted alone	14	5	19 (21.6%)
Interviewee acted in association with another health care worker	40	7	47 (53.4%)
Interviewee was assisted by a partner, friend or relative of deceased	9	1	10 (11.4%)
Partner, friend or relative of deceased was aware of the euthanatic procedure	9	2	11 (12.5%)
Nature or existence of collaboration unknown	8	–	8 (9.1%)

cussion' (see Table 7-3). These categories are also relevant to describing the nature of the collaboration between the interviewee and others in each episode. The cases summarised in Table 9-1, as occurring in association with another health care worker, or with active assistance from a partner, friend or relative, are cases where the collaborator or assistant was either involved on a 'hands on' basis, was 'active at the scene' as a knowing accomplice, or otherwise 'indirectly facilitated' the death.

'Hands on' involvement, as discussed in Chapter 7, includes such actions as accessing veins, injecting drugs, or preparing a concoction. 'Active at scene' involvement refers to someone who is complicit in the procedure and actively participates in it, usually by co-ordinating, giving directions and providing moral support. 'Indirect facilitation' includes supplying the drugs used in the death, writing 'lethal' prescriptions, giving specific advice about drug combinations, and being 'on call' should anything go wrong. The 53 per cent of cases in which an interviewee was assisted by another health care worker represent, therefore, examples of genuine collaboration, with both parties performing actions that brought them into (at least one of) these three categories.

The specific examples of involvement described in interview provided a basis for understanding the forms that collaborative euthanasia can take. But what of interviewees' knowledge of the wider community of 'euthanasia doers'?

Knowledge of the wider 'euthanasia community'

The semi-structured interview format gave each interviewee the opportunity to outline, in general terms, the extent to which they were aware of colleagues who had participated in assisted death, and vice versa. As might be expected, given the recruitment strategy described above, virtually every interviewee who admitted to participating in assisted death knew of others who were similarly involved.

Occasionally, an interviewee was reluctant to disclose the full extent of their knowledge, even in non-identifying terms. One well-connected interviewee observed that there were 'enormous resources for euthanasia' in community care teams, but added, 'I don't feel willing to discuss this with you; I feel protective of people on care teams, so there's information for you to get there, but you're not going to get it from me'.

Not surprisingly, 'revisionist' interviewees (see Chapter 6), and those who were most 'liberal' in their personal philosophy, tended to be best informed about the practice of illegal euthanasia by colleagues. But there were wide variations in knowledge. Merril, a doctor who had prescribed drug overdoses approximately forty times, knew of only one other physician who was involved, and to whom he had admitted his own involvement. 'This is a very private matter', says Merril, '[a] very private matter'.

By contrast, Kyle stated that six doctors had told him of their involvement, and claimed to know fifty physicians who 'have been or would be willing to be' involved in assisted suicide. Kyle himself had prescribed drug overdoses on 'probably around fifteen' occasions, and also shared his 'recipe' with two other physicians. Russell, a hospital physician, estimated that he had mutually disclosed involvement with ten to fifteen colleagues during 'one-on-one conversations'. He admitted to consciously hastening a patient's death on an estimated thirty to forty occasions over a ten-year period (this estimate was limited to AIDS patients).

There were no significant differences between San Francisco and Sydney/Melbourne data in interviewees' knowledge of euthanasia involvements. Warren, a psychotherapist living on the other side of the Pacific from Kyle and Russell, claimed that he could come up with a list of sixty names 'who have at one time or another been complicit in ethical murders', including GPs, psychiatrists, nurses and care team volunteers.

Even ignoring these unverifiable estimates, it is nevertheless possible to sketch out each interviewee's knowledge of the wider 'euthanasia community', relying solely on detailed accounts of involvement, and clues derived from the referral-based recruitment strategy. Jane, for example, was an activist Australian doctor (see Chapter 1), who lived in City 2. Jane had strong connections with a group of activist, male doctors in City 1. Jane was never asked to identify them, but there is considerable evidence that she knew at least two or three of the interviewees in City 1. In addition, Jane knew a specialist in City 3 who performed euthanasia, apparently with assistance from a Catholic nun (the actions of this specialist were confirmed in detail in another interview). Jane knew of at least three doctors in her own city who were involved, although she did not closely associate with them. Similar 'thumbnail sketches' emerge from each of the other interviews with health carers who had participated in assisted death.

Figure 9-1 illustrates some of the connections between interviewees and selected third parties in two Australian cities. It is an intentionally conservative diagram, constructed without breaching confidentiality, based on evidence of specific collaboration, and/or mutual knowledge of involvement. I have been reluctant to assume mutual knowledge, even between interviewees who clearly knew each other, socialised together, and admitted—individually in interview—to euthanasia. It is clear, however, that at least in the HIV/AIDS sphere, assisted death is a co-operative enterprise, facilitated by a network of friendships and professional connections which are themselves grounded in HIV medicine and/or the gay (and lesbian) community.

Figure 9-1: Knowledge of involvement of colleagues in assisted death in two cities

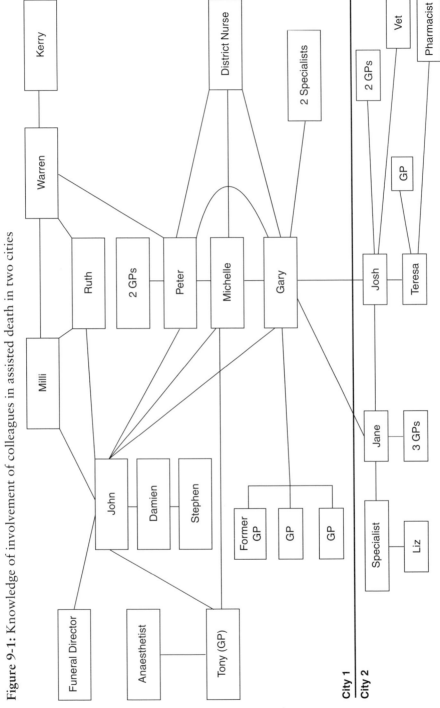

How does the underground work?

'Angels of death'

A startling insight into the extent (and possibilities) of co-operative euthanasia emerges from the interview with John, a funeral director. John plays a pivotal role in the euthanasia network in one city. His discount funeral service attracts considerable business from the gay community. He refers clients with AIDS who want an assisted death to trusted doctor friends in the network who have experience in this area. In turn, John is the undertaker of choice for AIDS-related death, especially assisted death.

John's interview was remarkable for its frank portrayal of the euthanasia referral process. A former nurse, John was first confronted with the treatment that the funeral industry was dishing out to men with AIDS when his lover, who was ill, went along to organise his funeral. 'We were greeted with a woman who could "cry on demand"', John recalls. She was 'terribly sympathetic', but 'the minute the word *AIDS* was mentioned', everything changed: 'No, you can't have an open coffin, you couldn't prepare the body, it wasn't to be touched'. 'People were being stigmatised in life', John says, and now 'they were being stigmatised after death . . . and I thought it was a pretty unhealthy way for the industry to be reacting . . . nine years down the line with all the medical knowledge that had been acquired about AIDS'. John saw the opportunity and went into the funeral business himself.

According to John, clients 'frequently' question him outright about 'whether I know a doctor . . . who will assist them, or they'll indicate that they've spoken to their own doctor, who is opposed . . . and won't discuss it'. 'So I'll give them the name of two or three general practitioners who I know are open minded [about euthanasia] . . . I'll also advise them to speak to their [community nurse] about it'.

M [Are there many community nurses that you know of who are open to assisted suicide?]

J Three or four, which is enough to help [the client] along.

M And how many doctors?

J I [can] probably think of ten.

M So would you say that there's an informal network?

J Yeah, I would certainly say that, in fact at one stage the group was given the nickname 'Angels of Death'.

M 'Angels of Death?'

J Yes [laughs] . . . [An] informal network of people who . . . co-operate and help, facilitate [euthanasia] under the right circumstances . . . I think it's comforting for some of the community out there just to be able to discuss it, it's probably discussed more than it's actually carried out. But those that want it carried out know that it's going to be carried out professionally, and at [the] time that's right for them.

The conversation then focused on the nature of the referral process.

M So if you refer someone you leave it up to the doctors or [community] nurses . . . to make the assessments?

J Yes . . . it then becomes a matter for the doctor . . . Sometimes the doctor will contact you and say, 'I've spoken to [John Doe] and it's not right at this point, but it might be further on down the track; we'll keep you informed' . . . Sometimes [the client] will ring back and say, 'I've spoken to doctor so-and-so and it was great, thanks very much', and then a few weeks will [go] by, a few months, and [the client] will ring up and say *it's going to happen* and [he] sort of puts you on standby for the weekend [laughs].

Later in the interview, John added that sometimes he would bump into doctors socially who would remark, casually, 'I probably need you on Friday night, hope you're not doing anything'. 'You just know', said John, 'nothing more needs to be said'.

This process was confirmed by interviews with health care workers who had used John's services. Gary, a GP, observes: 'It's an odd sort of thing, but I give [him] a call a day or two before and say, look, you know, four o'clock on Saturday we've [got] this job for you. Can you, you know, arrange your timetable?' 'It's not usual [for] funeral directors [to be] given the exact time', Gary adds, 'so it makes their job a bit easier and they can arrange things'.

Peter, a nurse, reflected on one episode involving John in the following terms:

We went in at midday and [the patient] took a while to die . . . he died about two, and the funeral director was just sitting by the phone, at home, this old gay man, waiting by the phone, and he was getting a bit toe-y because it was two o'clock and nothing was happening. So he was about to ring us, but I rang him and told him the job had been [done].

John estimates that assisted death accounts for no more than 10 per cent of his client base. Asked more specifically how many times he would have organised a funeral with the knowledge or strong suspicion that a health professional had intentionally short-ened the patient's life, John answered 'probably only fifteen or twenty a year, it's not that many'. Asked how many times he would have assisted a client's death by putting them in touch with a 'sym-pathetic' doctor, John replied 'probably ten or twelve times, I don't know, [it's] hard to say because it's just something you do for clients'.

As the interview progressed, it became apparent that John's involvement extended beyond making pre-euthanasia referrals, and disposing of bodies after the event. In a non-HIV context, John had been personally involved in euthanasia on two occasions, adminis-tering a lethal injection and an infusion respectively.

John had also participated in the deaths of two AIDS patients. On one occasion 'it was taking so long . . . [that] a pillow had to be held over [the patient's] head while they were unconscious and that was really distressing for the people who were there'.

M Were you in the room?
J   Yes, I helped the person do it.

On the second occasion a friend had asked John to give the final injection, which he did. A doctor was present and signed the death certificate. John then took the body away in the unmarked station wagon his business used for transfers. On a previous occasion when John was directly involved, 'the company that [he] was working for did the funeral'.

John was the only funeral director interviewed in this study, and it is difficult to know whether his collaboration with 'activist' HIV/AIDS health care workers is unique or not.[4] Interestingly, John recounted how on one occasion he supplied a lethal quantity of drugs to a friend with AIDS who lived in another state. After the friend's death, from suicide, John flew interstate to clear away the 'evidence', and ended up having a conversation with the funeral director who had carried out the cremation. Casually, the funeral director asked

John if it had been an assisted death, adding 'if ever you need me next time give me a call'.

Co-operative euthanasia in the community

Outside of hospital, the euthanasia process often begins with the referral of a patient to an activist doctor for assessment. Subsequent stages of the process involve obtaining the euthanatic drugs, carrying out the euthanasia procedure, de-briefing, and concealing any suspicious evidence. Networking and collaboration between health professionals are evident at all stages.

Referral: The initial referral may come from a funeral director, although usually it would come from a hospice or community nurse who has an ongoing relationship with the patient, or from another general practitioner. Michelle, a community nurse, explained how in one case she played a liaison role, 'bringing the parties together'. More specifically, she introduced the patient to a doctor who was prepared to assist, and was present in a non-specific capacity at the death itself. Peter, a nurse, asserts that: 'If someone walked in right now and said "I want to kill myself, I've got AIDS and I'm terminal", I would know . . . [which] GP or practice to refer them to . . . to give them a good assessment and [to] do the job if that's what got to be done'. This does not mean that the process of enlisting support for euthanasia is blatant or explicit. Bill, a hospice nurse, commented that it was largely an 'unspoken thing' and that 'I like to keep it vague'. He explained how he might remark to the doctor that the patient's medication did not appear to be working, adding, 'I think we're going to need something stronger; what do you think about Seconal [secobarbital]?' To an AIDS doctor, Bill explained, 'Seconal is like [a] big flag word' that indicates 'this person really wants to kill themselves'. Tentative approaches like this flush out those who are prepared to participate or co-operate in the euthanasia process, leading, in turn, to new collaborations.

Referrals may come from doctors who prefer not to explore the issue of euthanasia with a patient personally. While he didn't think he had a 'reputation' for euthanasia, and rarely spoke about it with colleagues, Harvey, a GP, received a large number of euthanasia referrals, and complained about it in interview. 'Offensive might be too high a word', he said, '[but] because I'm supposedly left wing and civil libertarian . . . people dump the hard stuff on me'.

Assessment: Once a health professional has taken responsibility for exploring the euthanasia option with a patient, that person may nevertheless seek a second opinion, or some assurance from a third party that it is appropriate to proceed. On an ad hoc basis, health carers may advise the patient to undergo psychiatric assessment, particularly if the patient appears depressed. Helen, a community nurse, referred patients in this way if they appeared depressed to a 'pathological' degree, even though she felt she had 'good assessment skills' and that a certain component of depression due to AIDS was 'not unreasonable'. One interviewee, a psychiatrist who had pre-scribed lethal doses of medication, described how he also performed pre-euthanasia 'assessments' at the request of colleagues. Another interviewee, an ex-priest, was regularly asked to assess potential candidates for assisted death. He agreed that he had carved out a (non-paying) 'ministry' in this area, which fitted in well with his therapy practice.

Since it operates informally, the assessment process (if there is one) may be rudimentary and utterly unsatisfactory. It may be little more than a brief telephone conversation. Gary, a GP, reported that before being involved in euthanasia he would telephone the hospital physician who may have recently treated the patient before dis-charge, for confirmation that the patient's outlook was bleak. After receiving the physician's assessment, Gary might ask 'So if [the patient] died it wouldn't be such a bad thing?' and they might reply 'No, it wouldn't be such a bad thing at all, it would be quite a rea-sonable thing'. 'They generally know what we're talking about', Gary says.

An informal assessment process provides few of the safeguards of a legislated, statutory regime. On one occasion, a trained psychi-atric nurse was brought in to assess a patient who was thought to be depressed by those close to him. The patient got the all-clear, although he had only told his parents the week before that he was HIV positive. Euthanasia was then performed by a GP who had only met the patient for the first time the previous day.

The process of seeking reassurance or advice from other col-leagues known to be involved in, or sympathetic towards, eutha-nasia, was a recurrent theme in interviews. The informal 'peer review' process provides opportunities for the sharing of advice and, potentially, the sharing of resources (drugs). Sometimes interviewees described a 'team meeting' involving a doctor, nurse, the patient and the patient's lover. Networking frequently goes beyond deciding whether it is appropriate to perform euthanasia, and extends to seeking advice about drug dosage. Interviewees reported seeking advice from other GPs, hospital physicians and anaesthetists, pharmacologists, pharmacists and vets.

It is likely that the process of informal review and assessment plays an important part in cementing feelings of solidarity, and in affirming the values of euthanasia participants. Potentially it provides opportunities for new colleagues to participate in the process at some level, and for the expansion of co-operative networks. These processes invite further research.

Obtaining drugs: As described in Chapter 10, interviewees obtained drugs from a variety of sources. They capitalised on connections with pharmacists, and colleagues who were prepared to prescribe or chart lethal quantities. Other strategies included the illegitimate use of legitimately supplied medicines, 'hoarding' practices and theft. It is important to emphasise how networking can facilitate the euthanasia process, despite the various limitations individual practitioners may place upon their own involvement. Doctors who do not have a long or close relationship with a patient may nevertheless be prevailed upon by a friend or colleague to write a prescription, donate syringes, or to provide Valium from their doctor's bag. Doctors who do not want to administer a lethal injection may nevertheless make themselves available to sign the death certificate after the event. A doctor who would never take the initiative may nevertheless respond to the 'crisis' that results when an overdose succeeds only in rendering the patient comatose.

Collaboration at the bedside: Even the most activist health professionals were grateful for the support of colleagues when performing procedures at the bedside. A common example of shared involvement was for one health care worker to access the patient's vein, while another injected the drugs. Frequently it is the nurse who takes the leading role. 'Nurses are usually better at finding veins', said one nurse, 'the doctors I've worked with . . . have so much riding on it that often when it comes [to] the point of putting the needle in . . . they get a bit nervous, a little bit edgy'. The same nurse, who found performing euthanasia 'very sad', 'very dramatic' and 'very stressful', added that 'it's good to have a second head to talk [to]' when an initial dose has been ineffective in causing death. In these circumstances, bedside collaboration may extend to strangulation and suffocation.

Another role that cropped up repeatedly in interviews, and which was frequently filled by nurses, was that of 'orchestrator' or 'general facilitator'. Although they might not administer the drugs, facilitators are complicit in the process, providing advice and re-assurance to the person who administers the drugs, as well as sup-port for lovers and friends. They co-ordinate participants and, as one interviewee observed, help to create an environment where those present will not 'freak out'.

As noted in Chapter 7, in one detailed account of involvement given by a GP, a judge was described as fulfilling this role. 'He was . . . running the whole thing, shepherding people here and there . . . being a support for everyone'. Members of the patient's family were 'all sitting around, holding [the patient's] hands, holding his feet, just being there with him'.

'I made it clear to everyone that this was actually murder', the interviewee recalls, 'and that anyone that was involved was actually an accessory [to murder]'. The judge also 'spoke up and said that . . . he was very aware of that . . . he made it clear what his position was and that he faced as much of a problem as I or anyone else in the room'.

Not long after, a veterinary drug was administered to the patient. 'He had a big smile on his face and he said goodbye to everyone, and then said "this tastes like blackberry" . . . went white [and] stopped breathing'.

After the death 'the family were incredible', the interviewee recalls. 'They thanked me profusely . . . it was actually a bit un-comfortable . . . I felt like some hero the way they were talking . . . it was a very moving situation and . . . [I] shed a few tears as I went and did the paperwork.'

On other occasions, the euthanatic episode will be a private affair for the patient, lovers and friends, although a doctor may be 'on call' in case anything 'goes wrong'.

Euthanasia networking extends beyond the death itself. If not present at the death, a doctor may be lined up to come around and sign the death certificate. Euthanasia-friendly doctors may counter-sign the cremation application. Stanley, who described himself as a therapist, noted that while he usually took on the facilitator role at the bedside, on other occasions he 'might be part of a tag team, where somebody else is the active agent and I have assumed the role of finding the body'. The allocation of roles is strategic, in order not to arouse suspicions and to minimise the risks for those involved.

De-briefing: Friendships and collegial relationships provide opportunities for participants to de-brief and find support after the death. 'People who know about it will often ring me up after the event and ask how it's gone . . . just to check on me, which is very nice', said one GP. Another spoke of discussing the event with 'close friends that have some professional involvement in the area . . . to get their reassurance that I've done the right thing'. A third spoke of 'a very personal chat with close friends'. A fourth interviewee, Nola, spoke of a 'breakfast club' made up mostly of female GPs. This 'club' reflected a variety of AIDS and cancer practices, and gave each doctor the opportunity to talk through their participation in assisted death.

The people to whom interviewees turned for support were not necessarily other participants, nor other health care workers. As dis-cussed in Chapter 1, Jane's 'support group' consisted of a group of other women with a public profile. Margaret's support group con-sisted of her own partner, a nurse, and a friend of her brother, each of whom were involved in the attempted euthanasia of her brother.

Making new connections: Several interviewees described their experiences of discovering that other colleagues were also involved in euthanasia. Paula, a general practitioner, attended weekly meetings and would hear about patients with AIDS who had died in a nearby hospital, in a hospice or in the community. As a result of 'code phrases', and other clues, 'I started to build up an idea of who perhaps did and [who] didn't'.

Later, one doctor broached the subject with Paula directly, asking her 'Oh, what do you use?' Surprised, Paula responded with 'Well, what do *you* use?!' They then exchanged recipes for lethal cocktails, Paula commenting that 'he had never heard of what I had used, and I had never heard of what he'd use'. Interestingly, the details Paula provided of this conversation helped to confirm that the doctor Paula spoke to was also an interviewee.

Co-operative euthanasia in hospital

Euthanasia is not limited to community settings, although the shared nature of institutional care, and the need to justify one's actions to colleagues, create a significant disincentive to euthanasia in hospital. In addition to legal considerations, interviewees cited the nature of supervision within hospitals and the general 'ethos' of hospital care, including conservative attitudes to pain management, as factors inhibiting their ability to even *discuss* euthanasia with patients and colleagues, let alone participate in it. The situation is summarised by Robert, a well-known AIDS researcher and physician. 'It's not difficult to prescribe injectable morphine and increase the doses and basically put people to sleep . . . but to actually give what we might call a lethal dose . . . is very rare in hospital practice.'

Nevertheless, euthanasia does occur in hospital, and the very presence of institutional constraints makes it all the more remarkable. As a 'traditionalist' (see Chapter 6), Robert may well be excluded from the practices of more activist colleagues. Indeed, the extent to which interviewees were involved in assisted death within hospitals was a surprising feature of this study. The interviews reveal a range of social processes which make euthanasia in hospital possible. As seen below, these range from co-operative overdosing involving one or two functionaries acting at considerable personal risk, to entire hospital units where euthanasia is blatant and which foster, to some degree, a culture of euthanasia.

Manipulating hospital procedures: In hospital, morphine and other potentially lethal drugs are administered by nurses, on doctors orders. Typically, a nurse must sign for the morphine that he or she accesses from the medicine cabinet, in the presence of a colleague. A colleague will also be required to witness the destruction of any 'excess' morphine from the vial which is left over, after the patient's order has been filled. Nurses may sometimes be authorised to administer additional, or 'breakthrough' doses of medication in response to a patient's continuing pain or discomfort.

Interviewees reported a range of ways in which these processes could be subverted. One nurse in a Catholic hospital explained that nurses on his unit felt comfortable playing 'fast and loose' with excess morphine, in order to help patients to 'spring the mortal coil'. Other nurses pointed out in interview that doctors may also participate in this process, ordering the nurse to administer the 'extra dose' which—importantly—will never appear on the patient's chart.

Language plays a key role in activating these processes. Although medical directives must be clear enough to be followed by 'sympathetic' colleagues or subordinates, the meaning is often deliberately ambiguous, reflecting the apprehension, or mixed feelings, of participants. Erin, a nurse, recalled a patient with chronic obstructive pulmonary disease who had been intubated three times and, now having caught TB, was terrified of being placed on a respirator again. Erin assisted the patient to die by dialling down the oxygen the patient was receiving, until he died of carbon dioxide narcosis. Later, he fended off an intern, who wanted to ignore the 'do not resuscitate' order above the man's bed, despite the fact the patient was now grey and clearly dead.

The physician in charge of Erin's unit was aware of Erin's involvement in this case. Several months later he approached Erin about another distressed patient they were caring for. 'Use as much morphine as you need', said the physician. 'I'll sign for it.'

Erin was taken by surprise.

'Do you know what I mean?' said the physician.

'I'm not sure', said Erin. 'Do you want me to make him comfortable, or do you want me to make him *ultimately* comfortable?'

'Yes', replied the physician, ambiguously.

The patient died that night.

The principal method for achieving death in hospital is overdoses of IV narcotics. At the level of language, this permits the intention to kill to masquerade as routine palliation. Russell, a hospital physician, observed that sometimes nurses will confront the doctor during (his) rounds, saying things like: 'I think all [the patient] needs is a morphine drip, why don't you have some compassion and just leave this poor kid alone?' Comments such as these would be spoken openly, Russell observed, and might lead to a discussion with nursing staff.

But what is the intention behind a seemingly innocuous discussion about a 'morphine drip'? In response to this question, Russell replied that it means 'don't torture the poor [patient], let them die slowly and easily and pain free *and let's speed the process up here*. 'It's spoken about pretty much the way people discuss whether to put the family pet to sleep or not', said Russell. 'People [know] that they are talking about death, and doing it from compassion.' Just as frequently, however, euthanasia remains an unspoken process between health professionals. A physician charts a dose which, in the patient's circumstances, is clearly extraordinary, and the nurse just 'knows'. 'You know that the four o'clock dose of morphine is going to be the last dose', said one nurse; 'it's not discussed, it's just done'.

Returning to the case of Erin, above, not long after the physician had asked Erin (albeit ambiguously) to perform euthanasia, a nurse colleague approached him with two vials of morphine. 'I've already signed these out to this patient . . . *in my name*', she said.

Erin was surprised to realise that his nursing colleague was also evidently aware that he had assisted the TB patient to die. 'I don't want to be an "angel of death"', he protested in interview. 'I don't think it's healthy for me . . . and I don't think it's healthy for the patients . . . *and this is a Catholic hospital*'.

This exchange provides a nice illustration of hospital collaboration, as well as the ambiguous language it is frequently couched within. 'She never used the word *morphine*', Erin recalls. 'She came after me and she said "I don't want to put you in an awkward position . . . but I think you can do what needs to be done . . . I *can't* do it, but I think it's in the patient's best interests".'

Erin's colleague had gone as far as she could: signing out in her own name a quantity of drugs sufficient for an overdose, and in so doing ensuring that Erin's name did not appear on the narcotics chart. Collaboration achieved the rest.

A culture of euthanasia? While it may be possible for individuals to co-operatively subvert hospital procedures in order to surreptitiously kill patients, to what extent does this occur blatantly, at a unit-wide level? Empirically, I cannot answer this, beyond pointing to some of the processes involved, as evidenced in interviews on both sides of the Pacific.

The dividing line between palliation and euthanasia can be hard to pick. The imperatives of pain control and palliation can disguise the fact that a patient is being intentionally drugged to death. At one end of the spectrum, a patient may become distressed, and medication will be escalated to control observable pain. Further along the spectrum, the patient may be sedated into a coma, although if medication were to be withdrawn, the patient would quickly become uncomfortable again. Further along again, medication may be escalated beyond what is needed for sedation, in order to depress respiration and hasten death over a period of time. At the far end of the spectrum, a massive 'lethal overdose' may be given by injection or as part of an IV cocktail.

Protestations aside, there is little doubt that hospitals do provide euthanasia, under the guise of sedation. The interviews with Zane, Russell and Liz, in particular, illustrate the differing degrees to which there was a 'culture' of euthanasia in three separate hospital units.

Zane, a quietly spoken palliative care physician, pointed out that 'the skill is to build up the dose rather than use one or two big doses'. He added that this avoided 'polarising' the nursing staff, and that 'the result is the same as if it happened in two hours'. Zane acknowledged that he was 'so dependent upon good personal relations'. Staff must be accepting of the doctor, of HIV patients, and of assisted death. 'If someone's out of step, then there'll only be conflict and complaints and everyone will step back for fear of being reported to some higher body.'

Key features of Zane's strategy involved admitting the patient at unusual hours, and capitalising on the changeover-of-shift period, where departing staff were briefing incoming staff, and were likely to be distracted. Seven o'clock on a Sunday morning was a good time because no hospital doctors or staff are around and 'you tend to have the older nursing sisters on duty at that time, the people you trust'. Another good time was after 9.00 p.m. on week days. Zane explained how he would capitalise on a 'crisis', driving the patient to hospital himself, and admitting the patient directly into his own unit. He would begin 'treatment' at around 9.30 p.m., close to changeover time, when staff are 'quite happy for you to do everything'. By the time the night staff are settled in around 11 p.m. or midnight, 'they don't know anything that's happened beforehand'. Other features of Zane's strategy involved avoiding the accident and emergency department, and always attempting to admit the patient into a single room.

Zane's strategy for hospital-based euthanasia illustrates the challenges faced by an activist physician who can afford to trust some, but not all, of his staff. Zane comments that 'the staff tend to trust you because they know that you've got a good relationship with the patient'. At the same time, Zane avoided the perceptions that would be created if he took the extraordinary step of administering medication personally. 'I don't handle the drugs myself . . . I only write the orders . . . so you have to have a staff who will accept administering these doses.'

In contrast to Zane, Russell worked in a unit where the intention to hasten death was more widely shared and accepted among nursing staff:

> We increase doses [of pain medication] knowing full well that it will kill the patient . . . there is a systematic increase, with less and less concern for 'is the patient getting pain control?' . . . it becomes more 'is the patient breathing?', so that's done on a very regular basis and people talk about it in hallways very openly: 'I think we're ready for the drip now'.

For 'legal reasons', the 'narcotic drip' will be documented in the patient's chart as being for 'pain control', rather than euthanasia. Russell stressed, however, that he had never made the decision to euthanise a patient himself, but only when the patient personally, or the patient's next-of-kin or someone holding a durable power of attorney, had first reached this decision. 'I assist, I don't decide', he said.

Russell admits that there has been a tremendous change over the past ten years in the way staff at his hospital approached death. 'Slowly people started talking about it in the health care team [and] it was actually very reassuring and very relieving to me that I wasn't the only one thinking and feeling this way.' Russell felt that members of his health care team shared 'similar values', and that this in turn reflected the response of the gay community to the death and dying issues raised by AIDS. 'The gay community [has] always felt disenfranchised from [the] mainstream . . . when it comes to marital status and morals and rights—we've always had to come up with our own standards of moral practice'. Russell considered himself a 'pretty moral, ethical physician' who had 'no problems sleeping at night'. Although unaware of the legal status of his actions, Russell added 'to be honest with you, I really don't care'.

The interview with Liz, a hospital nurse, suggested an even more radical culture of euthanasia within one hospital unit. The focus of Liz' interview was a detailed and confessional allegation of involuntary euthanasia. During the course of the conversation, however, Liz explained how the unit where she worked would 'book in' patients to receive a lethal infusion of drugs. Although the focus of the discussions was between the physician and the patient, nurses would be told that 'the cocktail is going up', and no attempt was made to hide its significance.

On one occasion, for example, an 'old man' with no family who was 'very quickly going downhill' said goodbye to his friends, and was admitted to hospital. 'He wouldn't have the infusion for about three days', said Liz. 'He watched telly, and ate and went outside and smoked, and sat in the garden and did all those sort of things, and then one morning he just said "today is the day" '. 'I was involved in putting that infusion up', said Liz.

Although she felt 'there is a place for [voluntary] euthanasia', Liz admitted that she 'avoided doing it', although others in her unit 'were more than happy to do it'. 'I mean, what do you say to the patient?', questioned Liz. 'You go to work, wash a few, knock off a few . . . here's your infusion, bye bye?'

Liz claimed that the therapeutics manual which the senior physician had written to assist staff working in the unit contained a 'written protocol' or recipe for a euthanasia cocktail. 'It was absolutely blatant', said Liz. She well remembers the directions the physician gave her in relation to one patient: 'Get [the infusion] up and get him out of here by sundown'. On another occasion, after indicating for her to turn up a morphine infusion, Liz remembers the physician scolding her by saying 'and make sure you do a good job of it this time'.

Ranging from the carefully-concealed to the blatant, the evidence of hospital euthanasia was an unexpected finding of this study. Interestingly, community-based health carers, even those with a long record of euthanasia involvement, were largely unaware of these processes. A recurrent theme in interviews with community-based doctors was their regret in being unable to respond to the anguished requests of their patients, following admission to hospital. Within hospital, however, physician-initiated euthanasia depends upon discreet partnerships with nurses who are willing to administer lethal infusions of drugs, on doctor's orders. For the legal protection of participants, these processes must masquerade as palliative care in the patient's medical record. The more people involved, the higher the risk.

Future research into these processes will not be easy. Hospitals themselves (and their research ethics committees) have a vested interest in minimising potential liability, maintaining a conservative and responsible public image, hosing down public fears, and discouraging 'prying eyes'. The interviews in this study were only achieved by direct approach to the health care workers concerned, usually at the suggestion of a third party with ethics oversight occurring at the university level. It is possible that the development of a 'euthanatic culture' within certain AIDS units is the product of witnessing over fifteen years of suffering, reinforced by the gay identities and personal values of health care workers themselves. Whether HIV/AIDS units are unique in this respect is an intriguing but unanswered question.

The implications of the euthanasia underground

The 'euthanasia underground' is an invisible community: a network constituted by the informal chain of associations between health carers who approve of, facilitate, and participate in, assisted death. Its structure and effectiveness are enhanced by the fact that it is partly a product of friendships and professional associations in the gay community, and within HIV/AIDS nursing and medicine. It is unknown whether (and if so to what extent) euthanasia networks exist generally, within other communities, localities, or organisations, or within the context of other diseases. At the very least, this study suggests that one would expect to find 'collaborative euthanasia' within larger cities where AIDS has had an impact.

The co-operative processes that constitute the euthanasia underground make assisted death easier to accomplish. The 'connectedness' of participants is, in effect, a technology which facilitates action at each stage of the process: obtaining and sharing technical advice, accessing drugs, performing bedside procedures, disposing of the body after death, and obtaining reassurance that one has done the right thing. The network creates a culture of assistance and support that legitimates the choice of assisted death, helps participants to do what is necessary and to cope with the emotions of involvement.

It would be wrong to assume that euthanasia networks are sophisticated in the sense of having any hierarchy, formal membership or defined roles. Security risks are minimised precisely through the lack of formal organisation and oversight, and by the partial knowledge of individual participants.

Despite its informality, the euthanasia underground is highly effective in facilitating the organisation and delivery of euthanasia services. The existence of euthanasia networks illustrates the failure of the policy of prohibition. This failure is made all the more obvious by the fact that those who end their patients' lives are not isolated and wild-eyed miscreants acting from the fringes of their professions. On the contrary, they are just as likely to be integrated within, supported and assisted by, a small cluster of colleagues and close friends whose shared values and allegiances make detection impossible.

It is in this context that one can better understand why some 'revisionists' oppose the legalisation of euthanasia (see Chapter 6). A law permitting assisted death under controlled conditions would impose a *competing protocol* for assessing when assistance was appropriate. Legalisation challenges the informal assessment mechanisms that already operate, impinging on established relationships, and introducing a level of oversight some regard as unnecessary.

On the other hand, despite the support that participants obtain from colleagues and friends, illegal euthanasia remains an extremely stressful enterprise. Some participants fear getting caught. The threat of criminal prosecution inhibits the sharing of information that would permit euthanasia to be performed quickly, gently and effectively. And the burden of secrecy is high.

Even if one assumes that assisted death is largely an AIDS-only phenomenon (which is unlikely), the scope, audacity and complexity of underground euthanasia highlight the crisis of policy. The medical profession has ignored these practices for too long, and society has been kept in the dark. The churches, prosecutors and legislators just don't want to know. But the closing times of life are too important, and patients deserve better.

Ultimately, the policy equation reduces to a choice between more of the same (the failed idealism of a law prohibiting assistance), and the pragmatism of a legislative regime that recognises the reality of the euthanasia underground, and seeks to regulate it. For social and moral conservatives it is an uncomfortable choice between seeking to channel underground practices into a controlled context, and reserving for oneself the luxury of condemnation.

It may be difficult to persuade those who believe that killing is always wrong that anything could improve on a policy of prohibition. Some may ignore the law, but wouldn't legalising euthanasia simply reward lawlessness? Let us assume, for the sake of argument, that those who take this view are right. Proponents of the status quo still face a serious public relations crisis, because—as the following two chapters will illustrate—the euthanasia underground is a disturbing place. Euthanasia is practised in an informal, intuitive and arbitrary manner. This is dangerous for patients. Abdicating responsibility, and hiding our heads in the sand, just isn't good enough.

10

Disturbing issues

Voluntary euthanasia and assistance to suicide are available in Australia today. The problem is that the practice is illegal and therefore only a few people can access it. You have to be affluent enough or lucky enough to have a relationship with the right doctor to be accommodated. Another problem is that it must be arranged and carried out in secret. There must be no witnesses. This means there are no controls or safeguards against mistake or abuse. From a public policy perspective, this situation is inequitable and dangerous.

Marshall Perron, Former Chief Minister of the Northern Territory, 24 August 1995[1]

As Perron recognises, a feature of covertly-practised euthanasia is the total lack of 'quality control'. Because it is practised in secret, little is known about the risks for patients, or the circumstances in which health care workers agree to participate. In this chapter and in chapter 11, I put on record some of the 'disturbing issues' that emerge from the euthanasia underground. They illustrate how the euthanasia underground is characterised, above all, by an *absence of professionalism*.

'Anti-professionalism' and the euthanasia underground

A 'profession' is a self-regulating organisation, characterised by specialised training leading to unique skills, and a tradition of disinterested service to others. As Beauchamp and Childress point out, in learned professions such as medicine 'the background knowledge of the professional derives from closely supervised training'.[2]

The surreptitious practice of euthanasia illustrates, in many ways, the very opposite of those attributes which characterise 'medical professionalism'. In the euthanasia underground there is no specialised training. Participants remain ignorant about what is needed to achieve a gentle death. There is a proliferation of what participants refer to bluntly as 'botched attempts'. Accountability is also absent. The medical profession for the most part turns a blind eye to the practice of illicit euthanasia by its members. There are no norms or principles guiding involvement. Rather, participation is shrouded in secrecy and deception, triggered by highly idiosyncratic factors, with evidence of casual and precipitative involvements. In place of a tradition of disinterested service to patients, there is evidence of a complete lack of 'professional distance', sharp conflicts of interest, and examples of euthanasia without consent.

These are serious charges. Nevertheless, the evidence for this 'anti-professionalism' comes from participants themselves, courtesy the pseudonymous interview format, which encouraged respondents to talk honestly and explicitly about their actions. This chapter focuses on one distinct dimension of 'anti-professionalism': the absence of a professional framework, or organised context, for the provision of euthanasia services. Because euthanasia is an 'under-the-table' procedure, there is no monitoring or accountability, no criteria guiding involvement, and few reliable strategies for achieving death. In the resulting environment, we see evidence of:

* frequent 'botched attempts' to perform euthanasia;
* evidence of coercion upon the patient, and/or the health care worker;
* evidence of rash or hasty involvement by doctors with little or no knowledge of the patient's circumstances;

    * evidence of euthanasia upon able-bodied patients who are
not in the terminal stages of illness; and

    * an all-pervasive culture of deception.

These disturbing issues cut both ways. Do the fragmented and idio-syncratic factors triggering participation in assisted death scream out for new forms of regulation, in order to reduce overall harm to society? Or does it merely demonstrate the true horror of delivering the power over life and death into the hands of doctors and nurses?

'Botched attempts' at euthanasia

> I've only had one real botch . . . it was horrible—it took four or five hours . . . it was like Rasputin, we just couldn't . . . finish him off . . . I tried insulin, I tried just about everything else that I [had] around and it just took forever . . . [It was] very hard for his lover. So um I sort of shooed the lover out of the room at one stage and put a pillow over his head, that seemed to work in the end [laughs nervously] . . . That was one of the worst [clearing throat] one of the most horrible things I've ever done (Gary, general practitioner).

Euthanasia has never been part of the medical school curriculum. Its illegality breeds what one interviewee called a 'code of silence', which forces each practitioner to rely on trial and error. Reliable knowledge about compassionate killing comes at a high price.

    Although bodies such as the AIDS Council of New South Wales have estimated that up to half of euthanasia attempts by people with HIV/AIDS fail,[3] the fact is that very little is known about the prevalence of 'botched attempts'.[4] Complications during the euthanasia process were a recurrent theme in interviews. Of the 88 first-hand accounts of involvement given by interviewees, 17 (19 per cent) involved 'botches'. It is worth remembering that many of the interviewees in this study were repeat players who had perfected their techniques, and thus their 'success ratios'. The rate of botched attempts may well be higher where health care workers are not involved.

Why euthanasia bids fail

There are a variety of reasons why euthanasia attempts fail. An important factor is that debilitated patients may still have strong hearts unaffected by the virus. Michelle, a community nurse, states, coarsely:

> Even if they've been sick for a long time, they're still young, relatively healthy young men with booming, bumping great 'Phar Lap hearts' that are really hard to stop . . . [in] a couple of situations I've been involved in it was just bloody awful because they just wouldn't die.

Practitioners regularly under-estimate the dosages needed to achieve death. As discussed in Chapter 7, euthanasia frequently involves overdosing a patient with morphine and other relatively accessible drugs for which there is a legal market. Many patients, however, are already receiving narcotics for pain relief, and some have a staggeringly high tolerance to morphine. Others have histories of intravenous drug use. Liz, a hospital nurse, tells of an episode of euthanasia which occurred, at the family's request, on an emaciated and demented patient in her unit. Liz was astonished at the man's tolerance to 'grams of morphine, not milligrams, [but] grams'. The patient was 'only about 5 foot tall' and it took about '13 bags of the cocktail to kill him'. 'The big joke was: what happens if he wakes up, he's going to think he's in Heaven, we better make sure . . . he's got [a] nice nurse on duty that night.'

Medical condition, body build, drug history and narcotic tolerance are all variables that must be factored in when developing a specific strategy to achieve death. One interviewee spoke of several acquaintances who had 'rung up the poisons bureau . . . and inverted their advice', ingesting the 'recommended' dose, only to wake up later or to be discovered alive by district nurses.

Martin, an HIV/AIDS community worker, recalls that on the first occasion he attempted to perform euthanasia, he followed advice given by an anaesthetist that '100 milligrams of morphine injected intravenously' would be sufficient. The patient, however, had been a runner and weight lifter, and 'had the respiratory system of a horse'. A second attempt using the same dose was also unsuccessful. For the 'next 108 hours that [the patient] lived', Martin recalls, 'we had great difficulty in getting [sufficient] morphine to actually contain his pain'.

Initially Martin and his friends used morphine prescribed for their own use. After that, additional morphine was stolen from the drugs cabinet of the AIDS ward of an inner-city Catholic hospital.

The patient, however, started fitting and vomiting up bile so intravenous Valium (diazepam) was administered, obtained from a community nurse who was 'on-side', who in turn had obtained it from a
sympathetic GP. A suction tube was used to prevent the patient
choking on the bile, but in the early hours of the morning he choked
on the tube and died.

'That's when I found out that medicine's a pretty inexact science,
I guess', Martin recalls, adding that when he later spoke to the anaesthetist about the incident, the doctor replied, 'well it works in geriatrics'. Disturbingly, two of the three occasions on which Martin has
been involved in euthanasia have been 'botched attempts', including
the death of his partner.

Complications in the euthanatic process are well recognised by
researchers who have interviewed participants in euthanasia. Reflecting on an interview-based project in the San Francisco bay area,
Jamison concludes:

> How does one accomplish an assisted death in the most 'efficient' and
> yet emotionally positive manner unless one has done it before or has
> well-developed models to use for this purpose? In this way, the lack of
> models, experience, and training makes this an act that must be con-
> stantly reinvented. Every experience is new, fraught with its own
> fears, hesitancy, and ignorance, and nearly every one who participates
> is an actor with an unrehearsed script.[5]

The consequences of miscalculation

'Botched' euthanasia attempts begin with an initial misconception
about the dose of drug required to achieve death. The realisation
that death is not occurring is incredibly stressful for participants,
who may feel that they are letting the patient down. Interviewees
reported feelings of panic and hysteria when faced by the prospect
of failure:

> The pulse started to disappear, and there was sort of a nod of
> acknowledgment that he was going, and then there was this all-of-a-
> sudden look of panic on the [face of the] person who was taking the
> pulse, *because the pulse started coming back* (Margaret, HIV/AIDS
> community worker).

Panic reactions manifest themselves in a variety of ways. Several interviewees reported desperate attempts to obtain assistance from a sympathetic doctor. Zane, a palliative care specialist, recalls: 'I had a frantic call around 2 a.m., [someone] saying "he seems to be getting lighter, he's waking, he seems to be moving a bit more and waking"'. In this case, Zane noted that the patient's partner was 'fearful and terrified' that the patient was going to wake up and find that 'he'd bungled his suicide attempt'. Zane bypassed the emergency department and admitted the patient directly to his own palliative care unit where he charted high doses of Hynovel (midazolam) and subcutaneous morphine every two hours. 'We'd made a conscious decision not to allow the patient to wake up', Zane recalls.

Many botched attempts do not end as smoothly as this. Where doctors are involved, a common reaction was to 'empty the doctor's bag' into the patient. Speaking of one failed attempt, Peter, a community nurse, says: 'The relatives left the room and the doctor and I opened the doctor's case and gave him everything in the case. It didn't work—he was still alive—and the doctor said "if you can get heroin, we'll give him heroin . . ."'.

When drugs fail, health care workers may resort to suffocation or strangulation. Three interviewees admitted to choking, suffocating or strangling a comatose patient, and several others reported incidents in which a third party had suffocated the patient. Off-tape, one community nurse stated that he had injected air into a patient's veins. Air embolism and suffocation using plastic bags were also documented in Jamison's study.[6] Among some in the HIV client and health carer community, suffocations are referred to metaphorically as 'pillow jobs'. 'I'll carry a lot of that to my grave', said Peter. 'I don't think you ever get rid of it.'

Loss of dignity is an undeniable feature of many botched attempts. Stanley, a therapist, recalls a scene where a patient self-administered 15 Seconal tablets, but failed to take an anti-emetic, to prevent vomiting. Desperate, the patient then ate his own vomit.

M   And you were there?
S   Yeah.
M   And did he die?

S   Yeah, not pretty, not happy, not without great consternation . . .
     i-i-it's a vision I still see in my head.

No less appalling was an episode recounted by Stanley involving a
patient who 'mentioned to his psychiatrist that he was thinking
about self-deliverance'. 'What planet [his psychiatrist] was from, I
don't know', Stanley recalls. Convinced that the patient was a risk
to himself, the psychiatrist arranged for the patient to be 'incar-
cerated into a mental facility where he received shock treatment'.
'There's nothing in the right to die movement', says Stanley, 'that is
as sick and perverse as . . . that!'

M   Where did you hear that?
S   Where did I hear?—I know the person.
M   You know the patient?
S   Yes . . . He called me. Actually, when I got there he didn't even
     know who I was because he had just undergone one of his shock
     treatments. It was a nightmare, it was SHOCKING, SHOCKING
     [very loud, emotional].
M   And this is a man dying with AIDS, in the terminal stages?
S   Exactly . . . right here in [this city].

Some examples

The narratives of involvement that I regarded as disturbing in this
study were rarely disturbing for only one reason. The following two
accounts of botched attempts are not the most sensational. They
were chosen to illustrate the different circumstances in which unsuccessful euthanasia attempts can occur, while introducing a variety of
other concerns explored later in the chapter.

Gordon was an experienced general practitioner called in to
'remedy' a botched euthanasia attempt. Gordon had been treating
the patient ('Stephen'), a 26-year-old, for a period of six weeks. 'He
had dreadful self-esteem and . . . was a very anxious, obsessive
person', says Gordon. He was an 'absolute misery-guts, I think he'd
never had a joyful experience in his life'. 'He just decided that he
wanted to die', Gordon recalls.

At the time, Stephen was estranged from his family (who had
rejected him because he was gay), and Gordon tried to help him to
sort out these issues, and to monitor his pain (which was minimal).

At one point Gordon arranged for Stephen to go into a hospice, which gave Stephen's 22-year-old partner a break. Stephen's partner went doctor shopping, obtaining prescriptions of Tryptanol (amitriptyline), an anti-depressant. Stephen also stockpiled morphine tablets obtained from the hospice. Gordon suspects that Stephen's decision to die was influenced by his friends: 'His self-esteem was so poor, I think he wanted to make other people happy'. Three of Stephen's friends were nurses, who spoke to some oncology friends about drug combinations.

On the night in question, Stephen invited his friends to dinner, before taking the Tryptanol, MS-Contin (a slow-release morphine), and Serenace (an anti-psychotic). 'I felt absolutely cajoled into this', says Gordon. 'I got the phone call about one or two in the morning. I remember having this shocking flu at the time . . . [and when I arrived], here were the nursing friends all expecting him to die'. Stephen was deeply unconscious, his pupils were dilated, and he was Cheyne-Stokes breathing.

Between 2 a.m. and 6 a.m. Gordon injected Stephen with 'everything from my doctor's bag, *and he still breathed*'. The reasons why Gordon chose to intervene are troubling:

> I realised well he's not going to survive, he's going to be dead anyway, I might as well speed it along . . . I think also because it was 4 o'clock in the morning, I had a cold, and I felt dreadful and I just wanted to get out of there . . . and I knew that if I didn't do something that they would find some other way to do it, and I was really concerned that . . . he didn't suffer.

Gordon reports that in the early morning, one of Stephen's nurse friends 'went to turn him and I think, and I'm not sure to this day but I'm almost certain that the nurse did a pillow job . . . I think that it was asphyxiation with a pillow'.

Gordon certified Stephen's death, and a funeral director arrived shortly thereafter as a result of prior arrangements. Stephen was cremated.

During the interview Gordon complained of being 'cajoled', 'assaulted', and 'abused' by Stephen's friends. He went on to describe the 'utter misery' of younger gay men: 'I've seen other people enjoy life and I know that this person could'.

Gordon is ambivalent about his future intentions, affirming that 'I won't take part in active euthanasia', and 'I'm not prepared to do something that's illegal'. Later, however, he said, 'If a Stephen happened again, in the middle of the night, I really don't know what I'd do . . . I'd be a bit more circumspect about the whole thing'.

How can we make sense of Gordon's story? Called out in the middle of a winter's night, suffering from flu and anxious to get home, a doctor pumps a comatose patient full of drugs in order to fulfil friends' expectations, all the while conceding that the patient had serious, unresolved emotional problems.

While some readers will regard this as unforgivable, it is important to emphasise that actions like these are not performed by the freaky fringe. On the contrary, these are the closely-guarded secrets of well respected health practitioners, people who—like Gordon—present impeccably, embody the demeanour of competent professionals and hold positions of status and leadership within the profession. The overwhelming majority of those interviewees who were implicated in 'disturbing' episodes were simultaneously gracious and dedicated professionals who inspired trust, and who genuinely cared about the suffering of their patients. It is difficult not to recall the interview with Richard, an opponent of euthanasia, who said: 'I don't idealise doctors'. 'They are fairly ordinary people with many of the same frailties which most people have, although hopefully accustomed to operating within a professional framework.'

A very different kind of botched attempt was recounted by Michelle, a community nurse, who estimated that she had been involved six to eight times in the previous four years. The patient ('James') developed PML (progressive multifocal leukoencephalopathy, a viral infection of the brain). 'Within three weeks', Michelle reports, 'he couldn't walk, [he] lost bodily function, he went mute, he disintegrated before our very eyes'. James had been a patient of Michelle's from a previous position. 'He was just gorgeous, and because I'm a nurse, there was that part of our relationship, but we also used to go to the footy, to the pub, and all that sort of stuff', says Michelle.

James had previously raised the issue of euthanasia with Michelle, who didn't have a problem with it, and had agreed to help. 'The night before, we all had tea together', says Michelle. 'We all had Kentucky Fried together and . . . he did some really stupid funny things.' 'I went home, and of course didn't sleep a wink', she adds.

The next day, Michelle arrived early, and a doctor who was also involved came around to James' house. 'We were . . . sitting around chatting, and then all of a sudden [the doctor] said to me, "Okay, let's get this show on the road; now are you sure?" "Yes I'm sure", all that sort of stuff, *because you don't just go in and whack a needle in and pump them full of drugs* . . . they [are] always made aware . . . that they can back out at any time'.

Michelle gave 'what I thought was the final dose', and waited for ten minutes until 'to all intents and purposes he was dead as a doornail'. The doctor left. But a couple of hours later James woke up. Matters were complicated by the arrival of James' family in the next room. It was a 'very, very small house', says Michelle. 'It didn't help with every bloody relative known to man who [James] hadn't seen in ten years rocking up on that very day'.

The family were sitting there 'fighting and carrying on'. There were tears, says Michelle, 'and . . . his niece rocked up, who is a registered nurse—fortunately only college trained and only experienced in geriatrics', and she was 'bawling over me everytime she saw me, you know, it was just dreadful'.

Michelle recalls, laughing, that she told the patient, 'when I get to heaven, I'm going to do it all over again . . . *I'm going to brain you for doing this to me*'.

After James woke up, Michelle rang the doctor, who 'was hysterical, he thought it was so funny'. 'I said "just get your arse around here, get your arse around here right now!"' 'He thought it was character building for me', says Michelle, '[but] I didn't think it was funny at all, because . . . [James] was my friend'.

The doctor arrived a second time, 'gave the appropriate drugs . . . pronounced him dead and signed the certificate and left'. The family was 'absolutely devastated', although the arrival of the doctor was 'a good look', because the family 'thought that he'd just come to . . . pronounce him dead and make sure it was all legal and fine'. Although this experience was '*really awful because I had to deal with all the family shit*', Michelle denied that she carried any baggage from her involvement, asserting that 'I do death well'.

Michelle's terse and crude manner in recounting her experience does little to inspire confidence. More troubling than this, however, is the shadowy role of the doctor. Absent doctors feature in several narratives, attending briefly to inject the patient, before fleeing the scene for personal and legal reasons. In Michelle's narrative, Michelle —a nurse—was the primary actor, injecting the patient, and only calling for 'medical back-up' when the patient woke up. That the doctor should find the 'botch' to be incredibly funny is inexplicable. Michelle's narrative also illustrates another recurrent theme: the practice of euthanasia under the very noses of relatives who have no idea what is taking place.

Precipitative involvements

As noted elsewhere,[7] a frequent precondition to interviewees' willingness to perform euthanasia was a personal knowledge of the patient through a long-lasting professional or personal relationship. That said, there are no rules in the euthanasia underground, and a disturbing theme in some narratives was the complete absence of any meaningful therapeutic relationship between euthaniser and patient. Interviewees reported feeling coerced or cajoled into hastening the death of patients they hardly knew.

Demanding death

Examples of rash or hasty involvement by health professionals often begin with a demanding patient, or demanding friends or family. Amanda, a community nurse, recalls one conversation:

> I was there for maybe an hour and [the patient] actually dismissed me at the end of the hour and said, 'look, this conversation is not getting us anywhere' . . . He said, 'I can't stand this anymore. I want to die and I want somebody to help me to do it and if you're not prepared to do that, then there is no point to the conversation going on'.

Similarly, Josh, a general practitioner, recalls:

> There was a guy who was shopping for a doctor to help assist him to die. He'd been given my name, he . . . put me on the spot . . . I'd never seen him before . . . He was telling all and sundry how we were going to assist him in suicide.

Doctors were resentful of patients who blithely assumed that they would assist in euthanasia. Josh, for example, returned to the incident described above later in interview, complaining about 'this guy that I talked about before who came in and expected almost instant euthanasia; you know, on tap; he was treating us like technicians'. Josh adds, somewhat naively, 'it's very easy for the person who's dying—they're actually not the one that [has] to carry the can at the end of the day. They're not the ones [facing] legal repercussions'.

Reactions like this are not surprising. Expectations of assistance from strangers suggest a reputation for being willing to perform an illegal act. Just as importantly, patient demands for euthanasia disturb the usual power (im)balance between doctor and patient, and deny doctors the opportunity of impressing on patients the need for secrecy. Doctors do not enjoy being treated like 'technicians'.

Gary, a general practitioner, tells of a 'recent' episode where the patient 'rang up and just wanted it done over the phone, basically'. He said 'we've heard you do this, I'm in hospital, I'm leaving tonight, can you come and do it?'

What is surprising, however, is that Gary—a GP with a high public profile, and experienced in HIV care—complied with the request. He went to the patient's home the next day and discussed the situation in the company of the patient's friends, admitting that 'it was difficult to get an appreciation of whether he was depressed or dementing'. Gary also 'had a chat' to one of the hospital physicians 'who seemed to think that death would be a nice thing'.

'I felt I was being pushed, rushed', said Gary. Nevertheless, he went to the patient's home. 'His lover was on the bed with him', Gary recalls, 'I injected him and that was quite quick and pleasant'.

Further information about this episode comes from an interview with a community nurse (referred to in this context as 'Gloria'). Unlike Gary, Gloria's involvement with the case extended over five days, although her role was more limited. 'I was pushed aside', Gloria says, 'I was like the middleman', liaising between the patient, the patient's lover and carers, and then Gary himself. 'It was difficult for the doctor', Gloria says, 'because he'd never met this man in his life before . . . the day of the event'.

Under further questioning, Gloria noted that the patient had 'only told his parents about a week before that he was HIV positive'. It also transpired that a nurse with a psychiatric certificate had been asked to do an 'evaluation', because 'for a minute there even the two people closest to him thought he might have been a bit depressed'. Gloria continues: 'Sunday was a bit iff-y, but by the time Monday came around it was quite apparent, like I said before, that the decision was an informed decision that didn't come from being depressed'.

Despite Gloria's assurances, readers may wonder whether this was not an example of euthanasia upon a depressed and vulnerable patient.

A variation on the theme of providing assistance to relative strangers is given by Joseph, a prominent AIDS physician. 'My hairstylist had a lover who was very sick', says Joseph, 'whose doctor wouldn't prescribe him anything . . . so he could end his life'. Joseph adds that he had followed the lover's disease process 'through the perception of . . . the stylist to the point where . . . [although] I don't like to prescribe things for people that I don't know . . . in this situation I felt rather comfortable doing it'. The hairstylist was 'traumatised' by his lover's deterioration and came to Joseph saying: 'I hate to ask you this but would you mind writing a prescription to help us?' Joseph recalls:

> I wrote a prescription to a patient who I had never seen and I sent it to him in the mail. I heard that next time I went in to . . . get my hair cut that it was the most beautiful experience that my stylist had ever had. It was Valentine's Day and they had a lovely meal with champagne . . . and they held each other and then . . . his partner took his pills and was released.

Joseph admitted that in this case 'there was no assessment involved whatsoever'. Although the lover's death was apparently both gentle and consensual, this account illustrates the complete absence of procedures or 'quality control' in the euthanasia underground.

Where euthanasia is non-consensual, there will, by definition, have been no opportunity for the health care worker to ascertain the patient's wishes accurately, and the doctor may also be vulnerable to pressure from others. In Tim's case, discussed in Chapter 8, a hospital discharged a patient into the care of an inexperienced doctor on a Friday afternoon. The patient had PML, and could neither move nor communicate. The patient's mother asked Tim to 'shorten' her son's life. Tim spent all of Saturday satisfying himself that the mem-

bers of the family were in agreement, before injecting the entire contents of his doctor's bag into the patient on the Sunday morning.

'It was simply me and the family', says Tim. 'I had no way of
communicating with [the patient] so in that sense I didn't have a
clear idea of what he wanted . . . At that point in time *I wasn't . . .
confident enough to approach someone else.*'

Opponents of euthanasia frequently assert that if euthanasia
were legalised, patients would feel coerced into seeking their own
death. In the euthanasia underground, however, there is also evidence
of coercion *upon doctors*, who support voluntary euthanasia in principle, but who lack stable criteria to guide their involvement. In Tim
and Gary's narratives the patients were all but strangers. In both
Gordon's and Zane's narratives friends imposed on the doctor to
'finish the patient off'. In Liz' case (discussed in Chapter 11) a nurse
felt coerced to follow a doctor's order by participating in what she
firmly believes was *involuntary* euthanasia.

Careful screening is surely an essential precondition to rational
euthanasia practice, even if performed illegally. Patients wishing
to die may be depressed, affected by drugs or facing other crises. If
euthanasia were regulated through statutory criteria, wouldn't the
community ultimately be better protected? Wouldn't there be less
scope for coercion upon doctors if there were transparent mechanisms in place through which terminally ill patients could plan
their dying?

'Pre-emptive euthanasia'

One of the challenges for euthanasia advocates, particularly if personal autonomy is the moral value which justifies legalisation, is to
define logical limits for the right to die. In the *Chabot* case,[8] the
Netherlands Supreme Court held that the 'necessity' defence[9] to a
charge of assisted suicide applied in circumstances where the patient
was not terminally ill, had no somatic illness, but was severely
depressed and had refused treatment. Since the terminally ill have
no monopoly on misery, opponents of legalisation are concerned at
the prospect of euthanasia becoming available to the disabled and
the dejected.

It was clear from interviews, and from the subsequent questionnaire, that patients with HIV (but not AIDS), do explore the

option of assisted death with their carers. Table 10-1 is based on the questionnaire responses of 26 interviewees who recorded the factors they saw as motivating the requests of patients with HIV for assisted death. As with Table 5-1 (factors motivating requests by patients with AIDS for assisted death), a wide range of factors are reported. These include current pain, discomfort and existential anguish experienced by the patient (items 3–6, 19–20), fear of dementia and of future disease progression (items 7–15), lack of hope, and depression.

Table 10-1: Factors motivating requests for assistance in dying by patients with HIV (but not AIDS) (as interpreted by interviewees) (n=26)

Factors motivating patients' requests for assistance to die	No. of interviewees who mentioned this factor
1. Strategy for coping now, want to feel in control of life, seeking assurance they will have an 'out' when they want it	7
2. Unbearable pain/discomfort	3
3. Loss of quality of life	2
4. Loss of independence and control	4
5. Can't cope any longer	1
6. 'Had enough', 'over it'	3
7. Fear of the future, of impending symptoms, disease progression, know what the future holds, have seen others suffer and don't want that to happen to them	11
8. Prospect of impending disability, realistic or imagined	1
9. Fear of dementia	4
10. Fear of losing control of bodily functions	1
11. Fear of losing control of life	1
12. Fear of loss of body image, cosmetic issues, 'walking skeletons'	2
13. Want to avoid being a burden	1
14. Don't wish to suffer during the dying process	1

15. Want to avoid seeing others show or try to hide their revulsion at seeing patient in terminal stages	1
16. Lack of hope, HIV seen as a death sentence	2
17. Alone, lack support	1
18. Depression	4
19. Multiple bereavement, friends and lovers have died	1
20. Seeing the suffering of family and friends involved in their care	1
21. Financially destitute	1
22. Personality disorder	1

The interviews revealed some, albeit modest, evidence of euthanasia upon able-bodied patients with HIV, who were clearly distinguished in the questionnaire from patients with AIDS. 'Pre-emptive' euthanasia in AIDS is clearly a matter of concern, in view of the success of protease inhibitors in improving longevity and quality of life. As seen in Table 10-2, several interviewees had prescribed or provided drugs for suicide purposes, although it is difficult to tell whether they were intended for immediate use. 'Stockpiling' lethal medications as an 'insurance policy' is a common practice.

Two interviewees were very clear that they had assisted patients with HIV to die. Peter, a nurse, had administered a lethal overdose (followed by strangulation) on at least one occasion, and claimed to have been involved three times. Jane, a general practitioner, had administered lethal IV drugs to a patient with HIV (but not AIDS) who was 'emotionally, spiritually and psychologically terminal—he was in a state from which no recovery was possible'.

The culture of deception

The practice of illegal euthanasia has spawned a culture of deception. Deceit is all-pervasive: it begins with the methods used to procure drugs; it permeates the planning and orchestration of the death itself; and extends to disposal of the body and associated paperwork. It permeates discussions between medical colleagues.

Table 10-2: Interviewees who assisted patients with HIV (but not AIDS) to die

Nature of assistance	Interviewees involved	Total
Promised to assist patient in future	Nola, GP (no action taken at time of interview)	1
Provided advice on suicide strategies, and/ or where to obtain drugs	Bill, hospice nurse Tony, GP (~5 times, but 'generally attempted to dissuade them')	2
Provided, or prescribed, medication, together with advice.	Damien, medical practitioner ('twice') Russell, hospital physician ('gave small doses of pain pills for later use—twice') Warren, psychotherapist (provided means to suicide ~20 times)	3
Active assistance to die	Peter, nurse (3 times) Jane, GP (once)	2

Obtaining the drugs

Outside of hospital, death is frequently achieved by an overdose of pain-killers or sedatives. Doctors may donate or personally administer these drugs from their doctor's bag or surgery. However, the doses required to achieve death frequently deplete the doctor's stores, and interviewees were aware of the risk of suspicion arising from unusual drug re-ordering patterns.

Analgesics, sedatives and anti-depressants may also be obtained through prescription. General practitioners may write scripts in the knowledge that the patient is hoarding the medication and will later self-administer an overdose. A similar process may occur when the person is an outpatient, or is discharged from hospital with a supply of medication. Tony provides a typical example: 'I wrote out a prescription [morphine and diazepam] which was appropriate to take over let's say a week or two weeks—of course that's not how it was administered!' Or, as Gary said, 'I thought an overdose of an anti-depressant would be best, so in the notes I wrote that he was

depressed and I gave him a prescription of [amitriptyline]—enough
to do the job'. The process is confirmed by Merrill, a physician practising on the other side of the Pacific:

> M   [But] what if, for example, the patient isn't in chronic pain and
> so Demoral [a barbiturate] is not really medically indicated?
>
> Mer . . . probably in that instance *I would develop some chronic
> pain* [very quiet].
>
> M   . . . [so] you're hoping to fudge the system to some extent?
>
> Mer To protect me and the patients.

Building a plausible (if fabricated) basis for prescribing euthanatic drugs is an important means of self-protection. Erin, a community nurse, observed that in his experience 'enlightened doctors'
would fabricate symptoms (e.g., insomnia) as a basis for prescribing
a sedating drug (such as Rohypnol), increasing the dose over time,
before switching to a stronger and 'more suitable' drug (such as
Seconal, a barbiturate).

Difficulties arise, however, when the charting of symptoms depends upon the clinical opinion of someone who won't co-operate.
Mark, a clinical psychologist, advised one patient who wanted to end
his life to tell the visiting nurse that he was suffering intractable pain.
In response, the nurse charted a (very conservative) recommendation
of two and a half milligrams of Valium (diazepam). In the absence of
a plausible chart entry, the patient's physician also felt unable to prescribe the morphine needed for the overdose. Later, Mark informed
the doctor that the patient was intending to kill himself, and requested a prescription of insulin. 'I could tell . . . that it was very
painful to [the doctor]', Mark recalls, 'he said, "you know there's
nothing in the medical chart that justifies [insulin], I just can't do it"'.

As it turned out, Mark found a bottle of potassium chloride in
a linen closet in the hall, and injected the patient with that. 'It
seemed like the only decent thing to do.'

For their part, patients can also become adept at 'conning' prescriptions from doctors who would not knowingly co-operate in a
suicide attempt. In Gordon's narrative, discussed above, the partner
of the young man whose suicide attempt was botched 'did a bit of
doctor shopping' on his lover's behalf. This involved going to a

doctor three times over a six-week period and saying 'I . . . need a repeat of [Tryptanol], I'm depressed and my partner's dying of AIDS'. The prescription was readily supplied. Who would question depression under these circumstances?

John, a funeral director, used a similar strategy, obtaining drugs in one State under different names, and posting them interstate to a friend who used them to suicide.

Several health professionals admitted to the theft of drugs. Martin, a community worker: 'It was stolen, yeah we actually stole [morphine] from the drug cabinet at [names the ward of an inner city hospital]'. Michelle, a community nurse: 'In the . . . first situation I [told you about, I was] the middleman if you like, yeah, like a drug dealer [laughs], yeah, I even um pinched the drugs'.

Not all thefts described in the interviews were for the purpose of euthanasia. Jane, a GP who estimated that she had given lethal injections on 50–60 occasions, admitted to the systematic theft of therapeutic retroviral drugs which at that time were only available to patients enrolled in drug trials:

M   Why was it necessary to steal?
J   Because [the drugs] weren't available at all.
M   They weren't approved by the Government?
J   . . . only in trials . . . We knew that the drugs we had weren't working. I mean a lot of these [new, retroviral] drugs are . . . returned to pharmacies and destroyed . . . I have a real problem with that. So if I had to steal it out of a hospital fridge I actually don't consider that as much of a problem.

The sharing or pooling of prescribed medications is another strategy for amassing a lethal quantity, whether as a 'contingency plan', or for a definite attempt. A couple of interviewees claimed that information and drugs were sourced surreptitiously through Australian State-funded AIDS councils and agencies. In San Francisco similar allegations were made about 'dedicated volunteers' associated with the Hemlock Society. Stanley, a therapist and experienced participant, noted that the final wish of some patients was to donate the drugs left over after their death to 'the underground, to assist other people who cannot or have not been able to 'score', as we say, their drugs'.

The San Francisco interviewees provided interesting speculation into the nature of this 'drugs underground'. One interviewee,
a community nurse, claimed to know the contact details of airline
workers who were prepared to act as couriers, taking a 'shopping
list' to Mexico, where drugs such as Seconal (secobarbital) and
other barbiturates could be obtained without prescription.

On one occasion, the same interviewee ('Bruce') mentioned to
some trusted colleagues that he needed a 'flight to Mexico'. 'People
laughed at the time', said Bruce, adding that not long after, as one of
the nurses was leaving the office, she handed him a note which said
'If you need to go to Mexico, here's the travel agent'. Bruce rang the
number written on the piece of paper, making contact with 'Pat',
a pharmacist who (separately from his pharmacy business) ran a
'drugs re-distribution network'. Pat collected drugs from people
who had died or who had drugs they would not use, and distributed
them to patients who lacked health insurance. Pat also had links
with doctors who would write prescriptions for euthanasia mix-
tures, provided the patient's name and social security number were
supplied. On this occasion Bruce obtained a prescription of Seconal
through Pat, mixed it up in the blender and left it with the patient to
self-administer. The next day he received confirmation that the
patient was dead.

As mentioned in Chapter 9, when a patient is in hospital, nurses
may salvage the 'excess' left in the vial or bottle after the charted
dose has been withdrawn. 'We've all done it', says Marjorie, a community worker and registered nurse. 'You're supposed to [adminis-
ter] a certain amount of morphine and the rest gets chucked out,
well you don't chuck it out—you give it to the [patient] instead'.

Experienced nurses can become skilled at 'conning' larger-than-
required drug orders from junior medical staff. 'Nurses run hospitals, you know', says Chris, a palliative care nurse, 'and one of the
ways they run hospitals is by manipulating medical staff . . . that's
not . . . a new thing . . . though perhaps we're more explicit about it
. . . now'. Chris, who worked in a large, inner city teaching hospital,
went on to explain that junior medical staff were rotated so quickly
through successive specialty units that the only people who 'ever
had any idea of what's going on are the senior nursing staff and the
senior medical staff'. As a result, particularly in the AIDS context,

junior medical staff become 'used to being told by senior nurses what to do'. Chris elaborates:

> Our residents get used to doing what we ask because they are only [on the HIV/AIDS unit] for ten weeks, and most of [the] drugs they've [never] seen before and they'll never see again. So they usually have *no idea at all* about the drugs that they're ordering.

The end result, in Chris' experience, is an environment where junior doctors chart whatever dosages the nurse requests. The dynamic is 'quite complex': you have a new intern who's

> one week out of university . . . he doesn't even know how to page somebody on the telephone . . . The senior medical staff don't care, but the nursing staff have to teach them how to do all of those things, because otherwise the patients suffer and none of the work gets done.

Asked whether he had ever manipulated junior medical staff to obtain drugs to hasten a patient's death, Chris responded, 'yeah, we've done that; yeah, I've done that, and the reason you can get away with it is because . . . they are [so] used to . . . doing what you tell them that they . . . don't necessarily kind of stop and think . . .'. He added, 'some of them do and they're always wrong' [laughing].

A common theme in interview was of patients being discharged from hospital in order to return home to die a pre-arranged, assisted death. Several interviewees had facilitated such a process by donating drugs such as Valium or potassium chloride, which are not locked up in some wards.

Planning and orchestrating the death

How do health care workers orchestrate the death and participate in it, while minimising the risk of being caught? The practice of hospital euthanasia was explored in Chapter 9. The risk of dissent increases with the number of health carers collaborating in hospital care. Individually, health carers may surreptitiously administer the 'excess drug' left in a vial over and above the charted dose. Symptoms may be fudged and noted in the medical record as a pretext for titrating doses of morphine and other drugs to lethal levels. Nurses may adopt hospice terminology, charting that the patient appeared 'changed' on a previous visit, so that the patient's subsequent death appears more 'natural'.

Where the 'euthanaser' holds a senior position, lethal doses may simply be charted and administered by nurses upon doctors' orders. Although wholesale co-operation between doctors and nurses in killing patients may be uncommon, evidence of explicit, and implicit, co-operation between hospital staff was a significant finding of this study. In Zane's case (discussed above), a patient who had bungled a suicide attempt was admitted directly into the care of 'experienced' palliative care nurses, who helped to complete the attempt.

Euthanasia may also occur in hospital without the knowledge of health care workers, although interviews suggest that this rarely works smoothly. In one case, friends of the patient tried to help him die by injecting insulin or morphine into his IV line. In another case, Joseph, an HIV/AIDS specialist, travelled overseas to attend the hospital death-bed of a former lover ('Adam'). The two had parted thirteen years before, and Adam was 'wasted and not at all the person that he used to be'. After embracing Adam, Joseph recalls, 'I said "I'm here, I'm here to take care of you", and a tear came out of his eye'.

Adam's brother had obtained barbiturates from a vet, and while the brother tried to distract the nurse, Joseph hooked up two syringes to Adam's IV line. 'I really screwed up the whole thing royally by pushing . . . the stopcock in the wrong direction', Joseph recalls. The contents of the second syringe spilled over his trousers: 'from the groin all the way down to my knees was soaking wet'.

As Adam's breathing slowed, Joseph 'started squeezing the tubing for the ventilator and that set off an alarm'.

> It was really like a comedy of errors . . . everybody came rushing into the room—all the doctors—and they were going to do resuscitation and I said, 'Please, Stop . . . can't we just take this off?' . . . Finally his doctor arrived. [The doctor was] sort of aware of what was going on and sort of nodded that . . . maybe they should just disconnect the ventilator, and over the next few minutes he just stopped breathing.

The illegality of euthanasia creates an environment in which health carers don't know whom they can trust. Language plays a crucial role in exchanging the information needed to ensure that euthanasia is successfully achieved, behind a veneer of innocence.

Mark, a clinical psychologist, recalled an episode where he contacted a patient's doctor about the patient's strong desire for assistance to die. The doctor replied that he would arrange for a visiting nurse to ring back with the four-digit code which would unlock the slow-release morphine pump connected to the patient, and permit the flow-rate to be re-set. The nurse rang two minutes later, emphasising that ' "You certainly don't want to go over 80 [units per hour]",—which I figured was *exactly the thing to do* [Mark laughs] . . . so I went to 200'.

Language plays a similar role when a doctor is writing a 'lethal prescription', but does not wish to admit to full participation in the patient's plan, or is merely suspicious of the patient's intentions. 'It's almost like they went to school to learn this vocabulary', says Stanley, a therapist:

> Physicians will say: 'here is a prescription for 25 Seconals: *Be sure that you don't abuse this because if you take too many of them you will die!*' So they're covering their arse, of course, but also giving the patient a little wink that they know what's going on.

One hospital physician described this process as 'doing a dance'.

Warren, who was also a therapist, was scathing in his criticism of the way in which euthanasia was 'discussed in the medical world, especially in hospitals'. These are practices which 'everybody knows are occurring, and nobody is willing to acknowledge or take responsibility for [them]'. This leads to 'a whole lot of extremely regrettable and damaging side-effects; people saying they're going to do things and then not doing them, people doing things and saying they didn't do them . . .'.

When euthanasia is performed at home, health care workers will remain permanently at the mercy of friends and family who were aware of the plan or who attended the death. In many cases the only precautions taken are to engage with those present to ensure they are in agreement. Doctors will stress that participation puts them at risk, and that the assisted nature of the death must remain a secret, not only to protect the doctor's career, but so as not to defeat the patient's life insurance policy.

Bob, a general practitioner, provides an example of 'euthanasia by family consensus'. The patient had intentionally been rendered unconscious with drug overdoses, no fluids were administered, and no effort was made to change the patient's position to avoid pneumonia. A hospital physician who was also involved, reassured the family: 'tonight he'll go to sleep, you know, he'll be resting, and *he'll go on his journey*—which was the word that everyone used after that . . . they were all very distraught'.

When the patient lingered on, Bob administered massive doses of morphine to speed up the process. 'Even though [the patient] was asleep and clearly comfortable', Bob recalls, 'I was getting calls saying "he needs another injection"'. The patient's parents were saying things like "Well what have you given him? How long will it be now?" The presence of a priest further added to Bob's discomfort.

Between themselves, Bob and his medical colleagues spoke in blunt terms. Bob reports: 'The patient wanted to be dead and . . . the family . . . agreed and they now wanted him dead as well, and I had been giving him enough medication to achieve that'.

Although they didn't speak like this initially, 'later on it seemed silly to pretend that we were doing anything else'. When speaking to the family, however, 'the metaphors continued and that was largely to protect me, given that there were so many people involved and there were some people who were having doubts'. One of the doubters was the patient's own partner, who wanted to respect his lover's wishes, but whose personal attitude was less clear. 'I am not sure how all the family is going to cope now that he is dead', said Bob, 'and that still concerns me'.

Other interviewees were less concerned at the prospect of dissent within the family of a deceased patient. Gary, a GP, reasoned that 'even if someone did feel like squealing I think the family pressure would make it very hard to do—they'd be *ostracised*'. He gave an example of a case in which the sister of the patient 'was really not pleased with the whole thing at all . . . but mum basically told her: "Shut up! This is what he wanted"'.

A number of interviewees gave uneasy accounts of euthanasia occurring in the bedroom while relatives elsewhere in the house were completely oblivious to it. In Gay and Margaret's accounts of involvement (discussed in Chapter 8), the administration of a drug overdose to Margaret's brother was kept a secret from his parents, whom Margaret felt she could not confide in because of their 'very strong Christian point of view'. Ironically, a couple of days later, Margaret overheard her parents expressing pro-euthanasia views.

In other cases, family members were sent home so that they would be absent at the time of death. Liz reports an episode where a hospital physician sent the patient's mother home and then charted a lethal infusion (see Chapter 11). While the exclusion of relatives from the euthanasia process was usually the patient's wish, it sometimes deprived close family members of the opportunity to say goodbye.

Some 'seasoned participants' had reflected upon the security risks involved with euthanasia, and developed strategies. Stanley, a therapist, had clear parameters for his involvement:

> I always do my homework . . . I make sure that . . . if anyone else is going to be in attendance, that . . . we spend a good deal of time together so that I have a sense [of] where their mind is, that they're not going to freak out, that this will be held in confidence, that they have no moral or ethical or legal issues . . . if there's any loose ends, I don't proceed. If I'm the person who is going to be the active agent, [I make sure I am] not the person who finds the body, I always leave the scene . . . and even if other people are in attendance I would never stay after the person is dead, it's just inappropriate.

Health carers can minimise the risks and stresses of active euthanasia by absenting themselves before the point of death. Patients may also insist that a doctor not be present at the time of death, in order to protect the doctor, who may already have taken a risk by providing or prescribing euthanatic drugs. Bert Keizer, a Dutch physician, notes that the need for secrecy compels the doctor to 'spend more energy trying to cover his [*sic*] tracks than helping the patient die in a decent manner. He will, for instance, avoid being there in person when the patient dies. But his presence is vital at such a difficult time'.[10]

In one incident, Paula, a GP, procured a lethal quantity of potassium chloride from a doctor colleague, drew it up into a syringe, and gave it to the patient and his partner. 'They just gave me the mobile phone and I . . . cruised around [the suburb] for an hour or so until I got the word to come back.' Paula returned to the house to fill out the death certificate.

The wisdom of Keizer's advice is well illustrated, however, by Paula's next account of involvement. Paula had agreed to assist the death of a man who in fact brought forward the date of his death by a week and a day to fit in with Paula's holiday plans! Paula obtained a palatable mixture of phenobarbitone (a barbiturate) from a chemist, and delivered it to the patient, expecting to get a call from the patient's partner during the night to say that he had died.

Instead the telephone call came around lunchtime the following day, a few hours before Paula was scheduled to catch her flight. Annoyed at having to fit an extra trip into her already-crowded schedule, Paula arrived at the patient's house to find four friends, three of whom she had never met before, huddled around the patient's bed. Paula's instructions to lay the body out had been ignored. The patient was curled up with crooked limbs and stiff joints, still wearing his glasses.

Paula emphasised the importance of confidentiality to the four friends, and then had to spend 'the rest of the afternoon trying to find an undertaker'. 'They made *me* organise that', said Teresa, 'which I was quite angry about, because they were sort of seemingly incompetent'. One option was a pauper's funeral, which would have required the police to be notified. Apart from this, the cheapest funeral Paula could find was cremation, at a cost of $1500. In the end the friends 'agreed to cough up' the price of the cremation, and Paula caught her plane.

Some months later Paula read an article in the press, written by one of the four friends, criticising her handling of the death. 'It went for a whole page', Paula recalls; 'I felt quite sick in the stomach. I thought "you bitch, you dog . . . we sat there in this group and . . . it was never going outside of that room, that was the arrangement that we had" '.

The article implied that Paula was incompetent because the patient had taken so long to die, and that the euthanatic drug should have been injected, rather than ingested. 'I really only glanced down the first column but it was more than I could cope with, and then I just felt that everybody in [the city] was reading [the newspaper] and . . . talking about me.'

The absent doctor is only one disturbing feature of this account. A man's time of death is brought forward to suit a doctor's holiday plans. The doctor supplies a lethal concoction, but otherwise leaves it to the patient to ingest. Later she resents the fact that responsibility for disposing of his body has devolved on to her. The dead man lies stiff and contorted on the bed, and no one wants to pay for his funeral.

Whatever the merits of legalised euthanasia, there is surely something to be said for remaining with the patient throughout the whole process. Harvey, a general practitioner who had performed euthanasia a dozen times, adopts an alternative approach:

> My policy is that if I'm going to do it I have to make sure that it's done properly, that's why I stay there [with the patient]. I wouldn't be into giving somebody an injection, and leaving them, waiting for the relative to find them, because that's a disaster if it's unsuccessful, so even though I find it very stressful I would make sure I stay [to ensure] it's done properly.

Disposing of the body

In the usual course of events, the product of illicit euthanasia is a dead body, flooded with lethal levels of drugs, which must be disposed of without arousing suspicion. Recent needle marks present an added risk. Gary explains:

> They don't ooze [blood] very much and the veins collapse after death, so . . . a pin-prick is all you'd see, you wouldn't see a gouge or a bruise, but . . . if someone went over the body with a fine-tooth comb they'd discover it.
>
> M If there is an autopsy, for example?
>
> Yes, that's right. If someone dobbed [a doctor] into the Coroner for some reason, then it would be detected, and that's one of the reasons we . . . don't use barbiturates because they would be easily detectable, we use Valium and morphine because people are often on Valium or morphine anyway, we use potassium [chloride because] when you die the cell walls . . . break down, especially the red blood cells, and potassium is just thrown out everywhere . . . Now, they can probably

do levels and find that they're very high, but probably not . . . It's not an unexpected death, it would require someone to notify the police, [and] that's why [we try] to burn [the deceased] as quickly as possible.

Elsewhere, Gary confirms the need for: 'cremation, cremation, cremation, as soon as possible: burn the evidence!'

Cremation was a recurrent theme in the interviews. Josh, who used a barbiturate as his drug of choice, admitted: 'Of course, the great worry here is toxicology'. Hardly surprisingly, Josh 'insists' on the patient being cremated. John, a funeral director, told of one case where the patient had told 'just about everybody' that he was planning euthanasia: 'who the doctor was going to be, and who was going to be there'. 'I thought if ever the shit was going to hit the fan, it would be that day', said John. 'It wasn't until the coffin was actually in the cremator that I breathed easily [laughs]. I thought [laugh] here goes the evidence . . . now there is no evidence, thank you very much!'

Peter, a nurse, describes the 'window period' between death and cremation in similar terms:

After death, prior to cremation, anyone can ask the question and the Coroner can intervene [to] test the body . . . for drugs, and then find out that they were killed, and then there's questions asked, and then you can be charged . . . *You sit in sweat waiting for cremation to occur* . . . All of the people you speak to, if they're being honest, will say the same thing, *we're all waiting for the smoke to go up in the crematorium.*

If the patient has previously advertised the time and manner of their death, this adds dramatically to the stress health carers feel during the 'window period'. In another case involving John, the patient 'rang everyone that he knew' from his hospital bed and said 'I'll be dead tomorrow'. Hardly surprisingly, hospital authorities refused to discharge him, and in fact organised a psychiatric evaluation. 'They tried to talk him into palliative [care]', said John, 'so he played the game with them and settled down and didn't mention it'. A few days later the patient was discharged, and euthanasia occurred as planned, although the funeral was 'brought forward very quickly' and was a much smaller affair than the deceased had originally planned.

Lying on the death certificate and cremation forms is a necessary part of post-euthanasia practice. The following exchange with Josh, a general practitioner, was typical:

M   You signed the death certificate?

J   Yes.

M   What did you put . . . as the cause of death?

J   Well I certainly didn't put 'Lethabarb' as the cause of death [laughter]. I am forced to lie. I said that he [died] of AIDS and disseminated Kaposi's Sarcoma . . . The cremation certificate [also asks] questions like 'do you know [if] there could have been any foul play? Could this death have resulted from poisoning?' and I have to lie there . . . I mean, you've got to protect yourself.

Typically, the doctors interviewed in this study recorded the patient's most recent AIDS-related infection or cancer as the cause of death. 'If you look at someone who's died of AIDS . . . there's no doubt in your mind about the cause of death', says Mark. 'I mean, just the physical appearance of the body: I don't think Coroners want to do autopsies on people who have AIDS, I think they're afraid of them, I mean they can cut themselves while they're doing an autopsy and get HIV.' Michelle, a community nurse, was even more cavalier. 'Once you put HIV and AIDS [on the death certificate], they don't care . . . they're so *stupid*'.

Several interviewees were dismissive and even contemptuous of the possibility of police investigation. Asked whether she feared prosecution, Jane, a GP, responded 'Go for it, go for it, everybody! Good luck!' Another said:

I can't imagine the Office of Public Prosecutions getting extraordinarily excited about somebody who was going to die in four or five days time. It's possible, but it would be a nightmare to try . . . you [would] get half a dozen conflicting stories: 'Yes, the doctor was there'; 'No, he wasn't'; 'Yes, he gave an injection'; 'No, he didn't'. None of the stories would tally and it would be extraordinarily difficult to make sense of it.

The role played by John, a funeral director, in assisting AIDS euthanasia within one city was detailed in Chapter 9. In John's

State, when a deceased is to be cremated, the doctor who signed the death certificate must also fill out a cremation application form. Furthermore, a second registered medical practitioner is required to examine the body, and to confirm that—having made inquiries— there are no suspicious circumstances. John estimated that on half the occasions he needed a cremation form counter-signed, he used a 'sympathetic' doctor who was part of the euthanasia 'network'. The doctor would fill out the form, no questions asked, without viewing the body. 'I'll just whiz up [with the documentation], and he [the counter-signing doctor] . . . just signs it and away we go', said John, adding that 'he knows what's gone on anyway, because the network works quite well'.

Another interviewee confirmed this process, noting that John used 'doctors who we also know—gay doctors' to counter-sign the certificate, and that they 'don't look too close'.

On the other occasions John needed a cremation form counter-signed, he used a 'regular' doctor whose surgery was located near John's mortuary. While this presented the theoretical possibility that the doctor might discover signs of a euthanasia death, John took comfort in the fact that 'the odd needle mark on the arm is not going to worry anybody', since people with AIDS have frequently lived with an IV infusion before death.

Deception permeates every aspect of illicit euthanasia practice. By all accounts, health care workers are remarkably accomplished in their deception. Deceptive practices contribute to the *invisibility* of euthanasia, and help to perpetuate the myth that because euthanasia is prohibited, it never occurs.

Illegal euthanasia illustrates dramatically what we might call 'medical anti-professionalism'; that is, an absence of appropriate training, an absence of oversight, an absence of accountability, and an absence of principles guiding involvement. Unlike therapeutic medical procedures, which are carried out within an organisational, and intellectual, framework, euthanasia is carried out informally, in an idiosyncratic environment largely lacking in norms or controls.

A further dimension of medical professionalism, apart from training, monitoring, and accountability, revolves around the notion of 'disinterested service': the patient-centred ethic. The following chapter explores how this dimension of medical professionalism has also become degraded in the euthanasia underground.

11

More disturbing issues

Do I believe that you can have legal euthanasia without any abuses? No. Do I believe you can have legal euthanasia without more abuses than we already have? Yes.

Peter Singer, bioethicist[1]

The disturbing issues presented in this chapter and in Chapter 10 reflect the relative absence, within the euthanasia underground, of those characteristics which make up the notion of 'medical professionalism'. Chapter 10 focused on the relative absence of an intellectual framework and organised context for euthanasia. We turn now to another dimension of 'anti-professionalism', exploring how the patient-centred ethic, and the notion of 'disinterested service' that is characteristic of medical professionalism, have been undermined and corrupted in the euthanasia underground. As a result, we see evidence of:

* non-consensual euthanasia;
* a lack of professional distance by persons performing euthanasia;
* the 'cowboy syndrome', as evidenced in cavalier speech, attitudes, and actions; and
* burn-out.

As noted previously, these issues cut both ways. One view is that the onus is now on opponents of euthanasia to demonstrate (if they can) how patients are better protected under the current policy of prohibition than they would be if euthanasia were flushed out into the open and regulated in an explicit way. Another view is that prohibitionism is still the best policy, but that more should be done to track down and punish the offenders. A third view is that there are, in fact, benefits in having euthanasia remain 'symbolically' illegal, provided that this does not inhibit doctors from following their conscience in 'hard cases'. As discussed in Chapter 6, this option is favoured by some activist doctors themselves, who recoil at the prospect of new legislation or guidelines impinging upon their clinical judgment.

It is the uneasy hypocrisy inherent in the third view which invites the most vigorous response. Accountability is the foundation of an ethical profession. While I do not question the sincerity or compassion of those who participate in euthanasia, the *judgment* of participants certainly invites harsh criticism.

Euthanasia without consent

Past the door marked 'the terminally ill' are an endless number of other doors—the chronically ill, the demented, the crippled, the deformed, the chronically depressed, the terminally sad, the heartbroken, the hopeless, the unloved, the lonely, the simpletons, the economically unviable. Not to mention the passageway leading to the doors marked 'infants and children'.

Michael Gawenda[2]

The argument is commonly made that if voluntary euthanasia were legalised, it would lead to a 'subtle transformation of ethical sensibility',[3] and eventually, to a dramatic increase in non-consensual killing. Bernadette Tobin warns that euthanasia legislation would 'certainly over time embolden doctors to act on ascribed "autonomous wishes", that is to say, on "what the patient would have wanted if only he [or she] were able to tell us" '.[4]

In the form that it is usually put, the 'slippery slope' is really only a half-argument because it fails to factor in the existence of the euthanasia underground that *already* exists. Opponents of legalisation tend to play down or ignore the euthanasia underground precisely because it devalues the 'benefits' of a prohibitionist euthanasia policy. Some may feel that illicit killing is the price society pays for doing the 'right thing', or that it is just deserts for those arrogant enough to flout 'God's law'. The uncomfortable truth is that the law's ban on euthanasia merely drives it underground, thereby creating the conditions for a culture of 'anti-professionalism'.

While voluntary euthanasia was the dominant form of euthanasia practised by interviewees, there were admissions of non-consensual and even involuntary euthanasia. This is clearly a matter of concern. But the underlying issue remains: if euthanasia (including non-consensual euthanasia) is already happening, then what has prohibition accomplished? We are forced to re-evaluate our assumptions about how law can best protect the vulnerable, while minimising suffering.

A number of interviewees expressed views in favour of non-consensual euthanasia, usually making indirect appeals to perceptions of common decency and compassion:

> I had a demented aunt. She was demented for seven or eight years, in a nursing home, virtually catatonic . . . I went out there with my partner to visit her . . . She's sitting in a chair with a table up front of her, and every so often she would fall forward and hit the bridge of her nose on the edge of the table, and they had taped a piece of foam rubber [on it to protect her]. My partner looked at me and he said: 'you know, we wouldn't treat urchin cats and dogs like this, we would put them out of their misery; the whole place, just warehoused with people like this . . .'

While most of us would fear the prospect of ever becoming Mark's aunt, a policy of compassionate, non-consensual euthanasia is an alarming response, as the interviews confirm.

Non-consensual euthanasia

In a number of anecdotes, interviewees performed euthanasia on a patient whose desire to die at the time of euthanasia was *unknown*. I refer to these as *non-consensual* euthanasia deaths. In some cases the patient was mentally incompetent, and euthanasia was carried out at the family's request. In other cases, although the patient had apparently expressed a desire to die to a third party (e.g. a family member), the interviewee obtained no independent evidence of this before hastening the patient's death. Examples of non-consensual euthanasia emerge from the discussion of 'precipitative involvements' in Chapter 10, and elsewhere throughout this book.

One very unusual attempt at non-consensual euthanasia involves Anne, a counsellor in the Jungian tradition. Anne recalled a former client who had 'talked very actively about suicide', prior to disclosing his AIDS status to his family, who were thereafter 'extremely supportive'. The patient's deterioration was 'particularly slow' and painful to watch. After his admission to hospital, the patient continued to choose vigorous drug therapy. Eventually this was withdrawn, but the patient took a 'very, very long time to die: day after day after day after day'.

Finally, Anne got a desperate message asking whether she could do anything to hasten his death. Readers may or may not regard Anne's actions as a contributing factor to the death, although they do illustrate the 'arbitrary quality' of the timing of death (see Chapter 6).

'We assembled around his bed at two o'clock', recalls Anne.

> He was only semi-conscious. I spoke very loudly and I said that it was me, Anne, that we were around his bed, that we were going to say goodbye to him and we were going to encourage him to 'cross over' . . . I was amazed [at] the courage of his family, his partner broke down and wept, and said 'I'm saying goodbye, you must now move on, because I am going back to the farm to look after the goats; the goats are running wild and I need to get back to the farm and so this is my goodbye'.

> The mother did likewise . . . she said goodbye very clearly . . . that it was time that he moved on, that he journeyed on. The father—this was very difficult for the father—he said exactly the same . . . so in each case we said our goodbyes [although] we didn't choose the word 'die'.

Anne then directed the members of the family to sit in the room at the end of the patient's bed so that he didn't die alone, 'but there was to be no further communication with him, they weren't to touch him, and he died a couple of hours after that'.

At this point in the interview, Anne wept silently, composed herself, and added, 'the family was at great peace; I was a wreck. I think it was a form of euthanasia, I didn't use medicine [but] I took on a power [crying] I did it with great humility . . . at the request of the family'.

Involuntary euthanasia

For all its grey edges, non-consensual euthanasia is a world away from cases where the patient has not only *not* requested death, but *evidenced a desire to go on living*. Two interviewees gave detailed reports that fall into this category.

The first account involved Harry, a general practitioner, who in conjunction with a hospital physician, had been looking after a wealthy patient with AIDS. The patient's boyfriend, a nurse, was also the sole beneficiary of the patient's estate, following a late change to the patient's will. After the patient's discharge from hospital, Harry visited him at home and noticed that he was receiving an 'extremely high dose' of morphine (several hundred milligrams) through a syringe driver.

By one o'clock the next day the patient was dead. There were allegations that the boyfriend had overdosed his partner because 'he wanted the money'. A former boyfriend 'claimed to this day that it was a murder'. The police investigated and Harry was interviewed, although he told police that he had 'no evidence whatever' to confirm this allegation. Harry neglected to inform the police about the high dose of medication administered to his patient, faltering somewhat during interview and stating that 'it wasn't outrageous . . . it wasn't . . . a lethal dose'.

The second account was very much more detailed. Liz, a hospital nurse, made discreet arrangements to be interviewed in a department store coffee shop. Her whole interview was confessorial in nature, and revolved around a patient she had nursed in a specialist AIDS ward in a city hospital. The patient 'had about a hundred T-cells', so he 'wasn't close to the end of his life', although he had slowly lost control of his bodily functions, required a catheter, and could no longer move his arms. The patient also had neurological problems: a number of scans, lumbar punctures and other tests had been carried out.

Throughout the period of his admission, the patient's mother had stayed with him, washing him and feeding him. 'This man was determined to live', said Liz, 'he was determined to get better, but the physician . . . didn't . . . see it this way . . . It got to the point that one Thursday, the physician . . . came into the unit and said, "This has got to stop, send mum home to have a shower" '.

'Once mum had left the ward', said Liz, the physician charted an infusion of midazolam, morphine and Tegratol (carbamazepine) 'designed to kill' the patient. According to Liz, the physicians's words were 'get it up and get him out of here by sundown'.

Feeding the patient breakfast earlier that morning, Liz recalled that he had said, 'Hey, do they know what's wrong? When am I going home?' 'It was obvious to me that he wanted to go home', said Liz. 'He wanted us to make him better, he didn't want to die . . . it was like the physician had found that he couldn't solve the problem *so there was only one way out of the problem.*'

Liz approached two registrars who were working on the unit. ' "What are we doing to this man?" ' she asked. ' "We're *killing him*" ', and they said: ' "no, it's come to the point that he's going to die, and if we don't step in he's going to have a very bad death. He's going to fit" '. 'And I thought they knew something magical', said Liz, 'that he'd reached a certain point and [that] all HIV patients fit before they die'.

Liz admitted that at the time of this incident she was not an experienced nurse and had not been nursing on that unit for long.

> I actually went out to the ladies, and I was sitting there and I was crying and I was thinking 'what can I do?' I wanted to run down to . . . the Director of Nursing, but I thought, my God, if I do that, this is going to open up a hornet's nest and I was frightened . . . It makes me so angry because I . . . wasn't strong enough to say 'Hey, I'm not doing this, absolutely not' . . . I just felt like I was on my own . . . they couldn't see what it was . . . it was *murder.*

Liz made it clear during the interview that euthanasia had occurred on other occasions in the unit but 'always . . . with the patient's consent'. Indeed, this physician's willingness to participate in euthanasia was confirmed by another interviewee, who spoke of him in glowing terms. On this occasion, however, it was—in Liz' words—'definitely without the patient's consent, [there was] no discussion . . . with the patient's family; it was done in a situation when the family was sent away . . .'.

The lethal infusion was drawn up by Liz and another nurse. The patient had 'two or three' infusions running already, because 'we were treating him with many different drugs, so [the family] didn't really notice that another bag was there'. Since the patient was comfortable, Liz ran the infusion very slowly, turning it down as the patient became 'increasingly drowsy'.

Later, the physician walked into the room just as the patient moved his hand a little. 'That's focal fitting', said the physician, 'turn it up'. During interview, Liz vehemently disagreed with this assessment. 'It wasn't focal fitting, there is *no way* . . . but instead of upsetting the family . . . I turned it up . . . [but] when he left I turned it back down again.'

Liz' shift ended at 1 o'clock that afternoon. The nurse on afternoon shift 'had long been involved in this sort of thing and they just turned the infusion up'.

The patient died nine hours later, and his bed was vacant the next day.

> M So we're talking about an organised, orchestrated attempt to kill a patient involving at least a couple of nurses, a couple of registrars and a senior physician?
>
> L Yes.
>
> M And this was an instance where it happened without the patient's consent?
>
> L Yes.
>
> M . . . Sometimes . . . palliative care nurses or physicians [will] talk about . . . increasing the doses [of medication] when a patient is [within a few hours of death] . . . And they [also] talk about the principle of double effect—the drugs shorten life but they're also therapeutic . . . You're not confusing this situation . . .?
>
> L Oh, no no way [indignant].
>
> M This is totally different?
>
> L Absolutely . . . I know what this is, I said what it was, it wasn't therapeutic at all.

Under continued questioning it became clear that Liz' objection to the whole process was not based on any deep religious or ethical opposition to euthanasia *per se*. As discussed in Chapter 9, Liz alleged that the unit where she worked accepted patients who had 'booked in' to receive a lethal infusion of drugs, and Liz had willingly participated in voluntary euthanasia on prior occasions.

What upset Liz about this incident, however, was that the patient—who may have been mentally incompetent anyway—*evidently wanted to go on living*. Furthermore, the patient's mother was kept completely in the dark about the physician's intentions. 'He had a little dog and, you know, that was his life, he lived with his mum . . . he didn't want to die, no way at all'. 'They were such a close family . . . just working class people . . . they just thought . . . this doctor knows what he's doing . . .'.

'I just feel I let them down', Liz explains; 'he may have died in another week . . . another month . . . but [it] was enough for the family just to [sit] there with him, it's all they wanted'.

Liz saves her strongest criticism for the physician, who has since moved on from that unit. 'The doctor played God, *he thought he was God . . . he'd decided this was the time for this patient.*'

> L I used to say to the Registrar [who was also involved in this inci-
>   dent] 'I'll see you in Hell' . . . I really think that's where we're off
>   to: me and my friend [another nurse who was also upset by this
>   incident] . . . the physician, and the registrar.
> M You don't seriously think that?
> L Oh, I used to, I don't know if I do anymore, as I said . . . I sort of
>   block it off, I don't want to think about it.

It is difficult to evaluate Liz' story. She was an inexperienced nurse disagreeing with the assessment of an experienced physician. It's not hard to imagine how the physician, drawing upon long experience and deep reserves of medical chauvinism, might demolish this nurse's testimony.

On the other hand, the interactions between the various players were hardly compatible with palliative care. Liz had nursed the patient intensively before his death: he was young, his body was not 'wasted', and 'we were able to control his pain quite easily with oral medication'.

The charge of involuntary euthanasia is all the more worrying, coming from a nurse who had no misgivings about participating in voluntary euthanasia. What comes across most strongly in interview is her sense of isolation and bewilderment: 'it was like I was the only person there that could see clearly what was happening', she said. 'It was murder.'

Conflicts of interest

Some may regard the killing of one's patient as inherently in conflict with the role of a doctor or nurse. The issue of remuneration for euthanasia services, however, provides an added dimension. One Australian doctor volunteered in interview that he didn't 'get paid lots of money for bumping [patients] off', but conceded that he treated euthanasia as a 'long consultation', and received payment under the Medicare scheme. 'It usually takes a while by the time I . . . talk to [the patient] about it, do it, write the death certificate, talk to family and friends, ring up the funeral director—*it can be a couple of hours out of a day.*' By contrast, another Australian doctor referred to euthanasia as 'a non-Medicare rebateable aspect of medical care'.

One American interviewee, after recovering from the shock of being asked, agreed that he charged *up to but not including* the 'last visit', adding, somewhat indignantly:

> But you know what? . . . As I said to you, most of these people are my friends and I would have done it [anyway] . . . it's not a question of 'well, Gee, what's in it for me?' I mean, what's in it for me is the *honour* of being present, it's much more than money can buy.

Ogden, reporting on a private conference of right to die activists in Seattle in November 1999, notes that payment for services was a topic of 'guarded discussion' by participants. Some 'deathing practitioners provide their services for free, while others accept donations "up to several thousand dollars" '.[5]

There was no evidence in the present study that interviewees benefited financially to any appreciable degree from their involvement in euthanasia. It might readily be argued, however, that to receive remuneration for supplying euthanasia services places doctors in a position of conflict of interest, particularly when the process is illegal and surreptitious, with doctors acquiring reputations and accepting 'referrals'.

Others may argue that to treat euthanasia as a medical procedure, deserving of time and professional attention, would improve the quality of the process, and ensure that death was swift and gentle. This aim might best be achieved by treating euthanasia as a legitimate (if stringently regulated) medical procedure, rather than as an ad hoc favour.

If medical practitioners can have a financial interest in euthanasia, then so can funeral directors. There seems little doubt that John's openness to assisted death and his capacity to dispose of bodies without attracting attention carried with it the financial advantages of being 'undertaker of choice' among key participants in the AIDS euthanasia network in one city. On the other hand, while John may have derived a modest income from euthanasia deaths, all funeral directors ultimately make their living from death and it does little justice to the man who was interviewed to characterise him as a ruthless 'profiteer'.

More worrying perceptions arise from John's admission (discussed in Chapter 9) that he was the primary actor in at least four deaths, and in one case, having given a lethal injection, proceeded to take the body away *in his capacity as a funeral director*. Even here, though, one should remember that John's direct involvements were immensely personal occasions involving close friends. It is unknown whether he in fact rendered an account on any of these occasions. On the basis of impressions gained in interview, it would be grossly inaccurate to characterise him as offering a 'one-stop shop': death and burial at a discount price! Even so, lurid interpretations such as this illustrate the perceptions that euthanasia advocates invite upon themselves when participation in euthanasia is not strictly quarantined from business activities.

The 'cowboy syndrome': cavalier speech and attitudes

Euthanasia is a strange business. For the most part, interviewees spoke with compassion and conviction, and their testimony was genuinely moving. Sometimes, however, the brazen language, flippant attitudes, and seeming lack of emotion of some respondents, were quietly sobering.

Death need not necessarily be sombre and humourless, and indeed, the practice of celebrating a person's life with a pre-death 'wake' (see Chapter 7), challenges the myth of death as a solemn event. Nevertheless, the cumulative impact of the language chosen by a small number of interviewees undermines perceptions of their professionalism and integrity. Some comments, flippant in tone, are probably best regarded as examples of the interviewee 'showing off' in interview. Michelle, for example, describes her patient as 'this gorgeous gorgeous gorgeous human being', enthusing that 'the needle went in and the drugs went in and he was dead in five minutes and it was all *absolutely gorgeous*'. Later in interview, she asserts smugly, 'I do death well'.

Sometimes the odd slip of the tongue lends an inappropriately theatrical flavour to the euthanasia scenario. '*At high noon*', says Gary, 'I just went around [there and] . . . I just injected him'. On another occasion Gary describes his arrival at a patient's home to perform euthanasia in the following terms:

> He'd [had] sex [the] morning that we finished him off . . . he met me
> at the door and gave me a kiss and invited me in and said, 'Oh well,
> let's get on with it', and then marched off. I mean, that was difficult,
> in a sense.

Later in the interview, however, Gary admitted that performing euthanasia 'does get easier with time'.

A common belief shared by 'revisionists' in this study is that the quality of a person's life is more important than longevity. Speaking of the practice of giving pain relief to terminally ill patients, Stephen, a nurse, said, 'a couple of hours, a couple of weeks or a couple of months extra, that's the dividing line and . . . it doesn't make that much difference'. Similarly, speaking of the moral dilemma that arises when a dementing, possibly incompetent patient expresses the wish to die, Gary surmises, 'I suppose it depends on the degree of dementia, but if we're talking of a matter of days or weeks, [it] hardly seems to matter'. He adds: 'I can't imagine the Office of Public Prosecutions getting extraordinarily excited about somebody who was going to die in four or five days time, you know'.

Attitudes such as these overlook the fact that time of death *does* matter. A precipitative death can rob patients and their loved ones of opportunities for achieving a sense of completion, expressing love, giving blessings, and saying goodbye.

Of the many comments and anecdotes that left us unsettled, it is difficult to choose which one 'takes the cake'. Was it Gordon, who admitted that one reason why he tried to 'finish off' a depressed patient after a botched suicide was that fact that he had flu, 'felt dreadful and . . . just wanted to get out of there?' Or was it Paula, whose patient was forced to bring his death forward to fit in with her Christmas travel plans, and who was resentful of the interruption on the day of her departure occasioned by the need to organise the funeral? Was it Michelle, naively rejoicing in a successful procedure? Or Chris, who describes his feelings on hearing that his father had started breathing again (despite being overdosed with morphine and pethidine): 'fuck, when is this man going to die?'

Burn-out, and lack of professional distance

Unlike cancer, the burden of the AIDS epidemic has focused on a relatively small population of health care workers. One interviewee estimated that the care of patients with AIDS in the general practice setting in inner Sydney was focused on a couple of dozen doctors who had 'specialised' in AIDS care and were known to have an interest in it.

For those with high HIV case loads, the stresses of practice are magnified by the higher proportion of very ill patients, the frequency with which suicide talk arises, and the need to respond to it. If one adds to that the stresses of involvement in illicit euthanasia, then the potential for burn-out, impaired judgment and lack of professional detachment become immediately apparent. Richard, a 'traditionalist' interviewee who disapproved of euthanasia (see Chapter 6), saw the seeds of these problems in the tendency for participants to put their perceived duty to patients above their duty to themselves. To avoid depression and burn-out, doctors need to become more sophisticated in policing the boundary between professional commitment and personal involvement: 'one's duty is initially to oneself, otherwise it's very hard to be a good practitioner'.

The personal cost of involvement in illegal euthanasia was a central theme in interviews, and one emphasised throughout this book. 'I hate it', says one doctor, 'my partner hates it, because [she] knows that I'm going to be really horrible to be around . . . afterwards'. Another emphasised the 'emotionally demanding and draining' nature of involvement, adding, 'there's only a finite amount of times you can do it' and 'I think I've almost reached the expiry date'. These are typical comments.

On the other hand, a number of interviewees admitted that stress levels do decline as one gains experience in euthanasia. One hospice nurse, who could no longer estimate the number of times he had assisted a euthanasia death, reflected that while he 'unloaded a lot in the beginning', it was less of an emotional burden now, because he felt his intentions were compassionate. 'I feel very comfortable', said one hospital physician. 'I have no problems sleeping at night.'

Several community-based interviewees felt the same way. 'I'm fairly much at comfort with myself and my conscience', said one. 'It's not one of [those issues where] I'm overwhelmed and have layers of guilt'. 'It does get easier with the time', adds another GP. 'After doing several . . . You get over it quicker'. The same doctor notes: 'I suppose that could be an argument for the thin edge of the wedge . . . that . . . maybe now it's just a short leap to me actually *enjoying this*, but I think that's going a bit far'.

Stanley, a therapist with a long history of involvement, claimed that 'I've never been burned out in this business . . . because I think death is a natural thing'. In his experience, the people who tend to suffer burn-out are those who 'think that death is unnatural', who are trying to 'avert [it] at all costs'. In Stanley's experience, 'dying people are a joy to be around'; it is the survivors who 'tend to be completely fucked up'.

Despite these comments, a significant theme in interviews was the pain and stress of participation in assisted death. As noted in the previous chapter, stress levels are amplified even more when the euthanasia procedure is botched. Peter, a community nurse, remarks:

P You've got to resort to some other form of, you know, bringing death on, and . . . it's very very hard to do.

M Such as?

P Strangulation, or suffocation.

M Which must be extremely stressful to you?

P   . . . I don't think you ever get rid of it. There may be people you've spoken to who will comfortably say [that they are] all-together about it; I know them in a different light, and I know that they all carry lots of sadness and lots of stuff inside them about what's happened.

As a key player in the 'euthanasia underground' in one city, Peter is in a unique position to know what he is talking about. Warren, a therapist, is similarly well placed:

They're working too hard, the level of burn-out among gay doctors is colossal, they've had to resort, I think, to a kind of 'clan-ishness' and a kind of brotherhood . . . which feels good until you realise how much of an exclusive world they've had to construct for themselves.

Warren goes on to mention the 'guilt and personal blame, exposure to blackmail, [doctors'] inability to discuss [the issue] with their own lovers . . . which is, I think, an enormous strain'.

A final factor which ratchets up stress levels is the fact that doctors and nurses are frequently killing their friends. While the distinction is at times a rubbery one, each first-hand account of involvement in assisted death was categorised according to whether the euthaniser admitted to acting in a 'personal' capacity, to assist a lover or friend to die, or whether their involvement was 'professional', in the sense that the interviewee was providing a 'medical service' to a pre-existing or a new patient. As shown by Table 11-1, in nearly a third of cases (29.6 per cent), the interviewee was acting in a 'personal', as distinct from 'professional' capacity. Typically, on

Table 11-1: 'Professional' vs 'personal' involvement in 88 first-hand accounts of involvement in PAS/AVE

	HIV/AIDS anecdotes (n=75)	Non-HIV/AIDS anecdotes (n=13)
Interviewee involved in a 'professional' capacity	55	7
Interviewee involved in a 'personal' capacity	20	6

these occasions, interviewees were assisting in the death of friends, lovers and former lovers.

The risks of burn-out demonstrate the need for greater levels of institutional and personal support for health care workers (see Chapter 6). We should not forget, however, the potentially detrimental consequences for patients themselves. For those already active in the euthanasia arena, there is the risk that burn-out and mental stress will cause health carers to subtly favour the euthanasia option out of their own need not to witness further patient suffering.[6] This risk is magnified in the euthanasia underground, where any independent assessment of whether the patient is competent, depressed, demented or vulnerable is purely optional.

Disturbing issues 'above-ground'

This chapter has focused on some disturbing themes that emerge from the euthanasia 'underground'. One should not assume, however, that legitimate, 'above-ground' care is without its own share of disturbing issues. Two themes stand out from the interviews. The first is the cruel indifference some health care workers display towards the pain and distress of patients. Such cruelty fuels the euthanasia movement. Seeing instances of inadequate care played a critical role in the development of pro-euthanasia attitudes in some interviewees. The second issue, already mentioned in Chapter 6, but worth re-emphasising, is the degradation of 'amateur' suicide.

Mark, a clinical psychologist, tells of a patient ('Ben'), whose partner had died naturally at home. Mark attended the home, and was present while Ben attempted to report his partner's death. The Coroner's office was closed, and the police, the hospital and everyone else all advised Ben to call '000'. Ben eventually did this, explaining that there was no emergency, and that his partner had died in his sleep four hours ago.

'Ten minutes later a fire truck, police car, a paramedic unit all come screeching out in front of the house', recalls Mark. There were 'four or five firemen all dressed up in thick rubber boots and yellow rubber coats and fire hats . . . carrying boxes of medical equipment'. They came 'bursting into the house'. Ben had a durable power of attorney for his partner which contained a signed 'do not resuscitate' order. Despite protestations, the medics 'attached all kinds of medical equipment to him, gave him oxygen . . . heart paddles, the whole business'.

'*The corpse was cold*', explained Mark, 'but they were convinced that they would be liable if they didn't attempt resuscitation'. It is not difficult to imagine how incidents like this breed contempt for the standards (and standard-bearers) of orthodox medicine.

John, the funeral director, has featured prominently in this book, and it is worth recounting a painful episode he told at the very end of his interview. John was, at this time, working as a nurse on night duty in an oncology ward, tending a man in his late seventies who had cancer and diabetes. 'Because [of] his diabetes', John explains, 'he had gangrene'. The patient had been given pethidine so that he could withstand the pain of changing the dressing on his toe. While this was being done, however, the patient's big toe on his right foot 'literally fell off into the dressing'.

The man was in great pain, and John rang the registrar to request more pain killers. The registrar refused. John says, 'I told him he was a cruel mongrel and that he really should get over to the ward [to] check the patient out [and] perhaps he'd change his mind'. 'I ended up getting the nursing supervisor to get him to come out of the quarters to check the patient out.'

In the end, the registrar ('a little smart-arse registrar full of his own importance and [with] no compassion') still refused to chart a higher dose of pain killers. John recalls that 'his excuse was: "I'm a Christian—if I give this man any more drugs we will be killing him and *you don't understand that, nurse*" '.

'I just thought then that it was one of the cruellest things I've ever seen happen', John says, 'from a profession supposedly there to help people, but they've gotten their help mixed up with the prolonging of life'. 'That's where I first formed my opinions of things', says John.

This is not a unique story. Other interviewees shared similar stories of pain, medical indifference and clinical disrespect. 'How cruel and uncaring we can become in the name of life', says Kyle, a family physician, sharing a similar story, post-interview, of how his mother died.

If inadequate care, particularly pain relief, generates pro-euthanasia attitudes, so does the reality of 'amateur' suicide. Nearly 17 per cent of the anecdotes recounted by interviewees in this study

concerned suicide. Terri, an experienced palliative care nurse, wrote
to the interviewer post-interview to report on a terminally ill patient
with AIDS who discharged himself from hospital, took an overdose
of Warfarin (an anti-blood-clotting agent), and slit his wrists in the
bath. The attempt failed. The patient was rushed to hospital. His
wrists were stitched and he was sent off to a specialist AIDS ward.
Although he received counselling, the patient considered that he had
no quality of life. He wanted to die, and his family supported him
in this.

Following his discharge from hospital, the patient enjoyed a
meal and drinks with his family. 'They laughed, talked, and remi-
nisced together.' Then the patient told his mother, father, sister and
brother to go for a walk with the dog. They were told that he would
be dead when they returned. While they were away, the patient
jumped out of the window of his high-rise flat.

According to Terri, this successful 'splatter suicide' came about
because the doctors who had been asked to assist the patient to die
had refused, for legal reasons. Some readers will see in this kind
of incident the justification for a legalised euthanasia regime, as a
response to human desperation. Others will see, perhaps, a need for
counselling, or better palliative care, but little more. In the writer's
view, 'amateur' suicide is a social reality likely to be at least partly
influenced by the relative availability of euthanasia. It is a disturbing
issues that must be factored into the debate.

Implications of the disturbing issues

The disturbing issues presented in this chapter and the preceding
one are not, as some would suggest, the work of a freakish fringe, of
pariahs and outsiders, ill-trained rookies and medical school failures.
In large part, the admissions featured here are the secrets of respected
and experienced professionals, the media-savvy, the specialist edu-
cators, published researchers with national reputations. They are
issues from the heartland of HIV/AIDS medicine, and not some
insignificant and easily excisable part of it.

Evidence that there is a euthanasia underground, and of what
goes on within it, adds important new dimensions to the euthanasia
debate. Foremost, it challenges the assumption that the legal prohib-

ition on euthanasia is working. In reality, prohibition neither effectively inhibits the practice of euthanasia, nor adequately protects the vulnerable patients who most desire it. Regrettably, the informal criteria supplied by the conscience of the doctor or nurse involved are not an adequate screening mechanism.

Advocates of legalisation, for their part, can take little comfort from the issues canvassed in these chapters. These are, after all, the stories of those *who most support euthanasia practice*. Some are on the verge of burn-out, some talk like cowboys, and some actively oppose legalisation because it would cramp their style. If nothing else, the disturbing features of euthanasia practice cry out for a regulatory response. But where will it come from? From the police, who in many jurisdictions, with some justification, have avoided stomping, jack-boot style, over issues of such moral and personal complexity? From professional medical bodies, whose level of engagement with these issue rarely reaches beyond the occasional 'symposium' in a medical journal? From politicians, running scared from the torrent of letters unleashed by the mainstream churches?

The difficult issues do not end with questioning law's prohibition of euthanasia, or doctors' acquiescence in its *ad hoc* practice within the 'medical brotherhood'. The social harm of the 'euthanasia underground' must also be balanced against the risks of abuse under a legalised regime. It would be naive to suppose that a legalised regime would do away entirely with demand for illicit euthanasia in cases not satisfying statutory criteria. Any legalised euthanasia regime will also carry its own share of risks, as opponents of legalisation are swift to point to (and inflate).

Both advocates and opponents of assisted death care about dignity at the end of life. The challenge for opponents, however, is to show how the law's prohibition of voluntary assisted death remains the best policy, despite evidence of underground euthanasia within a culture characterised by the lack of medical professionalism.

12

De-mystifying
euthanasia practice

I think the reality is we've got to accept it's happening . . . it is
happening quite widely [at] different levels, [in] different ways.
We've got to accept that its occurring, [we've got to] pull our
head out of the sand . . . start talking about it amongst each other.

Peter, community nurse

We can't have an informed debate about euthanasia policy until we
de-mystify the social practices that surround end-of-life decision-
making. In many ways, we have had an impoverished euthanasia
debate. Beginning with the Remmelink Report in the Netherlands,[1]
there have been a number of studies quantifying the practice of
assisted death. These have led to heated debate about statistics, and
speculation about 'slippery slopes'. For their part, the media have
depicted a polarised and ideologically-driven divide between militant advocates and uncompromising opponents of legalisation. The
popular debate over euthanasia policy has focused disproportionately upon one set of actors (namely, doctors), and there has been
insufficient discussion of 'bedside issues' by those familiar with the
personal dynamics of terminal care.

The themes and issues presented in this book provide powerful
arguments both for and against a policy of legalisation. The purpose

of this chapter, rather than taking sides and producing yet another manifesto, is to emphasise the tensions evident in the interview data, and to draw out their importance to the euthanasia debate. In particular, I will be drawing together the most salient themes from previous chapters and interrogating some taken-for-granted assumptions and misconceptions about euthanasia practice. Ultimately, a 'de-mystified' perspective on euthanasia is one which acknowledges the complex, multi-faceted and highly personalised context within which end-of-life decisions are made.

Who's dying, and why?

A recurrent argument favoured by opponents of euthanasia legislation is that the legalisation of assisted death will prompt a subtle shift that leads insidiously towards the non-voluntary euthanasia of the elderly.[2] In Australia this fear was well caricatured by placards carried by demonstrators at various points during the debate, bearing messages such as 'Euthanazia: No Thanks!'[3] The assumption that the 'target group' for euthanasia is decrepit or geriatric patients, who lack the vitality to adequately represent or assert their own interests, is not true of AIDS euthanasia, and has led to some important aspects of euthanasia practice being overlooked.

The interviews revealed episodes of euthanasia involving patients who ranged from late teens to middle age. Euthanasia is not simply an issue about geriatric care. It is an issue faced by the dying of all ages, all of whom share an interest in a decent demise. A frequent comment made by interviewees was that patients with AIDS are young, articulate, politically aware and keen to maintain control over their disease process. 'The HIV/AIDS community has really changed the face of death', said one, because 'they're young and they want to take control of their lives'.

Several important consequences follow from this. The first is the horror of 'botched attempts'. 'Disease-ridden young boys with AIDS' are, in the words of one community nurse, 'very hard to kill'. The human spirit is resilient: overdoses of analgesics or opiates frequently fail. Experienced nurses and doctors may feel driven to resort to suffocation, strangulation.

In AIDS euthanasia, voluntary choice is a very strong and re-current theme. On the one hand, interviewees reported that by not ruling out euthanasia as an option, they were better able to explore and alleviate the issues of fear and loss of control that were frequent motivations for euthanasia. A more sobering theme, however, was that a minority of patients may not wait until they become decrepit or debilitated before seeking euthanasia assistance. Evidence of 'pre-emptive' assisted suicide and euthanasia by those with HIV but not AIDS hardly qualifies as an expression of empowerment and raises serious concerns: about the quality of available health care, the criteria which 'trigger' illicit involvement, and the real motivations behind requests for assistance.

The interview data highlight the risks of taking euthanasia requests at face value. Suicide talk and euthanasia requests are com-plex messages. The interviews with nurses, in particular, illustrate how euthanasia talk may distract health carers from the real issues the patient is confronting.

Pain management is a hotly contested site within the euthanasia debate. Voluntary euthanasia draws strongest emotional support when marketed by advocates of legalisation as a merciful act of last resort for intolerable pain and suffering.[4] The focus on pain by advo-cates enables them to avoid the sense of unease many would feel if euthanasia were to become more widely available for reasons un-related to pain. Conversely, if euthanasia is (largely) about merciful relief from pain, then opponents are free to ignore the wider issues of dignity, autonomy, control and existential exhaustion. The focus on pain permits opponents of legalisation to medicalise the debate (by directing attention to technical expertise and palliative care), and also to foreclose it (by insisting that pain can be resolved, using the latest palliative care techniques).

Unresolved pain was an important theme motivating patient euthanasia requests (see Chapter 5). But pain is a slippery concept, and perceptions of pain are frequently a melange of emotional, spiri-tual, social as well as physical factors. Pain may be exacerbated by the anguish of family disagreements, fractured relationships, unre-solved sexuality, and disclosure issues. Perhaps rarely, euthanasia talk may become a platform for acting out one's anger towards others.[5] While intolerable pain is a 'respectable reason' for desiring euthanasia, few would regard euthanasia as an appropriate way to resolve these other issues.

But pain and suffering are not the only factors generating demand for euthanasia. An extraordinarily wide variety of other issues may also be implicated (see Chapter 5). Frequently, suicide talk is a metaphor for regaining a sense of control over life; an insurance policy rather than a cemented intention. Requests may reflect the patient's fear of further deterioration or particular symptoms, rather than their present experience (see Table 5-1). Some patients are depressed, and some may indeed have a treatable depression. Interviewees spoke of patients who, following treatment for depression, experienced further life that was meaningful and fulfilling. Assessing a patient's mental status is important when a patient requests euthanasia. But this may be extraordinarily difficult when patients are on heavy sedation, in pain and distress, or suffering organic conditions that mimic depression.

Neurological complications are increasingly common in AIDS, and fear of future dementia, or insight into the dementing process, was the 'last straw' for some patients. One interviewee reported urgent requests from a patient who was becoming progressively more demented, who begged her, 'help save me from playing with my shit'. Where the patient's capacity for an autonomous choice is in doubt, health carers are understandably cautious to assist, despite the cavalier opinion of one interviewee who stated that 'if we're talking of a matter of days or weeks, [it] hardly seems to matter'.

A subtle and disturbing issue which emerged from some interviews was that patients may, perhaps rarely, feel 'locked into' honouring a publicly-uttered decision to die, made to friends or family, even when they later change their mind. There were examples in interview of patients 'fitting in' with the travel plans of the euthanising doctor, or of relatives, in planning their death. It would be naive to assume that a patient's desire to die will never be influenced by factors that are extraneous to the patient's condition. Health care workers may project their own sense of horror and repulsion, in subtle ways, on to the patient, thereby reinforcing patients' sense of futility. This raises difficult issues. Being a sounding-board, and providing 'emotional accompaniment' are a part of care-giving, and these benefits could hardly come from an emotionally remote carer. But risks may arise when care workers are themselves burned out, or fail to recognise the fragility of their patients and the extent of their influence over them.

Euthanasia requests cannot be disassociated from the patient's individual circumstances: the 'bedside context'. Participants in assisted death realise this, as the integrity of their connection with the patient is often the ultimate justification for illicit assistance. There is a desperate need for more research which explores the personal dynamics and nuances of bedside care, drawing on nursing and palliative care perspectives in particular. Advocates of assisted death assume that it is possible to distinguish between euthanasia requests that are a mis-expression of an underlying, unresolved need, and those that reflect a personal philosophy or choice, despite optimal care. The stakes are high. Interviewees gave examples of patients who had earlier demanded euthanasia but who then went on to find meaning through the natural dying process. Similarly, there were examples of patients who had contemplated suicide, or survived the attempt, but who valued the life they went on to live. The enemy, in the end, is a simplistic view.

This catalogue of concerns must make frustrating reading for those who see euthanasia as a simple issue of patient choice, and cannot understand all the fuss about 'patient safeguards'. Stanley, a therapist, says: 'I believe in self-determination: some people are going to mess up, some people are going to make mistakes . . . but . . . I'd rather err on [the side of self-determination]'. For some, safeguards are an obstacle to patient autonomy, an invitation for 'compassionate totalitarians' to dominate weak and frail patients at the very time they most need to have their autonomy respected. On the other hand, while interviewees were alive to the risks and ambiguities of euthanasia requests, it is significant that they did not regard all such requests as misplaced or inappropriate. Many of those who explored the subtleties and complexity of euthanasia talk in most depth had also participated in episodes of assisted death.

Some important challenges emerge from interviewees' exploration of euthanasia talk. Firstly, an extraordinarily wide variety of factors do, in fact, motivate patients to explore assisted death as an option. These data challenge assumptions about what are the conventionally-accepted 'good' reasons for euthanasia intervention;

for example, a terminally ill patient suffering intolerable pain and suffering. They also force us to consider whether there can be any logical basis for limiting euthanatic intervention to patients with a terminal illness. The terminally ill, even those with AIDS, do not, after all, have a monopoly on suffering.

Secondly, given that the meaning of a euthanasia request is so deeply bedded to individual life circumstances, a further challenge arises over how to accurately assess and confirm whether the patient is requesting assistance for the 'right' reasons, in such a complex environment. In view of the complexity and ambiguity of euthanasia talk, the onus really rests on euthanasia advocates to show how a legislative protocol could adequately take account of the difficulties nurses and other care givers identify. The Northern Territory's *Rights of the Terminally Ill Act*, for example, embodied the assessment that euthanasia is a permissible choice for terminally ill patients who are experiencing pain, suffering or distress to an extent unacceptable to them, where no reasonable treatment (other than palliative care) is available. A statutory protocol was embodied in the Act to confirm these elements and to exclude depression.[6] The stricter the process for screening out wrong reasons, however, the more difficult it becomes for patients to have their 'right' reasons vindicated.

The design of any 'safe' euthanasia regime creates a sharp conflict between the 'hands off' and the 'hands on' camps, between those reluctant to dictate how doctors should exercise their professional skills, and those in favour of supervision and oversight. The spectre of a swat team of lawyers, ethicists, psychiatrists and general do-gooders descending on the patient in a paternalistic frenzy to second-guess the patient's decision fills many with horror. On the other hand, is it safe to leave it up to the individual doctor or nurse? What record do health care workers have in assessing when it is appropriate to intervene?

Who's killing, and why?

The voices of medical practitioners have largely dominated the euthanasia debate in Australia, and probably elsewhere. Doctors' opinions are regarded as pivotal, as reflected in a succession of Australian and American studies showing significant levels of involvement in assisted suicide and/or euthanasia, as well as a comprehensive fragmentation of attitudes towards the ethics of involvement, and the question of legalisation (see Tables 3-1, 3-2).

Our study certainly confirms the involvement of doctors in assisted death, including general practitioners, hospital physicians, psychiatrists and palliative care specialists. But nurses are also implicated, both in community and hospital settings, in collaboration with, and independently of, doctors. The interview sample also included counsellors, psychologists and community workers, whose involvement in assisted suicide and euthanasia matched or exceeded in some cases that of doctors, and who performed a role not dissimilar to community-based nurses. Their voices are rarely heard in the euthanasia debate.

A recurrent theme in interviews was that the law's prohibition of assisted suicide and euthanasia inhibits free discussion of end-of-life decision-making generally, and assisted death in particular. Interviewees are afraid to talk, they feel 'very, very isolated'. In a typical comment, Bill, a hospice nurse, observes: 'you can't talk about it openly . . . it's too dangerous to talk about'.

Important consequences follow from this. Firstly, when health care workers do attempt to educate their patients or colleagues about drug strategies, or co-opt their colleagues to assist, everything is couched in double-speak. Information about gentle and effective euthanasia strategies is poorly transmitted: every participant becomes a pioneer. Misled by myths about 'successful' drug strategies, and hampered by difficulties in accessing appropriate quantities of drug, health workers 'botch' the euthanasia process, over and over again. Secondly, the culture of silence is also reflected in a complete absence of stable criteria for involvement in assisted death. There is no discussion, no consensus: assistance is provided for widely varying and idiosyncratic reasons.

Thirdly, this 'conspiracy of silence' (as one interviewee termed it), is a significant stressor for those who do choose to participate in assisted death. Emotional exhaustion and burn-out further jeopardise the intuitive assessment process that health care workers rely upon. Fourthly, the absence of uninhibited discussion and genuine dialogue means that euthanasia remains hidden from public view. To research it, you need anonymous surveys, interviews camou-

flaged with pseudonyms and guarantees of confidentiality. Researchers themselves face ethical dilemmas, and even prosecution.[7]
The resulting knowledge vacuum perpetuates the gaping chasm
between community assumptions about end-of-life care, and the
truth of the matter.

Health care worker involvement in assisted death spans a broad
range of actions. These include referral and informal assessment of
patients, prescribing, providing, stealing and administering drug
cocktails, directing the euthanasia procedure, and concealing evidence. A variety of euthanasia strategies exist, including sudden overdoses, the gradual escalation of drugs to lethal levels, and the sudden
withdrawal of the medicines or technology required to sustain life.

The disturbing practices described in previous chapters illustrate the absence of those attributes that make up the notion of
'medical professionalism'. The culture of silence spawned by the
illicit nature of euthanasia results in a culture of trial and error, of
backyard or 'coat-hanger euthanasia'.[8] The assessment process was
at times pitifully inadequate, or non-existent. Interviewees admitted
to assisting the deaths of people with whom they had no prior therapeutic relationship: people they had never met, or met only on the
day of the death. The interviews document examples of able-bodied
HIV patients who were assisted to die, examples of non-consensual
euthanasia, and allegations of involuntary euthanasia. The interview
with John, a funeral director, illustrates in forensic detail the blatant
subversion of the legal processes attending death.

The practice of euthanasia is concealed and protected by an all-
pervasive culture of deception. In hospital it is a culture characterised
by the manipulation of ward procedures, fudged symptoms and
double-speak. Less visibly, death is hastened through a combination
of heavy sedation and denial of fluids. In the community it is a
culture also characterised by fudged patient symptoms, deliberately
ambiguous language, the mis-prescription or theft of drugs, and by
false declarations on death certificates.

In presenting evidence of illicit euthanasia practice, I do not
suggest that every episode of assisted death was, by definition, disturbing. In many cases, patients were reported to have died a gentle
and peaceful death in circumstances where all concerned felt that

this was appropriate. Even so, there are no processes for examining the wisdom of involvement. Patients are utterly dependent on the personal values and integrity of the health care worker.

End-of-life decision-making is characterised by a wide variety of attitudes and practices, as illustrated by our three categories: 'traditionalist', 'conservative' and 'revisionist'. These categories build upon each respondent's moral attitudes, level of involvement, attitudes towards legalisation and perceptions of the professional role (see Chapter 6). Revisionist interviewees were vocal advocates for euthanasia who had re-imagined their professional role to include, in appropriate circumstances, killing. While revisionists represent the clearest challenge to current professional and legal norms, a significant number did not support legalisation. This dichotomy suggests interesting possibilities for further quantitative research.

Conservative interviewees, by contrast, have little invested in the euthanasia debate and are essentially 'advocates for life'. An important finding, however, was that a conservative ethos does not necessarily preclude involvement in assisted death. Survey studies may under-estimate the true levels of involvement in assisted death, especially where conservatives 'quarantine' involvement to their personal, as distinct from professional, lives.

Ambivalence was an important theme emerging from this study: feelings of ambivalence experienced both by those who had participated in assisted death, and those who had not. Some interviewees were haunted and scarred by their involvement. More alarmingly, perhaps, certain of the 'revisionists' had adjusted better and were unable to recall the many occasions they had assisted patients to die.

Investigating illegal euthanasia

In this book I have attempted to showcase the possibilities of a qualitative, interview-based approach to researching illicit euthanasia practices. AIDS provides an appropriate context for such a study. As even the staunchest opponents of euthanasia acknowledge,[9] AIDS generates misery and degradation the equal of any other disease in living memory. It is the disease that most justifies euthanasia in the public mind and, not surprisingly, is a major site of euthanasia practice.

Interview-based investigations are intensive and time consuming, placing obvious limitations upon the number of HIV/AIDS carers interviewed in each city. Nevertheless, there was evidence of euthanasia in each city where interviews were conducted. In Sydney, Melbourne and San Francisco, there was evidence of an informal chain of associations facilitating the organisation and provision of euthanasia services. Collaboration was evident in the way patients were referred to euthanasia-friendly doctors, in the way drugs were obtained, in bedside procedures, de-briefing, and concealment of evidence. The backbone of this underground network was community-based nurses and doctors, whose relationships with each other were strengthened by shared HIV specialisation, and/or involvement in the gay community. There are important opportunities for future research into the extent and nature of collaborative euthanasia practice, including the participation of the funeral industry in discreetly cremating evidence of assisted death.

One possible response to the claims made in this book is that they reflect 'AIDS exceptionalism'. The interviewees were all urban health professionals with a significant HIV/AIDS focus. It is possible that the politically activist ideologies or ethical frameworks of the interviewees meant that they were more likely to approve of euthanasia, and to participate in it, than health care workers generally. More generally, it may be true that those who work in AIDS receive more frequent requests for euthanasia, develop more intense relationships with their patients over a longer period of time, or feel a special sense of kinship with HIV patients by virtue of shared gay identity.[10] Survey research certainly suggests disproportionately high rates of involvement among AIDS physicians.[11] But it also demonstrates significant levels of involvement across the board (see Chapter 3).

At the very least, the interview findings substantiate the reality of illicit euthanasia by those working in HIV/AIDS medicine. The existence of a relatively tight community of AIDS-specialised health care workers also assists in drawing attention to the network of associations that characterise the euthanasia underground. Whether these social relations are unique to AIDS, or are evident elsewhere, is a question that deserves further study.

The picture of euthanasia that emerges from the present study is one of complexity that cannot be captured by generalisations. A focus on aged and mentally vulnerable patients assists opponents of assisted death in arguing the risks of a 'slippery slope' if euthanasia is legalised. In AIDS, however, we see a demand for assisted death in patients who are in the prime of their lives. The importance this group places upon maintaining control over the disease process has had an important impact on euthanasia practice. On the one hand, while the presence of a 'euthanasia escape route' may comfort some patients, 'botched' attempts, and 'pre-emptive' euthanasia must also be recognised and factored into the policy debate.

The popular debate about euthanasia tends to focus on pain control. Interview research, however, shows that euthanasia requests are complex messages. Pain is but one of many factors motivating the desire to die. The conflicts over euthanasia are unlikely to be resolved by new analgesics, or multidisciplinary techniques. Furthermore, euthanasia talk illustrates the risks of a simplistic libertarian response.

The popular debate also assumes that euthanasia is an issue of what doctors should and should not do. The interviews confirm, however, that doctors are but one of a variety of professional groups heavily involved. The euthanasia underground is not the exclusive preserve of the 'medical fraternity'. The assumption that, in the absence of legalised channels, euthanasia will default to the wisdom and supervision of doctors is utterly fallacious.

The attitudes and practices of euthanasia participants are complex. There is no simple dichotomy between those who practise euthanasia and wish to legalise it and those who don't. Many (but not all) participants have mixed feelings about their involvement; ambivalence and anguish are common. Some seasoned participants oppose legalisation for fear it will undermine their clinical prerogative.

Popular discourse superficialises euthanasia as either 'ultimate abandonment' or 'merciful release'. The interviews, however, depict a more complex landscape: a place where individuals triumph over disease by regaining control of their final moments and where patients dehumanised by suffering ultimately find meaning and peace. But it is also a realm where intentions go unscrutinised, where ends justify means, and where lack of knowledge results in primitive killing. Judged on our data, activist doctors, nurses, therapists and community workers receive a mixed report card. In the absence of regulation, they are the high priests and priestesses of the back-rooms, mixing an incomplete and hidden body of knowledge with good intentions and periodic recklessness.

13

Euthanasia policy:
hard questions,
hard consequences

*Every time I wake up there is that horrible feeling. But now it's
more bearable as I remember your promise, 'I will help you'. I
only have to hold on for a short while. Just another few days. But
then I think about you: how terribly you'll be judged and perhaps
sentenced for what you did for me.*

*For me all is finished now. It makes me happy in a special
way: a sad way but peaceful at the same time. And in one way or
another it feels like pure justice. I am empty now, all is finished.
Long ago I used to watch telly with my boys. Each night 'Pipo-
the-clown' was on. And each night Pipo said what I am saying
now: 'Goodbye flowers, bye birds, bye fish, goodbye people'.*

Letter from Mrs B. to Dr Chabot, September 1991[1]

The euthanasia debate is bitter and controversial because both
sides have important points to make. People value the right to make
decisions about their own bodies. When it comes to their dying, they
want their death to keep faith with the way they have lived.[2] As
Justice Brennan of the US Supreme Court pointed out in the
Cruzan decision: 'Dying is personal. And it is profound. For many,
the thought of an ignoble end, steeped in decay, is abhorrent. A
quiet, proud death, bodily integrity intact, is a matter of extreme
consequence'.[3]

260

But people are also concerned about the consequences of a society that reaches out to embrace death. They fear that a 'subtle transformation of ethical sensibility'[4] will occur and that, in so many gradual and indirect ways, we will begin to push the dying, the sick, the vulnerable and unproductive towards death, instead of grappling with the more difficult (and costly) challenges of palliative care and human anguish.

This book provides ammunition for both advocates and opponents of a legalised euthanasia regime. One can argue that the interviews are a grim testimony of what happens when health care workers arrogate to themselves the right to kill patients. On the other hand, AIDS illustrates the reality of the suffering that creates the demand for euthanasia services, and shows how that demand is being met in a largely haphazard way in an unregulated environment. In this way it plays into the hands of those who argue that prohibition has failed, and that patients are best protected by making euthanasia visible, and conditionally permissible.

Slippery slopes and consequences

While there are many arguments against euthanasia, for policy makers the consequences of any legal intervention are of central concern. John Keown, a well-known English critic of the Dutch model, warns of the 'slippery slope' effects of decriminalising voluntary euthanasia. He argues: 'non-voluntary euthanasia is now widely practised and increasingly condoned in the Netherlands. For inhabitants of such a flat country, the Dutch have proved remarkably fast skiers'.[5] Pollard and Winton, while acknowledging the limitations of palliative care in controlling emotional anguish which is unrelated to pain, assert that:

> If a law were to allow the subjective concept of emotional distress as grounds for killing, it would be open to inevitable, uncontrollable, and probably undetectable abuse . . . Killing the failures of medical or social care would be negative in that it would not contribute to finding solutions to their problems.[6]

According to these and similar 'slippery slope' arguments, euthanasia is an alarming policy response to suffering and illness, which both celebrates failure and invites abuse.

The risk of a 'slippery slope' deserves serious attention. Never-theless, it remains to be demonstrated.[7] As yet there is no empirical foundation for the claim that the Dutch policy of conditional decrimi-nalisation has resulted in a higher percentage of assisted deaths than in largely prohibitionist countries like Australia or the United States, less still that legalisation causes higher rates of non-consensual eutha-nasia.[8] About the only thing that is clear, as Griffiths points out, is that more is known about euthanasia in the Netherlands than in other countries.[9] All too frequently, Dutch practice has been used as ammunition for domestic debates, by commentators starved of the data required to draw any real comparison between euthanasia rates in the Netherlands and in prohibitionist countries.[10] According to Griffiths, Bood and Weyers:

> Those who invoke the hoary metaphor [of the slippery slope] to criti-cise Dutch legal developments rely on local taboos in their own coun-tries *as if they described actual practice* and contrast such a mythical situation with the actual empirical data that exist for the Netherlands. Meanwhile, the Dutch are busy trying to take practical steps to bring a number of socially dangerous medical practices that exist every-where under a regime of effective control.[11]

The reality of AIDS euthanasia should caution us against reck-less claims that a policy of decriminalisation (as in the Netherlands) *causes higher* rates of euthanasia, especially non-consensual, or in-voluntary euthanasia. Alarming things happen in Australia, San Francisco, and other places too. The difference may well turn out to be that legalisation merely makes euthanasia *visible*. We may even find that disturbing practices, including 'botched attempts', strangu-lations, and the practice of euthanasia in the absence of any prior relationship between doctor and patient, are disproportionately evi-dent in countries where euthanasia is more difficult to access, and where it defaults to an invisible 'underground'. There are important opportunities for future research here, although not, perhaps, if one's mind is already made up.

Critics of the Dutch should also remember that intentional killing already lies latent within English, Australian and American law, obscured only by ignoring the inevitable consequences of doctors' actions when life-sustaining treatment is withdrawn, or when life-shortening analgesics are administered (see Chapter 4). Slippery slopes, therefore, are a particularly precarious form of analysis.

All the same, the euthanasia policy dilemma does require us to weigh the potential for the abuse of sick and vulnerable patients, in an environment where the law permits assisted death, against the current indignities that result from unrelieved suffering (the absence of euthanasia) and illicit euthanasia. In considering this equation, we should not ignore the social ramifications of legalisation. As Elaine Thompson emphasises, euthanasia laws will change norms and behaviour. They will change values; it is foolish to think that they will have no impact on our thinking about the dying process.[12]

The interview data collected in this study have challenged my own views on euthanasia. Early on in the study, shocked by graphic descriptions of 'botched attempts', I favoured the view that legalisation is a conservative policy response which calls to account those members of the health professions who practise euthanasia. The unfettered discretion of doctors and nurses is a starkly inadequate model for assisted death. The euthanasia underground provides no framework to guide the illicit involvement of 'revisionists', and none of the accountability that a statutory protocol would aim to provide. Legalisation, on the other hand, recognises the demand for illicit assistance and aims to provide a safety valve. It seeks to subject euthanasia to the rule of law, and to integrate protective procedures into euthanasia practice.

All of this may, of course, be quite wrong. Even so, the portrait of illicit euthanasia presented in this book casts a new onus on opponents of legalisation to demonstrate why, and how, the policy of prohibition best secures the shared goal of dignity at the end of life.

Euthanasia policy is not a choice between having no euthanasia and making euthanasia legal. It is a choice between driving it underground, and seeking to make it visible. Euthanasia is a 'pretty sleazy business at present', remarks Philip Nitschke. 'It's a matter of who you know.'[13] Opponents of legalisation must respond, therefore, to the policy challenge the euthanasia underground represents.

Five responses to the euthanasia underground

Attack (or ignore) the messenger

For some, it will be tempting to attack the methodology of this study, and similar studies, the truthfulness of interviewee reports, to claim that data were exaggerated, the wrong questions were asked, or that answers were misunderstood. There are precedents for this. In Australia, opponents have accused euthanasia advocates of 'irresponsibly worrying patients' with 'suburban myths' about euthanasia,[14] or attacked funding bodies for funding 'ideologically motivated' research.[15] Evidence of illicit euthanasia does, after all, undermine the logic of the argument that we are necessarily better off banning euthanasia. Ogden writes that 'there are enormous difficulties in designing adequate research on euthanasia. It is a lesser challenge to criticize the research conducted by others or to construct a hypothetical argument than it is to design and conduct superior studies'.[16]

More realistically, those whose minds are irrevocably made up may prefer to bury studies like this in silence (despite the considerable ammunition the interview data provide them). We might call this the 'ostrich' approach to euthanasia policy. It was well evident in the Australian Senate's hearings into the *Euthanasia Laws Act*, which overturned the Northern Territory euthanasia legislation.[17]

Death is confronting, and euthanasia is doubly confronting because it is also about killing. It violates our moral intuitions, which are, after all, based on an ethic which has served us well by prohibiting intentional killing. But if killing is always wrong, and if euthanasia policy can never be informed by consequences, then it is very difficult to have a debate at all. Nothing about illicit euthanasia will ever shock or unsettle us enough to think that maybe we would be wise to consider new ways of regulating it.

Good reasons for doing nothing?

Another response to evidence of underground euthanasia practices comes from Kevin Andrews, the Australian politician who introduced the *Euthanasia Laws Act* into federal Parliament. In his second reading speech to the Senate, Andrews said:

> One of the arguments is that it is happening already, so we should regulate it. This is like saying that some people will obtain high powered automatic guns, so we should regulate, not ban them. If a

person is willing to disregard a law which says lethal injections are never allowed, why would they be constrained by a law which says lethal injections are sometimes allowed? If some doctors are prepared to take the law into their own hands and reject the clear requirements for knowledge and consent, why would they change their attitude, especially when dealing with an incompetent patient?[18]

Andrews' response draws attention to an important theme in the data. As discussed in Chapter 6, fully one third of the thirty 're-visionist' health care workers interviewed were cool towards the prospect of legalisation because it represented a potential imposition upon clinical decision-making. This mind-set was well illustrated by Gary, a general practitioner, who gave six detailed examples of his involvement in interview. Speaking of regulation, Gary says: 'It should be in [the] hands of doctors—provided they have discussed it with another doctor and it is a reasonable thing to do and it is reported to a Coroner as euthanasia'. Significantly, Gary resists the suggestion that there should be any psychiatric evaluation, saying, 'I don't want anyone else involved'. It is not surprising that interviewees like Gary were enthusiastic about Dutch euthanasia policy, which leaves the assessment of whether a patient comes within the criteria for euthanasia largely up to the treating doctor.

If euthanasia were legalised, it is simply unknown whether the humbug of any resulting statutory protocol would prompt some to continue to provide illicit assistance in 'appropriate' cases that fell outside the legislative protocol. Illicit involvement is stressful, and outcomes are uncertain. A legislative protocol would provide a system of norms according to which doctors could justify their conduct, a platform for accessing gentle yet effective euthanatic drugs, and a legal shelter from the risks and burdens of illicit involvement. These advantages would undoubtedly be evident to participating doctors. Ultimately, however, the extent to which legalisation removes the incentives for participating in illicit euthanasia is an empirical question which could only be evaluated after euthanasia is legalised.

A different reason for favouring the current prohibition on euthanasia comes from Tony Abbott, another Australian parliamentarian who featured prominently in the debate over the Northern Territory's euthanasia law. Abbott asks:

How can the law improve what is currently left to the compassion and good sense of doctors, patients and families? Supporters and opponents alike must regard the first government approved killing since the end of capital punishment as an awful milestone in Australia's history because—for better or worse—men are walking where angels justly fear to tread.[19]

There is a greasy ambiguity in this statement. Is Abbott unaware that doctors *do* play God? Or is he suggesting that informal killing by doctors is fine, provided that we don't acknowledge it openly or attempt to regulate it? 'We might call this the Bendan Nelson argument', writes Peter Singer, 'after the former President of the Australian Medical Association who, while staunchly opposing any change in the law to allow doctors to assist patients to die, has said that in his own medical practice he intentionally ended the lives of terminally ill patients, and was right to do so'.[20]

We should not belittle the integrity of the relationships physicians forge over time with their patients. When doctors practise euthanasia, this usually acts as a crucial safeguard. But not always. Patients also need protection from the inexperience, enthusiasm and occasional recklessness of their carers. Gary, for example, typifies those doctors who believe that euthanasia should be legalised but with minimal external controls. He has been a vocal and articulate participant in the euthanasia debate. Yet even he admitted in interview to participating in the assisted death of a person he had not met before the event (see Chapter 10).

In medicine, as elsewhere, the law must respond to social need. Sometimes it *should meddle*. Arguing this obviously puts me on a collision course with those whose supremacist view of their clinical prerogative leaves little room for patient safeguards.

Prosecute the offenders!

Disquiet with the haphazard deaths that patients currently subject themselves to in the euthanasia underground may prompt some to favour a third option: to track down, prosecute, convict and punish those doctors and nurses who kill. A former Governor of Victoria observes: 'As the law stands, only the good sense of prosecuting authorities and juries stands between compassionate and courageous medical practitioners and convictions for murder'.[21]

To prosecute doctors, however, would also split the alliance between the churches and the medical conservatives, who together constitute the front line of resistance to legalising euthanasia. Criminal investigations and prosecutions would have extremely negative flow-on effects for patients. If euthanasia is to be 'stamped out', there would need to be a more muscular and intrusive policing of drug-prescribing and administration practices by doctors. In the resulting climate of fear and suspicion, it is not hard to imagine how doctors and nurses would be more reluctant to give adequate pain relief for fear of attracting attention to themselves.

Although advocated by some,[22] prosecutors are, in general, reluctant to punish health care workers who do not flaunt their involvement.[23] One has only to look at the extreme lengths Jack Kevorkian had to go to in order to become a martyr for the cause! Butch, a hospice physician, summarised the situation astutely in interview, saying that the authorities 'really don't want to get involved in this, they know that at some level [euthanasia] is happening', but 'it's a no-win situation to prosecute', unless there has been some 'extreme violation'. Quite apart from this, the discreet nature of the relationships which make up euthanasia networks suggest that it would be impossible to purge the health professions of those who participate in assisted death.[24]

Prosecuting rogue doctors is perhaps the most honest policy response for genuine opponents of euthanasia. But apart from the odd show trial, it is unrealistic. In the meantime, the law is held up to contempt.

In the absence of prosecutions, euthanasia advocates have resorted to a range of tactics to keep the issue in the public mind. In Australia, Philip Nitschke has built prototypes for euthanasia machines; more recently he has travelled between Australian State capitals, single-handedly staffing euthanasia advice clinics. Rodney Syme, president of the Victorian Voluntary Euthanasia Society, vowed publicly in the wake of the *Euthanasia Laws Act* 1997 that he would continue to provide assistance to patients.[25] At Easter 1998, in a newspaper article that provoked outrage, Syme re-interpreted the death of Christ as euthanasia by God the father to relieve Jesus' suffering.[26] Like Nitschke, Syme has sought to clarify the legal status of palliative care practices, by requesting Coronial inquests into the

deaths of patients who have died from the effect of increasing sedation given to control discomfort.[27]

Perhaps the most confronting tactic of euthanasia campaigners
is to use dying patients themselves. In 1999 the New South Wales
Voluntary Euthanasia Society produced a shock television com-
mercial featuring June Burns, a dying cancer patient and mother of
four, who told viewers 'I feel life is very precious and I've enjoyed
every moment of it and I wish I could go on but I can't and I'd like
to die with dignity'.[28] Eight months later June was reported to be
in remission, her doctors believing she could live for another two
years.[29]

Legalise and regulate

From a harm minimisation perspective, legalisation has several advantages: in the absence of any genuine commitment to prosecuting
offending doctors, it realigns medical practice with the law. It edu-
cates health professionals, and promotes a series of norms designed
to influence conduct. In this way it may reduce the incidence of illicit
assisted death, as well as suicide. By making assisted death a legal
option if things get too bad, patients may feel they have more
control over their disease process, and may in fact be *less* likely
to seek assistance as a 'prophylactic' against future suffering (see
Chapter 5).

If assisted death were to be legalised, it must be done in a systematic, rational way. Assisted suicide cannot reasonably be introduced without also legalising active voluntary euthanasia. One leads
logically to the other. In the United States context, Pellegrino points
out that in view of the failure rates for suicides, any law permitting
assisted suicide (for example, through 'lethal prescriptions') would
be 'disastrously ineffective' unless physicians were authorised 'to
administer the coup de grâce if necessary'.[30] He is right. This is self-
evident in the Australian context, where right to die activism has not
focused narrowly on assisted suicide. The 'absent doctor' was a disturbing feature in the accounts of some interviewees (see Chapter
10). The suggestion that doctors can avoid moral responsibility
by prescribing drugs and then leaving the dying process to the
untrained and debilitated patient, is simply pathetic, a point not lost

on the Dutch.[31] It should be seen for what it is: a form of medical abandonment.[32]

The main reason advocates of assisted death support physician-assisted suicide, but not active euthanasia, is because 'in assisted suicide, the final act is solely the patient's, and the risk of subtle coercion from doctors, family members, institutions, or other social forces is greatly reduced'.[33] While coercion may be a risk, it is not answered by a half-baked suicide statute. The risk of coercion is best minimised by a process of genuine assessment, involving independent review, regardless of who gives the final fatal jab.

Any responsible approach to legalisation must also safeguard the position of pharmacists who agree to fill a lethal prescription, and any nurses who assist at the bedside. Gentle yet lethal drugs must be accessible to precipitate the death.[34] Much of the stress and sadness of underground practices is the result of a knowledge vacuum. If euthanasia is to be legalised, then euthanatic strategies must find their place in the medical literature. This does not imply the creation of a new speciality, although some have seen a role for anaesthetists in this area.[35]

If legalisation makes good sense in policy terms, what form should legalisation take? There are a variety of possible models. Legislatures can enact a statutory regime incorporating a protective protocol, as occurred in the Northern Territory in 1995, and in Oregon in 1994. Alternatively, a right to die can emerge gradually from court decisions, whether those decisions revolve around the interpretation of the Constitution (as illustrated by two 1996 US Court of Appeal decisions),[36] or legislation (as in the Netherlands).[37]

There are subtle yet important differences between these models. In the Netherlands assisted suicide and euthanasia remain criminal offences, although in November 2000 the Lower House of the Dutch Parliament voted to amend the Penal Code to create an explicit defence where certain 'due care' requirements have been satisfied (see Chapter 4). Before this, the Dutch Supreme Court had recognised a defence of 'necessity' when life was terminated in accordance with certain criteria.[38] Although initially acknowledged in case law, guidance as to the scope of the necessity defence was also found in the statutory notification procedure that applied to

euthanasia deaths under burial legislation. The notification procedure included some 50 criteria which acted as guidelines for the
public prosecutor when assessing doctors' reports.[39] The Royal
Dutch Medical Association also issued guidelines which responded
to developments in the case law, and separate prosecutorial guidelines were issued following the *Chabot* case.[40]

Although popular with euthanasia advocates, the history of
Dutch euthanasia law illustrates the disadvantages of a regulatory
model that emerges from court decisions. Courts make poor social
policy planners. A 'common law' right to die will inevitably lack the
detail and fine tuning required to protect vulnerable patients and to
properly balance patients' wishes with public interests. On the other
hand, if courts were to 'legislate' a comprehensive framework for
euthanasia practice, they would be criticised for usurping the role
of the legislature.[41] The Dutch model has long been criticised for
its 'vague' and 'elastic' criteria.[42] It is, perhaps, no coincidence that
the criteria emerging from Dutch courts have been supplemented
and interpreted by other bodies, eager to settle on an appropriate
and stable set of criteria. The amendments to the Dutch Penal Code
reflect the most recent, and authoritative, consensus.

There is a subtle distinction between euthanasia laws which provide a defence to criminal liability for murder, and laws which set
out the pre-conditions to the lawful practice of euthanasia. There is
some support for the former approach. Brody argues that assisted
death should be seen as a compassionate response to medical failure
—'the failure of medical interventions to arrange a good death'. It
follows that 'assisting a death is an admission of incompetent medical practice until proved otherwise', with the result that assisted
death should only ever 'serve as a defence against a charge of homicide or of assisting a suicide'.[43]

There is some evidence that doctors' fear of prosecution, and
their desire to protect themselves and the patient's family from
investigation, have acted as a disincentive to reporting euthanasia in
the Netherlands.[44] If euthanasia is to become lawful, doctors deserve
unambiguous legal protection, and this is best achieved by a statute
which sets out the pre-conditions to lawful assistance in detail. The
recent Dutch amendments are a welcome reform.

Nevertheless, the Dutch model still places considerable reliance on the treating physician to determine whether the necessary conditions have been satisfied. In the *Chabot* case the Dutch Supreme Court stated that in cases where the patient's suffering was caused by a somatic illness (in contrast to existential misery or depression), there was no strict legal requirement for the treating physician to seek a second opinion at all.[45] While independent assessment is required under the new law, the safeguards fall short of those in the Northern Territory and Oregon laws. Euthanasia laws need robust safeguards because the stakes are high. We should not be overly concerned that independent assessment will intrude into the privacy and intimacy of the doctor/patient relationship. Patients regularly seek specialist assessment for a host of lesser conditions. Assisted death— the ultimate medical intervention—deserves rigorous safeguards.

If assisted suicide and active voluntary euthanasia are to be legalised, then democratic reform is also a worthy goal.[46] A legislated approach to euthanasia has a better chance of ensuring public accountability, and permits legislators to debate and build very specific safeguards into the statutory protocol regulating assisted death. Some of the necessary choices encountered in designing a statutory protocol are discussed on pages 274–9.

Influencing illicit practice: a fifth response

Even if assisted death is never legalised, there is still a further response to the euthanasia underground that deserves to be debated. Illicit euthanasia screams out for regulation, even informal regulation. If it is true—as survey studies suggest—that a not insignificant proportion of health professionals will continue to ignore the law's prohibition on assisted death, it is important that they should have the opportunity to calibrate their actions against some sort of benchmark, some minimum set of criteria. Innovative and valuable work, albeit in a slightly different context, has emerged from an initiative of the University of Pennsylvania Center for Bioethics, which collected representatives from medicine, nursing, psychology, hospice, patient advocacy, law, philosophy, clergy and bioethics, to consider what safeguards should be included in assisted suicide laws, assuming that these laws will be enacted.[47] The focus of these collaborators—both opponents and advocates of assisted suicide laws—was to ensure that physician-assisted suicide remains 'voluntary, regulated, and, most important, an option of last resort'.[48]

A challenge facing professional medical bodies, such as the Australian Medical Association, or specialist colleges, such as the Royal Australian College of General Practitioners, is to respond to the virtual certainty that many in their ranks are heavily involved in assisted death. Even if euthanasia remains a crime, a de facto standard, or framework for involvement, is better than none at all. It would be naive to hope for any institutional consensus on assisted death, but a statement of issues worthy of exploration with patients could at least direct doctors to matters that are frequently overlooked.

Among these issues would surely be: the problem of botched attempts caused by doctors' lack of knowledge about gentle yet lethal drugs; the risks of organic and reactive depression; the importance of continuity in the desire for assistance; the benefits of second opinions as to prognosis and mental state; alternative approaches to controlling pain and distress; and options for palliative care. The importance of assessing whether the patient is making a wise and informed decision (in terms of their own values and interests) requires health professionals to be alive to, and to adequately explore, the complex meanings of suicide talk. Doctors contemplating involvement in assisted death should be encouraged to explore practical issues with their patients: how to prepare one's affairs for death, and the impact of euthanasia upon partners, relatives, friends and health care workers. There are no doubt many other factors deserving attention.

Such guidelines could, if necessary, be deliberately vague, and need not advocate assisted death. But they should be specific enough to address the issues, risks and pitfalls which are present when health carers choose to assist.

Drugs policy provides a precedent for this kind of regulation. The intravenous injection of heroin is illegal, yet the risk of transmission of HIV and other infections through contaminated needles justifies policies which, on a facile analysis, assist drug users to break the law more safely. Needle distribution and exchange programs in Australia, 'which reflect a harm reduction approach to intravenous drug use, aim both to educate users about the necessity for safety in injecting and in sexual behaviour, and to facilitate safe behaviour by providing easy access to sterile injecting equipment and to condoms'.[49] A similar argument applies to the distribution of condoms to sex workers who are suspected of engaging in illegal acts of prostitution.[50]

Some may argue that any attempt to smooth out the highly idiosyncratic nature of illicit assistance through 'informal standards' is a last-gasp effort to promote euthanasia. This is an odd position for social and religious conservatives to take, however, in light of the disturbing issues documented in this study. At worst, it reflects a punitive lack of concern for those who are suffering most. It is akin to denying homosexuals, or women, the pill, because gay sex or pre-marital sex is always wrong, whatever the consequences in terms of transmission of HIV and other STDs, or ill-timed pregnancies. Euthanasia shares, in this respect, a tension between moralistic and consequentialist approaches seen particularly in the context of HIV/AIDS and drugs policy.[51]

Ultimately, if we really care about those who are dying, we must recognise the social cost of the principle of prohibition and influence doctors to do what they do carefully.

Fatal choices: designing a euthanasia protocol

What safeguards should be included in a statutory euthanasia protocol? The interviewees displayed little consensus on this question. Some saw no need to legalise euthanasia in order to protect patients from the risks of abuse. John, the funeral director, thought that the current system worked well because the risks of acting illegally forced doctors to carefully question their motivations. Russell, a hospital physician, agreed that 'the system is working fine the way it is', but later cautioned that any guidelines should 'make sure we don't have too much leeway'.

Few interviewees had given detailed consideration to what a euthanasia protocol might look like, although there was frequent, vaguely-expressed optimism in the Dutch model. Support for the Dutch model is certainly consistent with the concern of some re-visionists to minimise inroads into their clinical discretion.

Margaret, an AIDS community worker, thought that the issue of regulation involved 'a minefield of stuff'. Amanda, a community nurse, emphasised the need for a structure which ensured that 'there is no one person that makes [the] decision'. Peter, a nurse, favoured a 'tick sheet', with referral to a psychiatrist and other preconditions being ticked off sequentially. Bill, a hospice nurse who was troubled by his previous action in drugging a patient to death, reflected, 'I don't think the idea of hastening someone's death should be easy. I think there should really be a lot of anxiety . . .'.

In terms of precise safeguards, the responses of doctors were perhaps the most helpful:

> I think that the death certificate should say euthanasia or assisted suicide. I think it should be reported to the Coroner. I think that there needs to be further consultation with at least two doctors . . . I think that it should still be illegal but doctors should avoid prosecution, very similar to [the Netherlands] (Gordon, GP).

> I see that the Dutch system probably works—I don't know a lot about it—but I think there [should] be two medical opinions, I would actually go as far as saying that . . . it's worth getting a psychiatric review . . . [to] eliminate depression as a major influence (Josh, GP).

Later, Josh emphasised his preference for a 'medical model', which minimised bureaucracy and external inquiries.

A feature of the interviews was the evidence they provided of doctors ignoring their own suggested safeguards. Gordon, for example, had overdosed a patient without consulting any other doctor, and Josh without obtaining a psychiatric opinion. This illustrates the lack of accountability in underground involvement. Whether it shows that activist doctors would ignore the requirements and safeguards of a statutory protocol is a troubling question. We simply don't know.

Fundamental choices of reach and scope

There is a growing literature discussing 'safeguards' in euthanasia legislation.[52] Not surprisingly, no consensus emerges from it. Before one gets to the level of specific safeguards, however, it is clear that any legislative protocol must embody some fundamental choices about reach and scope. Perhaps the three most important choices are whether assisted death should be limited to patients who are: (i) competent adults; (ii) suffering from a terminal disease; and (iii) experiencing unbearable pain or suffering.

A patient who is both terminally ill and dying in agony represents the least controversial context for assisted death. Both terminal illness and unbearable pain and suffering were requirements under the now-defunct Northern Territory legislation.[53] The Dutch model, by contrast, only requires unbearable pain or suffering, although treatment possibilities for relieving that suffering must have been exhausted or rejected by the patient.[54] Oregon's 'Measure 16' does not require 'unbearable suffering', but does require an incurable and irreversible disease likely to cause death within 6 months.[55]

A 'terminal illness' is a somewhat elastic legislative criterion. By exercising their right to refuse life-sustaining medical treatment, patients may transform a chronic disability or illness into a terminal condition. On the other hand, is a persistently suicidal patient properly to be regarded as having an incurable illness, even if their life expectancy is as poor as that of a terminally ill patient?[56]

More fundamentally, as Kamisar points out, 'if either [respect for personal] autonomy or the merciful termination of an unendurable existence' is the basis for the right to die, 'why limit it to the terminally ill?'[57] Why not extend euthanasia as a choice for those whose chronic illnesses, injuries or disabilities (AIDS, spinal paralysis, advanced emphysema, amyotrophic lateral sclerosis, multiple sclerosis etc.) are the cause of chronic and intractable suffering? If self-determination and compassion are the controlling values, why limit assisted death to illness at all? Why not make it available to those who are constantly miserable?

Seen through libertarian lenses, the conflict generated by the euthanasia debate is between a 'communitarian' world view where social goals and values circumscribe aspects of individual freedom, and a more individualistic world view where personal choice within the private sphere trumps social values. The Dutch model for assisted death leans heavily in favour of individual autonomy. The *Chabot* case illustrates how a depressed and bereaved psychiatric patient could, by refusing psychiatric help, fulfil the criteria for unbearable suffering, with no prospect of improvement.[58] Dr Chabot says of his patient:

> In all times and cultures, there have been exceptional individuals who did not want to survive the death of a beloved one, be it a child or a spouse. They sought death in one way or another. I think this woman was one of those vulnerable persons . . . She did not want to feel better. She wanted to die . . . Her one and only value in life was her children, the cornerstone on which everything else was built. Once that stone was gone, the very idea of a future for her collapsed, became repulsive.[59]

Perhaps it is the fear of our own death that gives us alarm at the prospect that grief and loss, or a treatable psychiatric illness, could become grounds for euthanasia.

One reason, perhaps, for restricting assisted death to the context of terminal illness is that, because we value the sanctity of life ethic, an assisted death should only be entertained as a way of easing an otherwise horrible or lingering *death*, rather than as a way of escaping a *life* which would not otherwise be ending. The requirement for a terminal illness—which would exclude people with chronic conditions or disabilities—limits the collateral damage euthanasia causes to our intuitions about the value of life. On the other hand, the risk of artificially limiting the availability of assisted death may make any law less effective in combating illegal practices.

This compromise will not satisfy those who believe that if euthanasia is legalised at all, we will drift, insidiously, towards non-consensual euthanasia. One commentator warns that 'the notion of voluntariness will recede before the twin onslaught of compassion for, and non-discrimination against, minors, the intellectually impaired and those in a vegetative state'.[60] The Dutch Parliament, for example, debated legislation that would have permitted minors 12 to 16 to request physician-assisted suicide without parental consent, although this clause was removed prior to passage.[61]

If voluntary euthanasia is legalised, the question will inevitably arise whether the law should permit a person to 'pre-order' euthanasia by means of an advance directive, or to authorise a surrogate to make this decision, if incompetence precludes a rational decision during the terminal stages of disease. In November 2000, amendments to Dutch euthanasia law authorised advance directives ('euthanasia declarations'),[62] and this is a logical next step, considering that the right to *withdraw* life-sustaining medical treatment also encompasses advance directives and surrogate decision-makers. Furthermore, the common law also authorises the 'non-consensual' withdrawal of life support from incompetent persons when this is in their best interests (as when they are permanently comatose). Permitting the active killing of an incompetent person who is thought to be suffering grievously is not, therefore, as large a step as some assume.

Resolving these issues will always be difficult. Once the conceptual leap is made, and society permits some of its citizens to kill themselves, there may be pressures from some quarters to extend the right. However, slippery slopes are not self-executing. In each case, the quality of safeguards embodied in legislation, and the risks of abuse of the legislation versus the misery and suffering it was meant to avoid, must be confronted honestly, and debated publicly. Legislatures can make compromises which, even if they 'illogically' limit the availability of assisted death, can do so in an explicit attempt to balance the competing moral frameworks of our pluralist society. The primary aim of this book has been to point out the role of the 'euthanasia underground' in any ensuing debate.

Specific safeguards

There has been little research on the views of health care workers towards appropriate safeguards. A recent study of Australian nurses showed sharp divisions over whether assisted death should only be permitted when the patient was not suffering from treatable depression, was cognitively competent, in intractable pain, or only after palliative care options had been given.[63] In the writer's view, independent assessment is the cornerstone of a safe protocol; it is more important than preserving the clinical autonomy of the health care worker. The legal permission that would be given to doctors under euthanasia laws entails an expansion of medical power in a context where public interests are finely balanced and the risks are real. Independent assessment by specialists is hardly a novel concept in modern medicine. Society has the right to expect that those who choose to exercise this power will comply with legislative safeguards.

While a variety of health care professions are implicated in illicit euthanasia, the most obvious statutory model would make the carriage of the statutory process a matter for the treating physician. A doctor-centred approach makes obvious sense where euthanasia is limited to those with a 'terminal illness'. Clinical assessment of the patient's medical circumstances, by doctors, is inevitable.[64]

The treating physician's assessment of the patient's terminal condition should be subject to review. Due to the fluctuating final phases of certain diseases—such as AIDS—it makes sense for this second opinion to be given by a doctor who is a specialist, or who satisfies statutory criteria ensuring experience and expertise in the condition the patient suffers from.

The complexity of euthanasia talk demonstrates the need for psychiatric review to identify treatable depression, mental illness and dementia.[65] The psychiatrists, psychiatrically-trained nurses and therapists interviewed in this study understood the need for this requirement. Others, however, were confident in their own ability to assess patients, and stressed that euthanasia was the patient's 'right', rather than something the patient should have to convince others about.

The complexity of euthanasia talk also illustrates the need to ensure that options for palliative care are explored with the patient. By requiring investigation of palliative care options as a prerequisite to assistance, patients may, paradoxically, receive better care, and may be less likely ever to proceed with euthanasia.[66]

Physical pain and suffering cannot be quarantined from the patient's wider emotional and social circumstances. The involvement of a counsellor, psychiatrist or psychologist would permit patients to explore the conflicts that were evidently motivating the death wish in some of the cases described by interviewees: family and relationship conflicts, financial problems, disclosure issues, and deeply-hidden secrets relating to one's sexuality, or diagnosis.

The provision of assisted death to patients the doctor has only 'just met' was a particularly disturbing feature of some interviews. Nevertheless, since a treating physician may not wish to perform euthanasia, it is inevitable that terminally ill patients may end up 'shopping' for a doctor prepared to assist them. Quill and colleagues emphasise that 'physician-assisted suicide should be carried out only in the context of a meaningful doctor–patient relationship. Ideally, the physician should have witnessed the patient's previous illness and suffering'.[67] Miles fears that legalisation may 'empower not only physicians with good relationships, but also those with transient, inadequate, or troubled relationships with chronically ill patients'.[68] Continuity in the doctor–patient relationship is therefore an important safeguard, and legislators might properly require a minimum level of continuity between patient and physician. Sufficient time is also crucial to the quality of any independent assessment process: as Ryan recognises, 'often it is difficult and time consuming to tease out the complex motives behind the desire to end one's life'.[69]

If assisted death is to be justified (at least partly) on the basis of personal autonomy and choice, there must be clear evidence of a sustained desire to die, by a patient exercising free will. Recent research among elderly, terminally ill cancer patients, for example, suggests that the will to live is highly unstable, influenced by factors such as anxiety, depression and shortness of breath.[70] Continuity of desire is a crucial safeguard which would aim to screen out patients who were reacting to a temporary and resolvable crisis.

The approach to 'safeguards' adopted here means, inevitably, that the right to die cannot be an unfettered right, nor one that doctors could legally give effect to on an ad hoc basis. Opponents of legalisation will argue that no protocol can adequately protect patients. These criticisms may reflect deeper, religious or philosophical concerns. If the purpose of a statutory protocol is—at least in part—to encourage those who perform illicit euthanasia to channel their activities back within legal boundaries, then an unduly rigid and bureaucratic regime may be counter-productive.

In their own way, the words of Mrs B., at the beginning of this chapter, summarise the concern of opponents of euthanasia. That concern is that legalisation will encourage the self-annihilation of the bereaved and empty, those who have so lost a sense of their own worth that death feels like 'pure justice'.

It would be a tragedy if the long-term effect of euthanasia legislation was to push self-effacing and despondent patients over the edge, perhaps to relieve their loved ones from the worry of looking after them, or to conserve family assets. Professor Maddocks, an Australian pioneer in palliative care, states:

What I do not want . . . is to see a brisk new expectation arise in our society that a quick death is a noble one, that for the sake of the family, the health budget or the stress upon carers, it will be best to elect euthanasia. This is because I feel that some of the excellent sharing and exchanges of love that inspire and comfort the rest of us will be lost in accepting that fatal attraction, and our society will be the poorer for it.[71]

Callahan agrees, arguing that 'the greatest danger of [physician-assisted suicide] is the social legitimation of suicide as a way of dealing with the suffering and sorrows of life'.[72]

Guessing the flow-on effects of legalisation is a slippery business. The primary aim of this book has been to show that euthanasia is a present reality. The medical profession, and policy makers, must acknowledge this. As Dworkin, Nagel, Nozick, Rawls and colleagues wrote in their 'philosophers' brief' to the United States Supreme Court, 'the current two-tier system—a chosen death and an end of pain outside the law for those with connections and stony refusals for most other people—is one of the greatest scandals of contemporary medical practice'.[73]

Acknowledging the reality of illicit euthanasia opens up a space within which we can work towards minimising the harm and sadness caused by the poor judgment of both patients and their physicians. Euthanasia should be regulated, but even in the absence of legislation, there is important work for the medical and nursing professions to do, seeking to influence and improve the informal assessment processes that currently operate.

Legalisation is not, of course, a risk-free policy option. Professor Little warns that the 'subtle pressures which can influence informed consent for medical treatment could very easily enter the domain of euthanasia, interfering with extended and objective discussion'.[74] If this is true, how might it be demonstrated? One important avenue for future research is among palliative care physicians, nursing staff, and the terminally ill themselves, investigating bedside dynamics and relationships, and seeking to assess the extent to which patients really are (or would be) vulnerable to an early death as a result of subtle manipulation by health care workers.[75] How realistic is it to argue that euthanasia might become a 'persuaded act', performed disproportionately upon the weary-of-heart, who have lost their sense of personal worth, and who feel they are a nuisance? These are crucial concerns. But they can only be vindicated on the basis of evidence, rather than on speculation and religiously-motivated assertions.

This book has been influenced by a consequentialist, policy-oriented approach to euthanasia regulation. I have put the case for legalisation, while recognising just how difficult this debate has become. The legalisation of euthanasia would, of course, have a libertarian effect, by creating a space for personal choice. 'The essence of liberalism', Charlesworth points out, 'is the moral conviction that, because they are autonomous moral agents or persons, people must as far as possible be free to choose for themselves, even if their choices are, objectively speaking, mistaken'.[76] While threatening, perhaps, to the autocratic religions, or to those who see medicine as a strictly paternalistic enterprise, if personal autonomy is a worthy objective then there can be few contexts where its exercise is more important than in confronting one's mortality in the closing stages of life.

Appendix

The recruitment strategy and methodology adopted in this study

THE INTERVIEW FINDINGS presented in this book emerge from forty-nine detailed interviews I conducted with health professionals specialising in HIV/AIDS, principally in Sydney, Melbourne and San Francisco. As summarised in Table A-1, recruitment for the study took several forms. First, twenty interviewees volunteered to be interviewed following public invitations given within the context of five seminars, and conference presentations. Two further interviews arose when volunteers responded to a flyer distributed to the mailing list of an HIV interest group, and in one case an interview arose following a letter written to a community organisation.

Secondly, interviewees recommended to their colleagues and associates that they become involved. Early interviewees or intending interviewees acted as a screen, 'sussing out' the study, and satisfying themselves that I was 'trustworthy', before referring colleagues to me. Some interviewees played a pivotal role in referring me to other key players in the euthanasia network within that city, interstate, or internationally. Nineteen interviews came about this way. A snowball sampling technique such as this is particularly suited to investigating populations that are scattered, inaccessible, and lacking formal organisation.[1] While health care workers operate within organised and formal settings, euthanasia is carried out at an underground and informal level. In this sense, health carers who participate in assisted death are inaccessible, scattered, concerned about anonymity and fearful of exposure. The study also benefited from referrals by several physicians and members of AIDS community organisations who were not, themselves, interviewed. Six interviews came about this way. In one case, I approached an interviewee directly, without previous referral.[2]

Table A-1: Summary of recruitment methods

Recruitment Category	Total (n=49)
Volunteers	
– Volunteered following public presentations	20
– Volunteered in response to a flyer	2
– Volunteered in response to letter to community	
group	1
Referrals	
– Referred/recommended by interviewees	19
– Referred by non-interviewees	6
Approached directly by letter	1

Due to the form recruitment took, it makes no sense to talk of an overall 'response rate'. A feature of this study was that interviewees approached the researcher. The contacts made on occasions when I gave a conference or seminar presentation were particularly fruitful. Typically, they took the form of an introductory conversation or a business card being pressed into the hand, which I follwed up with correspondence explaining the aims of the study and the methodology, telephone calls and, eventually, a face-to-face meeting.

On occasions where an interviewee recommended another colleague, I encouraged the interviewee to invite the colleague to make contact with me voluntarily. Sometimes a significant period of time elapsed before this occurred (on one occasion, over two years). Due to the sensitive nature of the research, the focus was on facilitating interviewees to volunteer for inclusion in the study by telephoning or writing to me directly. Even so, I followed up referrals by letter or telephone if I thought it was appropriate. On three or four occasions, these approaches went unanswered, and were not pursued. On two occasions only, a person who had agreed to be involved backed out before the interview. One interviewee was a well known physician who had admitted in the media to hastening death, causing problems with his employer. Another was a community worker who explained that her husband was concerned about her legal liability.

No master list of interviewees was retained, in order to preserve anonymity, and to encourage frankness during the interview. All interviewees chose a pseudonym, although sometimes I re-assigned a different name to the interviewee, post-interview, to further secure anonymity. The interviews followed a semi-structured format (certain issues were raised with all interviewees), and in general were 70–90 minutes long. All interviews were transcribed, and those considered most important were coded and analysed using The Ethnograph,[3] a software package that facilitates cross-referencing between interviews, and search and retrieval functions using standardised codes. These codes were developed from the analysis of transcribed interview data.[4] As a result, the themes which emerged from interviews, and which form the basis for this book, were 'grounded' in interviewees' own experiences and perspectives.

Notes

Introduction

[1] A. McCall Smith, 'Euthanasia: the Strengths of the Middle Ground', 195.
[2] I. Kennedy, 'The Right to Die', in C. Mazzoni (ed.), *A Legal Framework for Bioethics*, p. 186.
[3] Russel Ogden's 1994 Vancouver study is an early exception: see *Euthanasia, Assisted Suicide and AIDS*, pp. 53–83. Several studies focusing on health care workers have included interview components. But the implications of personal accounts of involvement have not been explored in any level of detail. See, e.g. B. Black, J. Wallace, H. Starks et al, 'Physician-Assisted suicide and Euthanasia in Washington State', 919; P. van der Maas, J. van Delden, L. Pijnenborg et al, 'Euthanasia and Other Medical Decisions Concerning the End of Life', 669.
[4] S. Aranda & M. O'Conner, 'Euthanasia, Nursing and Care of the Dying: Rethinking Kuhse and Singer', 21; F. McInerney & C. Seibold, 'Nurses Definitions of and Attitudes Towards Euthanasia', 180.
[5] L. Snyder & A. Caplan, 'Assisted Suicide: Finding Common Ground', 468.
[6] R. Glover, 'Why the Vulnerable Flock to Dr Death', *Sydney Morning Herald*, 17 April 1999, p. S2.

Chapter 1

[1] Elaine Thompson, Associate Professor of Public Policy, University of New South Wales, speaking to a conference entitled 'Death and the State', the Centre for Public Policy, The University of Melbourne, 24 August 1995.

Chapter 2

[1] *Daily Telegraph* (UK), 21 July 1997, p. 1.
[2] 'Helping Patients to Die' *Age*, 25 March 1995, p. 1; C. Zinn, 'Australian Doctors Go Public Over Euthanasia', 895.
[3] R. Syme, D. Russell, P. Scrivener, N. Roth, A. Buchanan, D. Bernshaw, S. Benwell, 'An Open Letter to the State Premier of Victoria', 24 March 1995, p. 2.
[4] 'Charge Euthanasia Doctors, Says Right to Life', *Age*, 27 March 1995, p. 1.
[5] By a spokesperson for the Victorian Premier: 'Fury Over Assisted Deaths', *Sunday Age*, 26 March 1995, p. 3.
[6] 'Suicide Doctors Face Probe', *Sunday Age*, 1 April 1995, p. 1; 'Board Abandons Probe into Euthanasia Doctors', *Age*, 21 June 1995, p. 3; 'Police Probe on Euthanasia', *Age*, 22 June 1995, p. 3; 'Police Drop Euthanasia Inquiry', *Age*, 10 August 1995, p. 3.

[7] H Palmer, 'Dr Adams' Trial for Murder', 367, 374; C. Hawkins, *Mishap or Malpractice?*, p. 62.

[8] e.g. *Airedale NHS Trust* v *Bland* [1993] AC 789 at 867 per Lord Goff (England); *Compassion in Dying* v *State of Washington* 79 F. 3d 790 (1996), 822 (United States); *Auckland Area Health Board* v *Attorney-General* [1993] 1 NZLR 235 at 252, 253 (New Zealand). The principle also has specific legislative status in some States: e.g. *Consent to Medical Treatment and Palliative Care Act* 1995 (SA) s 17.

[9] H. Palmer, 'Dr Adams' Trial for Murder', 375.

[10] C. Hawkins, *Mishap or Malpractice?*, pp. 64–5. Devlin J, the presiding judge (later Lord Devlin), wrote a book about the case after Adams' death: P. Devlin, *Easing the Passing: The Trial of Dr John Bodkin Adams*.

[11] C. Dyer, 'Rheumatologist Convicted of Attempted Murder', 731.

[12] D. Brahams, 'Euthanasia: Doctor Convicted of Attempted Murder', 782.

[13] The Honourable Mr Justice Ognall, 'A Right to Die? Some Medico-Legal Reflections', 168–9.

[14] Editorial, 'The Final Autonomy', 758.

[15] Name withheld by request, 'It's Over, Debbie', 272.

[16] Ibid.

[17] See, e.g., Letters (1988) 259 *JAMA* 2094–8.

[18] W. Gaylin, L. Kass, E. Pellegrino, M. Siegler, 'Doctors Must Not Kill', 2139. Another wrote that: "the outrage of Debbie's case reminds us that we must never abandon the cardinal purpose of medical care—to save and sustain life and never intentionally to harm or kill. The other lesson of this case is that we must not destroy the virtue of that commitment by using medical art to prolong dying and puritanically refuse to relieve suffering": K. Vaux, 'Debbie's Dying: Mercy Killing and the Good Death', 2141.

[19] Ibid.

[20] G. Lundberg, ' "It's Over, Debbie" and the Euthanasia Debate', 2142.

[21] T. Quill, 'Death and Dignity: A Case of Individualised Decision Making', 693.

[22] Ibid.

[23] Ibid., 694.

[24] 'Panel to Decide: Should Doctor Who Aided Suicide be Tried?', *New York Times*, 22 July 1991, p. B1.

[25] 'Jury Declines to Indict a Doctor Who Said He Aided in a Suicide', *New York Times*, 27 July 1991, p. A1.

[26] *Vacco* v *Quill*, 521 US 793 (1997), available on the internet: <http://supct.law.cornell.edu/supct/>.

[27] T. Quill, C. Cassel, D. Meier, 'Care of the Hopelessly Ill: Proposed Clinical Criteria for Physician-Assisted Suicide', 1380.

[28] 'Panel to Decide: Should Doctor Who Aided Suicide Be Tried?', *New York Times*, 22 July 1991, p. B2.

[29] *Newsweek*, 8 March 1993, pp. 46, 48, quoted in G. Pence, 'Dr Kevorkian and the Struggle for Physician-Assisted Dying', 69.

[30] E. Pellegrino, 'Compassion Needs Reason Too', 874–5. Pellegrino argues that 'compassion is a virtue, not a principle', that 'compassion, too, must be subject to moral analysis', and that the moral psychology behind the act of killing does not justify the act: ibid. Against this, others argue that 'absolutist principles must always be chastened by mercy': K. Vaux, 'Debbie's Dying: Mercy Killing and the Good Death', 2141.

[31] 'As Memory and Music Faded, Oregon Woman Chose Death', *New York Times*, 7 June 1990, p. A1; M. Beck, K. Springen, A. Murr et al, 'The Doctor's Suicide Van', *Bulletin* (*Newsweek* insert), 19 June 1990, p. 80.

32 'Physician Fulfils a Goal: Aiding a Person in Suicide', *New York Times*, 7 June 1990, p. D22.

33 As reported by Beck, Springen, Murr et al, above n. 31, p. 81.

34 In the United States, an accused can be charged with a crime for which he or she is not subsequently tried. The charge may be used during subsequent plea-bargaining.

35 'Michigan Court Bars Doctor From Using His Suicide Machine', *New York Times*, 6 February 1991, p. A13.

36 'Kevorkian Assists in Death of his 17th Suicide Patient', *New York Times*, 5 August 1993, p. A14.

37 'As he Hoped, Kevorkian is Charged in a Suicide', *New York Times*, 18 August 1993, p. A12.

38 'Kevorkian, Pushing for Jail, Aids in Suicide in His Home', *New York Times*, 23 October 1993, p. A8.

39 Ibid.

40 'Kevorkian Takes Stand in Own Defence', *New York Times*, 28 April 1994, p. A16.

41 'Side Issue May Decide Kevorkian Verdict', *New York Times*, 29 April 1994, p. A14.

42 'In One Doctor's Way of Life, a Way of Death', *New York Times*, 21 May 1995, p. A14.

43 'Jury Acquits Dr Kevorkian of Illegally Aiding a Suicide', *New York Times*, 3 May 1994, p. A1; 'Special State Law Fails to Stop "Dr Death" ', *Australian*, 4 May 1994, p. 16.

44 'Jury Acquits Dr Kevorkian of Illegally Aiding a Suicide', *New York Times*, 3 May 1994, p. A1.

45 'Kevorkian's Trial Has Come to End, But Debate on Assisted Suicide Hasn't', *New York Times*, 4 May 1994, p. A16.

46 Ibid.

47 'Kevorkian Vows to Keep Fighting Laws Barring Assisted Suicide', *New York Times*, 18 December 1994, p. A43.

48 Ibid.

49 'Kevorkian: Trial or Witch-Hunt?', 2 April 1996, Last Rights Information Centre, US news bulletins (archives): <http://www.rights.org/deathnet/last_rights.html>; <http://www.rights.org/deathnet/bulletins.html>.

50 'Kevorkian Acquitted—for the Third Time', 14 May 1996, Last Rights Information Centre, US news bulletins (archives), above n. 49.

51 'Tonight on '60 Minutes': One Man's Final Seconds', *Age*, 27 November 1999; 'Kevorkian Charged with first-degree murder, freed on $750,000 bond', 25 November 1998, Last Rights Information Centre, US news bulletins (archives), above n. 49.

52 'Kevorkian Says his Role in Death was "Duty" ', *New York Times*, 23 March 1999, p. A18.

53 'Dr Kevorkian's Client', *New York Times*, 25 March 1999, p. A30.

54 'Kevorkian Appeals to Emotions of Jurors as they Begin Weighing Murder Charges', *New York Times*, 26 March 1999, p. A14.

55 'Judge Sentences Kevorkian to 10 to 25 Years and Denies Bail', *New York Times*, 14 April 1999, p. C14.

56 Ibid.

57 'Dr Kevorkian is a Murderer, the Jury Finds', *New York Times*, 27 March 1999, p. A1.

58 'Kevorkian Sentenced to 10 to 25 Years in Prison', *New York Times*, 14 April 1999, p. A1; 'Judge Shows No Pity and 'Dr Death' Gets 10 Years', *Sydney Morning Herald*, 15 April 1999, p. 10; 'Life for Doctor Death', *Sydney Morning Herald*, 17 April 1999, p. 36.

[59] 'In One Doctor's Way of Life, a Way of Death', *New York Times*, 21 May 1995, p. A14.

[60] 'A Matter of Life & Death', *Age*, 25 March 1995.

[61] 'Doctors Defy Death Law', *Sunday Age*, 13 April 1997, p. 1; 'Death Doctors Not Likely to be Charged', *Sydney Morning Herald*, 14 April 1997, p. 6.

[62] 'Nitschke Backs Register of Euthanasia Doctors, Nurses', *Weekend Australian*, 29–30 March 1997, p. 2.

[63] 'I Put Patient to Sleep: Nitschke', *Australian*, 18 April 1997, p. 1; 'Nitschke Patient Dies in Coma', *Sydney Morning Herald*, 18 April 1997, p. 5.

[64] 'Nitschke Builds a Coma Machine', *Australian*, 15 May 1997, p. 1.

[65] 'Nitschke Works on New Death Machine', *Sydney Morning Herald*, 20 September 1997, p. 11.

[66] R. Ogden, 'Non-Physician Assisted Suicide: The Technological Imperative of the Deathing Counterculture', *Death Studies*, 391–4; G. Alcorn, 'The Death Thing', *Sydney Morning Herald*, 18 December 1999, p. 9S.

[67] 'Live and Let Die', *Sydney Weekly*, 5–11 June 1997, p. 10.

[68] 'Right-to-Die Doctor Under Microscope', *Australian*, 7 October 1998, p. 3; Steve Dow, 'Live & Let Die', *Australian Magazine*, 7–8 August 1999, p. 33.

[69] 'Nitschke Reveals Patient Deaths', *Sydney Morning Herald*, 27 November 1998, p. 3; 'Doctor: I Helped 15 Patients Die', *Age*, 27 November 1998, p. 1.

[70] 'Nitschke to Open Clinic Despite Protests', *Sydney Morning Herald*, 26 April 1999, p. 3; Steve Dow, 'Live & Let Die', *Australian Magazine*, 7–8 August 1999, p. 30.

[71] 'Nitschke Floats Death Ship Option', *Australian*, 31 May 2000, p. 4.

[72] 'Lab to Test Poisons, Drugs for Euthanasia', *Australian Doctor*, 17 November 2000, p. 19; 'Drugs Will Get the Death Test', *Sydney Morning Herald* (on-line), 5 February 2001.

[73] 'Dr Nitschke's "Support" as Cancer Woman Dies', *Sydney Morning Herald*, 23 January 2001, p. 1. For legal reasons, Nitschke assembled a team of doctors to co-sign the prescription for sedatives, including former Federal health minister Professor Peter Baume.

[74] 'You Say You're Dying, but I Just Can't Trust You', *Weekend Australian*, 1–2 May 1999, p. 6.

[75] Criminal charges, while sporadic, do occur. In Western Australia the Director of Public Prosecutions is pursuing criminal charges against a Perth doctor, following the death of a woman with terminal kidney cancer, from the administration of a drug not used in palliative care: 'Two Accused of Wilful Murder for Sister's Hospice Death', *Sydney Morning Herald* (on-line), 13 April 2000; 'Euthanasia Election Debate as Approval Given for Clinic', *Sydney Morning Herald* (on-line), 16 January 2001. In Canada, the Supreme Court recently upheld the conviction of Robert Latimer for second-degree murder, after he placed his daughter Tracey, born with cerebral palsy, into the cab of a pickup truck and piped in exhaust fumes: 'Latimer Goes to Jail, Mercy-Killing Debate Goes On', 19 January 2001, Last Rights Information Centre, Canadian News Bulletins (archives): above n. 49.

Chapter 3

[1] 'The Death Thing', *Sydney Morning Herald*, 18 December 1999, p. 9S.

[2] *Auckland Health Board* v *Attorney-General* [1993] 1 NZLR 235 at 244 per Thomas J.

3 See, e.g., F. McInerney, ' "Requested Death": A New Social Movement', 137; and for discussion of the social forces underlying Oregon's assisted suicide legislation: D. Hill-yard & J. Dombrink, *Dying Right: The Death With Dignity Movement.*

4 G. Alcorn, 'Marshall Law', *Age*, 24 May 1995, p. 13.

5 M. Somerville, 'Sentencing Society to Ethical Death', *Age*, 13 November 1995, p. 13; see also M. Somerville, 'Legalising Euthanasia: Why Now?', 1.

6 Vatican—Evangelium Vitae, *On the Value and Inviolability of Human Life* (1995), para 66; see also para 67 ('The height of arbitrariness and injustice is reached when certain people, such as physicians or legislators, arrogate to themselves the power to decide who ought to live and who ought to die').

7 See T. Beauchamp, 'Public & Private: Redrawing Boundaries', 18.

8 See M. P. Battin, *Ethical Issues in Suicide*, pp. 201, 225.

9 e.g. B. Pollard & R. Winton, 'Why Doctors and Nurses Must Not Kill Patients', 426.

10 See B. A. Santamaria, 'Tacit Consent to Euthanasia', *Weekend Australian*, 1–2 April 1995, p. 28.

11 'Three in Four Back Euthanasia—Newspoll', *Australian*, 9 July 1996, p. 1. New Zealand polls suggest majority support at more modest levels: 'Majority of Kiwis Support Legal Right to Die', *New Zealand Herald*, 28 December 2000, p. A3 (61% in favour, 28% opposed to legalised euthanasia).

12 Harvard Program on Public Opinion and Health Care, 'Should Physicians Aid their Patients in Dying?', 2659.

13 'Public Support Rising for Assisted Suicide', 15 April 1996, Last Rights Information Centre, US news bulletins (archives): <http://www.rights.org/deathnet/open.html>.

14 R. Ho, 'Factors Influencing Decisions to Terminate Life: Conditions of Suffering and the Identity of the Terminally Ill', 25.

15 Seale and Addington-Hall's 1994 English study of the relatives of 3696 deceaseds found that 'about a quarter of respondents who answered the question felt that it would have been better if [the patient] had died earlier, and that a similar proportion of the dying people were said to have felt this'; 3.6% were said to have asked for euthanasia: C. Seale & J. Addington-Hall, 'Euthanasia: Why People Want to Die Earlier', 648.

16 M. A. Steinberg, J. M. Najman, C. M. Cartwright et al, 'End-of-Life Decision-Making: Community and Medical Practitioners' Perspectives', 131.

17 P. Baume & E. O'Malley, 'Euthanasia: Attitudes and Practices of Medical Practitioners', 137. Similar results were obtained in a 1994 English study: B. J. Ward & P. A. Tate, 'Attitudes Among NHS Doctors to Requests for Euthanasia', 1332.

18 See, more recently, 'Legalise a Lethal Dose, Say Surgeons', *Sydney Morning Herald*, 13 May 2000, p. 5. One study which suggests otherwise reported that over 93% of doctors would have ignored a patient's request for euthanasia, based on a case scenario involving a competent, 56-year-old man with a progressively debilitating disease: C. Waddell, R. M. Clarnette, M. Smith et al, "Treatment Decision-Making at the End of Life: A Survey of Australian Doctors' Attitudes towards Patients' Wishes and Euthanasia', 540. The authors speculate that this result shows that 'doctors believe that assisting a patient to die is an act that negates what they perceive to be the very essence of their profession'. It is possible that this study, contrasting sharply with previous studies showing higher levels of involvement in euthanasia, may simply reflect an understandable reluctance on the part of doctors to commit themselves to euthanising a hypothetical patient with whom they have no sense of relationship.

19 D. E. Meier, C. Emmons, S. Wallenstein et al, 'A National Survey of Physician-Assisted Suicide and Euthanasia in the United States', 1193.

[20] L. Slome, J. Moulton, C. Huffine et al, 'Physicians' Attitudes Toward Assisted Suicide in AIDS', 712.

[21] L. R. Slome, T. F. Mitchell, E. Charlebois et al, 'Physician-Assisted Suicide and Patients with Human Immunodeficiency Virus Disease', 417.

[22] 'Doctors Help in HIV Patients' Suicides', *Australian*, 17 November 1995, p. 3. 41 of 233 doctors (18%) acknowledged an involvement in assisted suicide or euthanasia; 53% were in favour of legalising assisted suicide, and 56% favoured legalising voluntary euthanasia: D. Fagan, 'Euthanasia: Report on 1995 Survey of Attitudes and Practices of Doctors who are Members of The Australian Society for HIV Medicine'.

[23] See J. Dombrink & D. Hillyard, 'Manifestations of Social Agency in the 1994 Reform of Oregon's Assisted Suicide Law', 141–2, 146–7, and, generally, D. Hillyard & J. Dombrink, *Dying Right: The Death With Dignity Movement*.

[24] D. Hillyard & J. Dombrink, 'Using the Law to Redefine Killing in Medical Settings', unpublished paper.

[25] P. Baume & E. O'Malley, 'Euthanasia: Attitudes and Practices of Medical Practitioners', 142.

[26] e.g. M. O'Connor, D. Kissane, O. Spruyt, 'Sedation in the Terminally Ill—A Clinical Perspective', 17; I. Byock, 'The Hospice Clinician's Response to Euthanasia/Physician Assisted Suicide', 1; B. J. Pollard, Letter to the Editor (1994) 161 *Medical Journal of Australia* 572; Dr Rodger Woodruff, 'Facts Needed to Balance Doctors' Euthanasia Push', *Age*, 30 March 1995, p. 12 (letter).

[27] 'Reply from Rodney Syme' (1999) 18 *Monash Bioethics Review* 35–6; B. Farsides, 'Palliative Care—A Euthanasia-Free Zone?', 149; B. Hart, P. Sainsbury & S. Short, 'Whose Dying? A Sociological Critique of the "Good Death"', 75.

[28] See e.g. George P. Smith II, 'Terminal Sedation as Palliative Care: Revalidating a Right to a Good Death', 382; T. Quill, B. Lo, D. Brock, 'Palliative Options of Last Resort', 2099; R. Syme, 'Pharmacological Oblivion Contributes to and Hastens Patients' Deaths', 40; J. A. Billings & S. Block, 'Slow Euthanasia', 21.

[29] See G. Craig, 'Is Sedation without Hydration or Nourishment in Terminal Care Lawful?', 198; P. Schmitz, 'The Process of Dying with and without Feeding and Fluids by Tube', 23.

[30] J. A. Billings & S. Block, 'Slow Euthanasia', 27; similarly, R. Hunt, 'Palliative Care—the Rhetoric-Reality Gap' 123–6; cf. J. Keown, 'Restoring Moral and Intellectual Shape to the Law After *Bland*', 484–5; D. Sulmasy & E. Pellegrino, 'The Rule of Double Effect', 545; T. Tannsjo, 'Terminal Sedation—A Possible Compromise in the Euthanasia Debate?', 13.

[31] R. Syme, 'An Act of Mercy for a Peaceful Exit', *Age*, 7 January 1997, p. A11.

[32] J. A. Billings & S. Block, 'Slow Euthanasia', 26–7; R. Ho, 'Factors Influencing Decisions to Terminate Life: Conditions of Suffering and the Identity of the Terminally Ill', 35.

[33] 'Right to Die Row Returns', *Age*, 2 November 1998, p. 1.

[34] 'Legislative Reform is Needed', *Age*, 7 April 1995, p. 16.

[35] e.g. J. R. Zalcberg & J. D. Buchanan, 'Clinical Issues in Euthanasia', 150; B. Pollard & R. Winton, 'Why Doctors and Nurses Must Not Kill Patients', 426.

[36] W. Reichel & A. J. Dyck, 'Euthanasia: A Contemporary Moral Quandary', 1322. In a more sarcastic vein, Tonti-Filippini writes: 'euthanasia would certainly improve the through-put rates—in the door and out to the morgue': N. Tonti-Filippini, 'Euthanasia Undermines Rights of Sick', *Australian*, 20 July 1994, p. 11.

[37] *Compassion in Dying* v *State of Washington* 79 F. 3d 790 (Ninth Cir. 1996); 1996 U.S. App. LEXIS 3944 at 119–20 per Reinhardt J (for the Court).

[38] J. G. Anderson & D. P. Caddell, 'Attitudes of Medical Professionals Towards Euthanasia', 106.

[39] Gino Concette, 'Life is not Ours to Choose', *Age*, 5 July 1996, p. A13; 'Vatican Condemns Territory Euthanasia Law', *Age*, 4 July 1996, p. A9; 'Ethical Dilemma: Churches United in Condemnation', *Australian*, 27 September 1996, p. 6.

[40] Australian Catholic Bishops' Conference, 'Pastoral Letter to the Catholic People of Australia', May 1995.

[41] H. Kuhse & P. Singer, 'Doctors' Practices and Attitudes Regarding Voluntary Euthanasia', 624–5.

[42] P. Baume, E. O'Malley & A. Bauman, 'Professed Religious Affiliation and the Practice of Euthanasia', 50.

[43] D. E. Meier, C. Emmons, S. Wallenstein et al, 'A National Survey of Physician-Assisted Suicide and Euthanasia in the United States', 1199.

[44] P. Baume, E. O'Malley & A. Bauman, 'Professed Religious Affiliation and the Practice of Euthanasia', 50.

[45] D. P. Caddell & R. R. Newton, 'Euthanasia: American Attitudes Toward the Physician's Role', 1671.

[46] J. Holden, 'Demographics, Attitudes, and Afterlife Beliefs of Right-To-Life and Right-To-Die Organization Members', 525.

[47] Ibid. 526. In Australia, Ho and Penney's 1992 study confirmed that highly religious people were less approving of euthanasia than non-religious people, although they put this down to underlying differences in level of conservatism, rather than religious belief per se: R. Ho & R. K. Penney, 'Euthanasia and Abortion: Personality Correlates for the Decision to Terminate Life', 77.

[48] e.g. Padraic McGuinness, 'Democracy and the Right to Die', *Sydney Morning Herald*, 6 July 1996, p. 33.

[49] Archbishop Sir Frank Little, 'There is Nothing Compassionate in a Doctor's 'Mercy' Killing', *Age*, 17 April 1995, p. 9.

[50] 'Assisted Suicide is not a Synonym for Homicide', *Age*, 17 May 1995, p. 15.

[51] B. Faust, 'Give Patients Free Will Over Life and Death', *Weekend Australian*, 10–11 June 1995, p. 26.

[52] R. Tallis, 'Is There a Slippery Slope?' *Times Literary Supplement*, 12 January 1996, p. 3.

[53] R. Goff, 'A Matter of Life and Death', 17.

[54] R. Hunt, 'Euthanasia: An Issue that Won't Die', p. 9.

[55] R. Manne, 'The Slippery Slope is a Life and Death Argument', *Age*, 14 June 1995, p. 18; see also R. Manne, 'Killing Made Easier', *Age*, 30 November 1998, p. 13.

[56] Max Charlesworth, *Bioethics in a Liberal Society*, p. 53.

[57] J. A. Burgess, 'The Great Slippery-Slope Argument', 169.

[58] See R. Magnusson, 'A Matter of Life and Death', *Sydney Morning Herald*, 26 March 1997, p. 21.

[59] <http://www.worldrtd.org/>.

[60] <http://www.compassionindying.org/>.

[61] <http://www.hemlock.org>.

[62] R. Ogden, 'Non-Physician Assisted Suicide: The Technological Imperative of the Deathing Counterculture', *Death Studies*, 388.

[63] Ibid.; G. Alcorn, 'The Death Thing', *Sydney Morning Herald*, 18 December 1999, p. 9S.

[64] G. Alcorn, 'The Death Thing', above n. 63.

[65] M. Somerville, 'Sentencing Society to Ethical Death', *Age*, 13 November 1995, p. 13. Few could have remained unaffected by a 1995 Dutch documentary, *Death on*

Request, screened in North America, Australia, England and other countries, which showed Dutchman Kees van Wendel de Joode, who suffered from a degenerative muscular disease, being put to death by his family doctor: J. Branegan, 'I Want to Draw the Line Myself', *Time*, 17 March 1997, p. 92.

66 For an Australian perspective, see D. Lupton, *Moral Threats and Dangerous Desires: AIDS in the News Media*; D. Lupton, 'Archetypes of Infection: People with HIV/ AIDS in the Australian Press in the Mid 1990s', 37–53.

67 See, generally, Graeme Stewart (ed.), *Managing HIV*.

68 The literature here is too extensive to cite, but see, e.g., R. S. Magnusson, 'Privacy, Confidentiality and HIV/AIDS Health Care', 51.

69 S. Sontag, *AIDS and Its Metaphors*, pp. 24–5.

70 The Honourable Justice Michael Kirby, 'AIDS: A New Realm of Bereavement'.

71 See C. Seale & J. Addington-Hall, 'Euthanasia: Why People Want to Die Earlier', 652–3.

72 B. Tindall, S. Forde, A. Carr et al, 'Attitudes to Euthanasia and Assisted Suicide in a Group of Homosexual Men with Advanced HIV Disease', 1069.

73 M. Cooke, L. Gourlay, L. Collette et al, 'AIDS Caregivers and the Intention to Hasten AIDS-Related Death', 69.

74 P. J. E. Bindels, A. Krol, E. van Ameijden et al, 'Euthanasia and Physician-Assisted Suicide in Homosexual Men with AIDS', 503. The 2.1% estimate for annual eutha- nasia deaths was made in the well-known Remmelink study: P. van der Maas, J. van Delden, L. Pijnenborg et al, 'Euthanasia and Other Medical Decisions Concerning the End of Life', 669.

75 M. Battin, *Ethical Issues in Suicide*, p. 215.

76 R. Ogden, *Euthanasia, Assisted Suicide & AIDS*; 'Mercy Killing Secret World Re- vealed', *Weekend Sun* (Vancouver), 12 February 1994, pp. A1–2; 'Suicide Study Attracts Continent Wide Attention', *Vancouver Sun*, 15 February 1994, p. B6; 'Van- couver AIDS Suicides Botched', *New York Times*, 14 June 1994, p. C12. Believed to be the first interview-based study into AIDS-related assisted suicide and euthanasia in North America, Ogden's study was based on accounts of involvement by physicians, social workers, counsellors, teachers and writers.

Chapter 4

1 Quoted in 'The Death Thing', *Sydney Morning Herald*, 18 December 1999, p. 9S.

2 J. Walters, 'Aid in Dying is Human, Humane', *Los Angeles Times*, 18 October 1992.

3 The Ad Hoc Committee of the Harvard Medical School, 'A Definition of Irreversible Coma', 339.

4 *Uniform Determination of Death Act* 12 Uniform Laws Annotated 443 (1995 Supp) (United States). In Australia see, e.g., *Human Tissue Act* 1983 (NSW) s. 33; *Human Tissue Act* 1982 (Vic) s. 41.

5 See, generally, R. Howard & D. Miller, 'The Persistent Vegetative State', 341; The Multi-Society Task Force on PVS, 'Medical Aspects of the Persistent Vegetative State', 1499 (Part 1), 1572 (Part 2).

6 *Airedale NHS Trust v Bland* [1993] AC 789 at 856 per Lord Keith.

7 *Matter of Quinlan* 355 A 2d 647 (1976).

8 *Cruzan v Director, Missouri Department of Health* 497 US 261; 111 L Ed 2d 224 (1990).

9 R. Veatch, 'The Impending Collapse of the While-Brain Definition of Death', 23. As Justice Stevens of the US Supreme Court stated in his dissent in the Cruzan case: 'For

patients like Nancy Cruzan, who have no consciousness and no chance of recovery, there is a serious question as to whether the mere persistence of their bodies is 'life' as that word is commonly understood . . . Life, particularly human life, is not commonly thought of as a merely physiological condition or function. Its sanctity is often thought to derive from the impossibility of any such reduction': *Cruzan v Director, Missouri Department of Health* 497 US 261 (1990), 345–6.

[10] N. Ford, 'Killing and Caring Don't Mix', *Sunday Age*, 29 October 1994, p. 14.

[11] P. Singer, *Rethinking Life and Death*, p. 52.

[12] *Airedale NHS Trust v Bland* [1993] AC 789, at 897.

[13] [1993] AC 789, at 858.

[14] [1993] AC 789 at 858–9 per Lord Keith, at 867–8 per Lord Goff, at 876–7 per Lord Lowry, at 883–4 per Lord Browne-Wilkinson, at 897–9 per Lord Mustill. For a recent Australian case in which doctors were completely wrong in their diagnosis of a PVS, see 'A Kiss from Man Doctors Wanted to Let Die', *Sydney Morning Herald* (on-line), 19 April 2000; 'Written Off by Doctors, Now Writing Notes', *Sydney Morning Herald* (on-line), 4 May 2000; *Northridge v Central Sydney Area Health Service* [2000] NSWSC 2141 (29 December 2000).

[15] [1993] AC 789, at 899. Each of the other law Lords' speeches reflected, or were consistent with, Lord Mustill's reasoning: see, at 869 per Lord Goff; at 858 per Lord Keith.

[16] For a contrary view, see J. Keown, 'Restoring Moral and Intellectual Shape to the Law After *Bland*', 485.

[17] [1993] AC 789, at 859 per Lord Keith, at 865 per Lord Goff, at 892–3 per Lord Mustill.

[18] [1993] AC 789, at 858–9 per Lord Keith, at 865–6, 873 per Lord Goff, at 887, 897–8 per Lord Mustill.

[19] [1993] AC 789, at 898 per Lord Mustill.

[20] [1993] AC 789, at 895 per Lord Mustill.

[21] [1993] AC 789, at 865 per Lord Goff.

[22] *Compassion in Dying v State of Washington* 79 F.3d 790, at 824 per Reinhardt J.

[23] *Vacco v Quill*, 521 US 793 (1997), 800–6.

[24] Cf, for a contrary view, J. Keown, 'Restoring Moral and Intellectual Shape to the Law After *Bland*', 484–5.

[25] T. Quill, B. Lo, D. Brock, 'Palliative Options of Last Resort', 2102; cf. T. Tannsjo, 'Terminal Sedation—A Possible Compromise in the Euthanasia Debate?', 15, 17.

[26] See, further, E. Winkler, 'Reflections on the State of Current Debate Over Physician-Assisted Suicide and Euthanasia', 313.

[27] As Justice Thomas of the New Zealand High Court has stated: 'In my view, doctors have a *lawful excuse* to discontinue ventilation when there is no medical justification for continuing that form of medical assistance. To require the administration of a life-support system when such a system has no further medical function or purpose and serves only to defer the death of the patient is to confound the purpose of medicine': *Auckland Area Health Board v Attorney-General* [1993] 1 NZLR 235 at 250 per Thomas J (emphasis supplied); see also at 253–4.

[28] See R. Cohen-Almagor, 'Reflections on the Intriguing Issue of the Right to Die in Dignity', 677.

[29] Cf. Callahan, who argues that 'It is a misuse of the word *killing* to use it when a doctor stops a treatment he believes will no longer benefit the patient—when, that is, he [*sic*] steps aside to allow an eventually inevitable death to occur now rather than later. The only deaths that human beings invented are those that come from direct

killing . . . In the case of omissions, we do not cause death even if we may be judged morally responsible for it': Daniel Callahan, 'When Self-Determination Runs Amok', 53.

30   [1993] AC 789, at 877.

31   England: *St George's NHS Trust v S* [1998] 3 All ER 673, at 685–6; *Airedale NHS Trust v Bland* [1993] AC 789 at 857, 859, 864, 882, 892. United States: e.g.: *Bouvia v Superior Court (Glenchur)* 225 Cal Rptr 297 (1986) (California); *Fosmire v Nicoleau* 551 NYS 2d 876 (1990) (New York). Canada: *Nancy B v Hôtel-Dieu de Québec* (1992) 86 DLR (4th) 385.

32   *Washington v Glucksberg*, 521 US 702 (1997), 725.

33   *Cruzan v Director, Missouri Department of Health* 497 US 261 at 279; 111 L Ed 2d 224 at 242.

34   *California Health & Safety Code* §§ 7185–7194.5. California was the first jurisdiction to enact 'living will' legislation, in 1977. For Australian examples, see, e.g., *Medical Treatment Act* 1988 (Vic); *Consent to Medical Treatment and Palliative Care Act* 1995 (SA).

35   California: *Probate Code* §§ 4700–4806. Australia: eg *Medical Treatment Act* 1988 (Vic) s. 5A; *Consent to Treatment and Palliative Care Act* 1995 (SA) s. 8.

36   *Vacco v Quill*, above n 23; *Washington v Glucksberg*, above n 32.

37   As Lord Browne-Wilkinson said in the *Bland* case, 'a mentally competent patient can at any time put an end to life support systems by refusing his consent to their continuation': [1993] AC 789, at 882.

38   See D. Sulmasy & E. Pellegrino, 'The Rule of Double Effect', 545.

39   P. Cotton, 'Medicine's Position is Both Pivotal and Precarious in Assisted-Suicide Debate', 363.

40   Ibid.

41   For a subtle and useful discussion on this point, see J. A. Billings & S. Block, 'Slow Euthanasia', 21. See also R. Cohen-Almagor, 'Language and Reality at the End of Life', 272.

42   T. Quill, B. Lo, D. Brock, 'Palliative Options of Last Resort', 2102; J. A. Billings & S. Block, 'Slow Euthanasia', 24, 27.

43   A contrary view, put by Smith, is that if 'terminal sedation' can be understood as part of a continuum of palliative care which is grounded in the voluntary choice of the patient—and disassociated from the stigma of euthanasia through reliance upon the principle of double effect—then dying patients are more likely to receive the pain relief they so desperately need. George P. Smith II, *Human Rights and Biomedicine*, pp. 204–6.

44   M. Perron, First Reading Speech to the *Rights of the Terminally Ill Bill* 1995 (NT), Northern Territory Legislative Assembly, 22 February 1995.

45   Marshall Perron, speaking to a conference entitled 'Death and the State', at the Centre for Public Policy, The University of Melbourne, 24 August 1995.

46   'States Grapple with Euthanasia', *Australian*, 26 May 1995, p. 1; 'Kennett Flags Right-to-Die Bill', *Age*, 26 May 1995, p. 1.

47   'AMA Push for States to Reject Euthanasia', *Age*, 26 May 1995, p. 6.

48   'Euthanasia Laws Facing Legal Challenge', *Australian*, 22 February 1996, p. 3. The case failed in the Northern Territory Supreme Court: *Wake v Northern Territory*, unreported, Supreme Court of the Northern Territory, 24 July 1996, Martin CJ, Angel & Mildren JJ; 'Supreme Court Rejects Challenge on Euthanasia', *Australian*, 25 July 1996, p. 7.

49   'Right-to-Die Law to Take Effect By May', *Age*, 21 February 1996, p. 3.

50 'Plea From the Grave', *Sunday Herald-Sun* (Melbourne), 8 October 1995, pp. 1, 4.

51 'First Death Under NT Mercy Law', *Age*, 26 September 1996, p. 1; 'Euthanasia Splits Nation', *Australian*, 27 September 1996, p. 1.

52 'Darwin Doctor's Deadly Device Makes a Macabre Display', *Sydney Morning Herald*, 8 July 2000, p. 15.

53 'Press "Yes" to Die Now', *Age*, 17 April 1996, p. A13.

54 'Mercy Death Renews Outcry', *Age*, 7 January 1997, p. 1. For a review of the cases of 7 patients who died, or took formal steps under the Territory legislation, see D. Kissane, A. Street, P. Nitschke, 'Seven Deaths in Darwin: Case Studies Under the Rights of the Terminally Ill Act, Northern Territory, Australia', 1097.

55 In October 1996 the NSW Parliament rejected euthanasia on a scale of four-to-one: 'Open House Slams Door on Euthanasia', *Australian*, 17 October 1996, p. 1; 'Historic Debate Full of Emotion', *Australian*, 17 October 1996, p. 4.

56 'Holy Alliance', *Weekend Australian*, 29–30 March 1997, p. 19; 'Andrews Alliance Ready to Fight On', *Weekend Australian*, 29–30 March 1997, p. 1; 'The Mandate of Heaven', *Sydney Morning Herald*, 31 July 1999, Spectrum, p. 6.

57 'Euthanasia Law Unclear and Unsafe: Senators', *Australian*, 7 March 1997, p. 4.

58 'Now More Want to Die', *Age*, 27 September 1996, p. 1.

59 'Euthanasia: Son Changes his Mind', *Australian*, 4 December 1996, p. 1; 'Political Pawn', *Weekend Australian*, 7–8 December 1996, p. 23; 'Dent Sees it as it Is', *Mercury* (Hobart), 5 December 1996, p. 18.

60 'Premiers Condemn Assault on Rights', *Australian*, 26 March 1997, p. 2; 'Kennett Spearheads Call to Allow Euthanasia', *Australian*, 14 April 1997, p. 3.

61 'Euthanasia Legal by 2007, Tips Perron', *Sydney Morning Herald*, 26 March 1997, p. 6.

62 A. Alpers & B. Lo, 'Physician-Assisted Suicide in Oregon', 483. For a comprehensive account of the processes surrounding the Oregon Act, see D. Hillyard & J. Dombrink, *Dying Right: The Death With Dignity Movement*.

63 The Act was initially declared to be unconstitutional on the ground that it offended the Equal Protection Clause of the Fourteenth Amendment: *Lee v State of Oregon* 891 F Supp 1429 (D Or 1995). This was overturned by an appeals court, which ruled that the plaintiff had no standing to bring the action. The Supreme Court refused to hear a further appeal.

64 'Physician-Assisted Suicide Law Faces Second Public Vote in November', 9 June 1997, Last Rights Information Centre, US news bulletins (archives): <http://www.rights.org/deathnet/bulletins.html>.

65 'Oregon Votes to Keep Assisted Suicide Law', 5 November 1997, Last Rights Information Centre, US news bulletins (archives), above n. 64.

66 'House Votes to Prohibit Federal Drugs for Assisted Suicide: 271 to 156' 27 October 1999, Last Rights Information Centre, US news bulletins (archives), above n. 64.

67 'Bush May Act on Assisted Suicide' 3 February 2001, Last Rights Information Centre, US news bulletins (archives), above n. 64. Regular updates are available from the site referenced above.

68 J. Griffiths, A. Bood, H. Weyers, *Euthanasia & Law in the Netherlands*, p. 99. For comprehensive accounts of the Dutch position, see Griffiths, Bood and Weyers, pp. 99–107, and D. Thomasma, T. Kimbrough-Kushner, G. Kimsma & C. Cieslieski-Carlucci (eds), *Asking to Die: Inside the Dutch Debate about Euthanasia*.

69 While termination of life upon request and assisted suicide will remain illegal under the new law, existing grounds for immunity (recognised in case law) will be imported into the criminal law (new sub-sections will be added to the Penal Code setting out

the defence): see Dutch Penal Code, ss. 293–4. For media reports, see 'Netherlands Moves to Legalize Assisted Suicide', *Washington Post*, 29 November 2000, p. A32; 'Dutch Parliament Passes Euthanasia Bill', *Sydney Morning Herald*, 29 November 2000.

70 For English translations of the Dutch law, see <http://www.minjust.nl:8080/c_actual/ persber/>, and click on press releases for 28 November 2000. The following discussion also draws on press releases and commentary linked as at February 2001 to the web site of the Dutch Ministry of Health, Welfare and Sport.

71 In *Chabot*, the Dutch Supreme court commented that 'A claim of necessity can therefore not be excluded simply on the ground that the patient's unbearable suffering, without prospect of improvement, does not have a somatic cause and that the patient is not in the terminal phase': John Griffiths, 'Assisted Suicide in the Netherlands: The *Chabot* Case', 237.

72 'Dutch Take Step to Make Assisted Suicide Legal', *Los Angeles Times*, 29 November 2000, p. 4.

73 Ibid.

74 The authors of the study stated that the patients whose life was terminated without an explicit request were 'close to death and were suffering grievously', and that in more than half of these cases the decision was discussed with the patient or the patient had indicated in a previous phase of their illness a desire for euthanasia if suffering became unbearable: P. van der Maas, J. van Delden, L. Pijnenborg et al, 'Euthanasia and Other Medical Decisions Concerning the End of Life', 669.

75 H. Kuhse, P. Singer, P. Baume et al, 'End-of-Life Decisions in Australian Medical Practice', 191.

76 'Choice Key to Law's Death Bill', *Dominion* (Wellington), 16 August 1995, p. 10; 'MPs Throw out Euthanasia Bill', *Dominion*, 17 August 1995, p. 1.

77 'Their Lordships on Euthanasia', *The Lancet* 430.

78 'Canada May Cut Euthanasia Penalties', *Australian*, 8 June 1995, p. 9; Special Senate Committee on Euthanasia and Assisted Suicide, *Final Report*, 6 June 1995: <http:// www.rights.org/deathnet/senate.html>.

79 *Re Rodriguez and Attorney-General of British Columbia* (1993) 107 DLR (4th) 342.

80 App. No. 10083/82 v *United Kingdom* (1984) 6 EHRR 140.

Chapter 5

1 K. Andrews, 'Are We Past Caring?', *Sunday Age*, 14 July 1996, p. 16.

2 S. Kalichman & K. Sikkema, 'Psychological Sequelae of HIV Infection and AIDS: Review of Empirical Findings', 623–5.

3 M. O'Dowd, D. Biderman & F. McKegney, 'Incidence of Suicidality in AIDS and HIV-Positive Patients Attending a Psychiatry Outpatient Program', 33; F. McKegney & M. O'Dowd, 'Suicidality and HIV Status', 396; J. Rabkin, R. Remien, L. Katoff et al, 'Suicidality in AIDS Long-Term Survivors: What is the Evidence?', 401. Suggested reasons for this may include AIDS-dementia and other neurological disorders, less distress and uncertainty following the onset of AIDS, and acceptance and refocusing.

4 T. Coté, R. Biggar, A. Dannenberg, 'Risk of Suicide Among Persons with AIDS', 2066; P. Marzuk, H. Tierney, K. Tardiff et al, 'Increased Risk of Suicide in Persons with AIDS', 1333.

5 F. Starace, 'Suicidal Behaviour in People Infected with Human Immunodeficiency Virus: A Literature Review', 67–9.

6 e.g. C. Alfonso, M. Cohen, A. Aladjem et al, 'HIV Seropositivity as a Major Risk Factor for Suicide in the General Hospital', 368.

[7] cf. Werth, who questions this assumption: J. Werth, 'Rational Suicide Reconsidered: AIDS as an Impetus for Change', 66.

[8] S. Schneider, S. Taylor, C. Hammen et al, 'Factors Influencing Suicide Intent in Gay and Bisexual Suicide Ideators: Differing Models for Men with and without Human Immunodeficiency Virus', 784.

[9] Ibid., 785.

[10] P. Marzuk, 'Suicide and Terminal Illness', 502.

[11] Similarly, Kleinman contrasts a narrow 'biomedical' model of *disease* with a broader, 'biopsychosocial' model encompassing the lived experience of the sick person: A. Kleinman, *The Illness Narratives: Suffering, Healing & the Human Condition*, pp. 3–6.

[12] M. Little, 'Assisted Suicide, Suffering and the Meaning of a Life', 291.

[13] A 'fracky neck' refers to a fractured femur. 'Brompton's cocktail' was a cocktail of opiates and analgesics which was used in the past for pain relief.

[14] Quoted in R. Tallis, 'Is There a Slippery Slope?', *Times Literary Supplement*, 12 January 1996, p. 3.

[15] See R. Syme, 'A Patient's Right to a Good Death', 204.

[16] See C. Seale & J. Addington-Hall, 'Euthanasia: Why People Want to Die Earlier', 647; see also L. Ganzini, H. Nelson, T. Schmidt et al, 'Physicians' Experiences with the Oregon Death With Dignity Act', 559.

[17] P. van der Maas, J. van Delden, L. Pijnenborg et al, 'Euthanasia and Other Medical Decisions Concerning the End of Life', 672.

[18] *Compassion in Dying* v *State of Washington*, 79 F.3d 790 (Ninth Cir. 1996); 1996 U.S. App. LEXIS 3944, at 3161–2. The decision was overturned on appeal; see Chapter 4.

[19] See, further, S. Miles, 'Physicians and Their Patients' Suicides', 1786.

[20] M. O'Connor, 'Nurses and Euthanasia—Some Issues', 34; R. Twycross, 'Where there is Hope, there is Life: A View from the Hospice' in J. Keown (ed.), *Euthanasia Examined: Ethical, Clinical and Legal Perspectives*, p. 143.

[21] C. Alfonso & M. Adler Cohen, 'HIV-Dementia and Suicide', 45.

Chapter 6

[1] Daniel Callahan, 'When Self-Determination Runs Amok', 55.

[2] H. Kuhse & P. Singer, 'Doctors' Practices and Attitudes Regarding Voluntary Euthanasia', 623–7; P. Baume & E. O'Malley, 'Euthanasia: Attitudes and Practices of Medical Practitioners', 137–44.

[3] This may not be entirely fair. Warren, a therapist, noted that assisting death was only a 'tiny but extremely distressing part of my work'. Other interviewees who supported legalisation acknowledged that primary control over the euthanasia process (under a legalised regime) would likely rest with doctors.

[4] See, e.g., S. Aranda & M. O'Connor, 'Euthanasia, Nursing and Care of the Dying: Rethinking Kuhse and Singer', 21.

[5] See also R. S. Magnusson & P. H. Ballis, 'The Response of Health Care Workers to AIDS Patients' Requests for Euthanasia', 312.

[6] D. Asch, 'The Role of Critical Care Nurses in Euthanasia and Assisted Suicide', 1374; see also R. Leiser, T. Mitchell, J. Hahn et al, 972 (letter); H. Kuhse & P. Singer, 'Euthanasia: A Survey of Nurses' Attitudes and Practices', 21.

[7] See F. Lewins, 'The Development of Bioethics and the Issue of Euthanasia: Regulating, De-Regulating or Re-Regulating?', 132; E. Willis, *Medical Dominance*.

[8] T. Walker, J. Littlewood & M. Pickering, 'Death in the News: The Public Invigilation of Private Emotion', 581.

[9] See C. Seale, 'Heroic Death', 597.

[10] As Seale states: 'In late modernity love is expressed through talk; if talk is absent there is nothing to reassure individuals that love is still there. Because unawareness involves silence it contains the threat of abandonment. Confessional talk provides more convincing proof of emotional accompaniment. With funeral rituals having lost much of their power, caring talk before death becomes, in the discourse of awareness, an act of anticipatory mourning that wards off the threat of abandonment and isolation, now feared far more than the older terrors of evil spirits': C. Seale, 'Heroic Death', 611.

[11] e.g. K. Pugh, I. O'Donnell & J. Catalan, 'Suicide and HIV Disease', 397; I. O'Donnell, J. Catalan & R. Farmer, 'Suicidal Behaviour and HIV Disease: A Case Report', 411.

[12] See also P. Marzuk, 'Suicidal Behaviour and HIV Illness', 367.

[13] S. Miles, 'Physicians and Their Patients' Suicides', 1786.

[14] HIV/AIDS health carers have reported examples of discrimination and stigma as a result of their work; e.g. L. Bennett, 'The Experience of Nurses Working with Hospitalized AIDS Patients', 133–6.

[15] R. Barbour, 'The Impact of Working with People with HIV/AIDS: A Review of the Literature', 221; D. Silverman, 'Psychosocial Impact of HIV-Related Caregiving on Health Providers: A Review and Recommendations for the Role of Psychiatry', 705; B. Kelly, L. Todhunter, B. Raphael, 'HIV Care: the Impact on the Doctor', 150.

[16] L. Bennett, 'The Experience of Nurses Working with Hospitalized AIDS Patients', 138–40; L. Bennett, P. Michie, S. Kippax, 'Qualitative Analysis of Burnout and its Associated Factors in AIDS Nursing', 181.

[17] N. Schram, 'Overwhelmed by AIDS', *Washington Post Weekly Journal of Medicine*, 18 June 1991, 14, quoted by the Honourable Justice Michael Kirby, 'AIDS: A New Realm of Bereavement', 12.

[18] M. Cleeman & E. Crock, 'Nursing People with HIV/AIDS—A Way of Life'.

[19] e.g. J. Werth, 'Rational Suicide Reconsidered: AIDS as an Impetus for Change', 65; T. Quill, C. Cassel, D. Meier, 'Care of the Hopelessly Ill: Proposed Clinical Criteria for Physician-Assisted Suicide', 1380; R. Ogden, 'Palliative Care and Euthanasia: A Continuum of Care?', 82; B. Farsides, 'Palliative Care—a Euthanasia-Free Zone?', 149.

[20] e.g. C. Cassel, 'Physician-Assisted Suicide: Progress or Peril?' in D. Thomasma & T. Kushner (eds), *Birth to Death: Science and Bioethics*, pp. 218–30.

Chapter 7

[1] R. Ogden, *Euthanasia, Assisted Suicide and AIDS*, p. 83.

[2] Stephen Jamison, 'When Drugs Fail: Assisted Deaths and Not-So-Lethal Drugs' in M. P. Battin & A. G. Lipman (eds), *Drug Use in Assisted Suicide and Euthanasia*, p. 223.

[3] M. Cooke, L. Gourlay, L. Collette et al, 'Informal Caregivers and the Intention to Hasten AIDS-Related Death', 74.

[4] But see Derek Humphry's *Final Exit* (paperback edition); M. P. Battin & A. G. Lipman (eds), *Drug Use in Assisted Suicide and Euthanasia*.

[5] In fact, Bob admitted in interview that having used all the morphine and syringes from his doctor's bag in the euthanasia process of this patient, he was unable to administer an injection during an urgent house call he had conducted just before the interview.

6 See D. J. Cook, G. H. Guyatt, R. Jaeschke et al, 'Determinants in Canadian Health Care Workers of the Decision to Withdraw Life Support From the Critically Ill', 703; E. Fox & C. Stocking, 'Ethics Consultants' Recommendations for Life-Prolonging Treatment of Patients in a Persistent Vegetative State', 2578.

Chapter 8

1 M. Foucault, *The History of Sexuality: An Introduction*, p. 59.
2 J. Gee, G. Hull & C. Lankshear, *The New Work Order: Behind the Language of the New Capitalism*, p. 11.
3 P. Ewick & S. Silbey, 'Subversive Stories and Hegemonic Tales: Towards a Sociology of Narrative', 198.
4 J. Beckford, 'Accounting for Conversion', 250.

Chapter 9

1 Quoted in 'C. Henderson, C. Ryan & T. Aubin, 'A Fight to the Death', *Who*, 23 February 1998, p. 35.
2 This was the only occasion on which several interviewees were concentrated within the same practice. Not all the doctors carried on full-time practice within that clinic.
3 Damian, for example, explained that part of his knowledge of euthanasia came from patients whose lovers had been under the care of another doctor. In the course of exploring with the client how the lover had died, Damian would be told confidentially that the lover's doctor had assisted their death.
4 The extent to which the funeral industry is complicit in burying and cremating the evidence of assisted death suggests interesting possibilities for future research.

Chapter 10

1 Marshall Perron, former Chief Minister of the Northern Territory, speech given at 'Death and the State', a conference organised by the Centre for Public Policy, The University of Melbourne, 24 August 1995.
2 Tom L. Beauchamp & James F. Childress, *Principles of Biomedical Ethics*, p. 7.
3 P. van Reyk, 'HIV and Choosing to Die' in Greame Stewart (ed.), *Managing HIV*, p. 161.
4 See S. Nuland, 'Physician-Assisted Suicide and Euthanasia in Practice', 583–4; R. Ogden, 'Non-Physician Assisted Suicide: The Technological Imperative of the Deathing Counterculture', *Death Studies*, 395.
5 Stephen Jamison, 'When Drugs Fail: Assisted Deaths and Not-So-Lethal Drugs' in M. P. Battin & A. G. Lipman (eds), *Drug Use in Assisted Suicide and Euthanasia*, p. 241.
6 Ibid.
7 P. H. Ballis & R. S. Magnusson, 'Treatment decision-making at the end of life: a survey of Australian doctors' attitudes towards patients' wishes and euthanasia' (letter).
8 For an English translation, see John Griffiths, 'Assisted Suicide in the Netherlands: The *Chabot* Case', 232.
9 According to the Supreme Court, the 'necessity' defence operates where a doctor is faced with conflicting duties: 'the duty to preserve life and the duty as a doctor to do

everything possible to relieve the unbearable suffering, without prospect for improvement, of a patient committed to his [*sic*] care': ibid., 236.

[10] B. Keizer, 'In Search of a Decent Death', *Guardian Weekly* (London), 13 April 1997, p. 24.

Chapter 11

[1] Quoted in P. Span, 'Philosophy of Death', *Washington Post*, 9 December 1999, p. C2.

[2] M. Gawenda, 'Change of Heart on Euthanasia', *Age*, 27 May 1996, p. A15.

[3] R. Manne, 'The Slippery Slope is a Life and Death Argument', *Age*, 14 June 1995, p. 18.

[4] B. Tobin, letter, *Australian*, 24 May 1995, p. 10.

[5] R. Ogden, 'Non-Physician Assisted Suicide: The Technological Imperative of the Deathing Counterculture', *Death Studies*, 396.

[6] This point is well made by Buchanan: 'If relatives or health professionals are chronically fatigued by care demands, or ambivalent about the patient in some way, their support will subtly diminish, leading the ill person to feeling they are a burden and come to believe they should "get out of the way"': John Buchanan in Simon Chapman & Stephen Leeder, *The Last Right? Australians Take Sides on the Right to Die*, p. 24. A recent study of informal care givers (rather than health care workers) in San Francisco suggests that this risk may be over-stated: M. Cooke, L. Gourlay, L. Collette et al, 'Informal Caregivers and the Intention to Hasten AIDS-Related Death', 73, 75.

Chapter 12

[1] P. van der Maas, J. van Delden, L. Pijnenborg et al, 'Euthanasia and Other Medical Decisions Concerning the End of Life', 669.

[2] B. A. Santamaria, for example, a long-time Australian commentator, writes: 'As the mass of old and sick people increases in an ageing society which will find it too expensive to keep them alive; as the pressure to balance budgets and to reduce, if not eliminate most social services progresses to its ultimate conclusion, the result is predictable . . . It can thus be guaranteed that voluntary euthanasia will end in the "execution" . . . of thousands of old and helpless people at the orders of anonymous medical bureaucrats': 'Euthanasia's Bell Tolls for Thee', *Weekend Australian*, 13–14 July 1995, p. 22.

[3] e.g. photograph accompanying articles in *Age*, 2 July 1996, p. A3.

[4] Professor Peter Baume, a former Australian federal Parliamentarian argues, 'It is simply not possible for me to care for someone in agony of body and spirit, with unrelieved distress, to ignore their repeated requests for assistance, to ignore their pleas that they be allowed to die, and still to say that I am a caring person or a good doctor': P. Baume, 'Voluntary Euthanasia and the Liberal Tradition', 9th Lionel Murphy Memorial Lecture, 30 November 1995, p. 5. Similarly, as the majority of the United States Court of Appeals for the Ninth Circuit wrote: 'Those who believe strongly that death must come without physician assistance are free to follow that creed, be they doctors or patients. They are not free, however, to force their views, their religious convictions, or their philosophies on all the other members of a democratic society, and to compel those whose values differ with theirs to die painful, protracted, and agonizing deaths': *Compassion in Dying* v *Washington* 79 F.3d 790, 893 (9th Cir. 1996).

[5] Jane gave an example of a 'particularly bitchy' patient who sent a 'really nasty letter' to an acquaintance, which he posted the morning that he died. The letter was along

the lines of 'by the time you read this I'll be dead, and here are all the things I've always felt about you'.

6 See, further, R. S. Magnusson, 'The Sanctity of Life and the Right to Die: Social and Jurisprudential Aspects of the Euthanasia Debate in Australia and the United States', 60–1.

7 Russell Ogden, who published a study of assisted suicide and euthanasia in the HIV/AIDS community in Vancouver in 1994, was requested by the Royal Canadian Mounted Police, British Columbia prosecutors, and the Coroner, to disclose the names of his interviewees. Later, when he was called to testify in an inquest before the Vancouver regional Coroner, he refused to identify his sources in connection with one case: 'Vancouver AIDS Suicides Botched', *New York Times*, 14 June 1994, p. C12. The Coroner held a finding of contempt in abeyance, pending further argument, but later accepted Ogden's submission that the public interest supported a privilege from disclosure (personal communication). See, further, T. Palys & J. Lowman, 'Ethical and Legal Strategies for Protecting Confidential Research Information', 39.

8 'Vancouver AIDS Suicides Botched', *New York Times*, 14 June 1994, p. C12.

9 e.g. B. Pollard, *The Challenge of Euthanasia*, p. 111.

10 See L. R. Slome, T. F. Mitchell, E. Charlebois et al, 'Physician-Assisted Suicide and Patients with Human Immunodeficiency Virus Disease', 420.

11 Ibid.; cf. D. E. Meier, C. Emmons, S. Wallenstein et al, 'A National Survey of Physician-Assisted Suicide and Euthanasia in the United States', 1193.

Chapter 13

1 Quoted in David C. Thomasma, Thomasine Kimbrough-Kushner, Gerrit K. Kimsma & Chris Cieslieski-Carlucci (eds), *Asking to Die: Inside the Dutch Debate about Euthanasia*, pp. 386–7.

2 See R. Dworkin, *Life's Dominion: An Argument About Abortion and Euthanasia*, p. 199.

3 *Cruzan v Director, Missouri Department of Health* 497 US 261 (1990) at 310–1 (Justice Brennan, dissenting).

4 R. Manne, 'The Slippery Slope is a Life and Death Argument', *Age*, 14 June 1995, p. 18.

5 John Keown, 'Euthanasia in the Netherlands: Sliding Down the Slippery Slope?' in J. Keown (ed.), *Euthanasia Examined: Ethical, Clinical and Legal Perspectives*, p. 289.

6 B. Pollard & R. Winton, 'Why Doctors and Nurses Must Not Kill Patients', 427, 428.

7 See, further, J. Burgess, 'The Great Slippery-Slope Argument', 169; J. Griffiths, 'The Slippery Slope: Are the Dutch Sliding Down or Are they Clambering Up?' in David C. Thomasma, Thomasine Kimbrough-Kushner, Gerrit K. Kimsma & Chris Cieslieski-Carlucci (eds) *Asking to Die: Inside the Dutch Debate about Euthanasia*, pp. 96–7.

8 The available evidence, in fact, points the other way. In 1997, Kuhse, Singer, Baume et al published survey results comparing end-of-life decision-making in Australia with the well-known Dutch study published by van der Maas et al in 1991: H. Kuhse, P. Singer, P. Baume et al, 'End-of-Life Decisions in Australian Medical Practice', 191. They estimated that in 1995/96 1.7% of Australian deaths were the result of active voluntary euthanasia (compared to 2.1% of Dutch deaths in 1991). They estimated that a further 3.5% of Australian deaths involved the termination of life without the patient's explicit request (compared to 0.8% of Dutch deaths in 1991).

9 John Griffiths, 'Assisted Suicide in the Netherlands: the *Chabot* Case', 247.

[10] Griffiths, Bood and Weyers point out that 'Dutch practice, about which a great deal is known, is used to condemn not so much the Dutch but, via them, proposals for liberalization elsewhere where very little is known about actual practice': John Griffiths, Alex Bood, Heleen Weyers, *Euthanasia and Law in the Netherlands*, p. 21.

[11] Ibid., p. 303 (emphasis supplied).

[12] Elaine Thompson, Associate Professor of Public Policy, University of New South Wales, speaking to a conference entitled 'Death and the State', at the Centre for Public Policy, The University of Melbourne, 24 August 1995.

[13] Steve Dow, 'Live & Let Die', *Australian Magazine*, 7–8 August 1999, p. 33.

[14] e.g. 'Specialists Blast Talk of Secret Euthanasia', *Weekend Australian*, 18–19 January 1997, p. 10.

[15] e.g. 'Euthanasia Survey Ideological: Ethicist', *Australian*, 25 February 1997, p. 6, reporting on a submission by Dr John Fleming, director of the Southern Cross Bioethics Institute in Adelaide, to the Australian Senate hearings on the *Euthanasia Laws Bill* 1996 (Cth).

[16] R. Ogden, 'Palliative Care and Euthanasia: A Continuum of Care?', 82.

[17] Senators' level of engagement with the policy implications of current illegal practices was embarrassingly inadequate: see Senate Legal and Constitutional Legislation Committee, *Consideration of Legislation Referred to the Committee: Euthanasia Laws Bill 1996*, March 1997, p. 128. Arguments by advocates of legalisation concerning current illegal practices were cited in the Report, but were not apparently addressed by opponents: ibid., pp. 62–3. The authors' submission on these issues was ignored.

[18] Kevin Andrews, *Euthanasia Laws Bill* 1996, second reading speech, Australian House of Representatives, 28 October 1996.

[19] T. Abbott, 'Act of Compassion or Merely Killing?', *Australian*, 27 September 1996, p. 13.

[20] P. Singer, 'Time Bids Farewell to the Politics of Fear', *Age*, 10 October 1996, p. A15; see also 'Euthanasia Is An Option, Says Nelson', *Age*, 22 May 1995, p. 5. Similarly, Faust puts her finger on the pulse when she writes: 'The Australian Medical Association doesn't like euthanasia because it might lead to increased State regulation of their highly individualistic profession': B. Faust, 'Give Patients Free Will Over Life and Death', *Weekend Australian*, 10–11 June 1995, p. 26.

[21] R. McGarvie, 'Euthanasia and the Issue of Consent', *Age*, 21 April 1995, p. 12.

[22] e.g. B. A. Santamaria, 'Tacit Consent to Euthanasia', *Weekend Australian*, 1–2 April 1995, p. 28; similarly, 'Death Doctor Not Likely to be Charged', *Sydney Morning Herald*, 14 April 1997, p. 6; 'Charge Euthanasia Doctors, Say Right to Life', *Age*, 27 March 1995, p. 1. Margaret Somerville, by contrasts, suggests that doctors who perform euthanasia should be charged with medical negligence: Brian Pollard, 'Distracters in the Contemporary Debate on Euthanasia' in John Morgan (ed.), *An Easeful Death? Perspectives on Death, Dying and Euthanasia*, p. 74.

[23] A. Meisel, J. Jernigan, S. Youngner, 'Prosecutors and End-of-Life Decision Making', 1089.

[24] 'Along with prostitution, drug dealing and, formerly, male homosexual acts, abortion illustrates the phenomenon of unenforceable laws', writes Beatrice Faust. 'Any law prohibiting the exchange of sought-after goods or services between willing buyers and sellers will be almost impossible to enforce': 'Bans on the Unbannable Devalue the Law', *Weekend Australian*, 7–8 June 1997, p. 25. The same might be said of euthanasia.

[25] 'Andrews Won't Stop Me, Doctor Vows', *Australian*, 26 March 1997, p. 2.

26 'The Father, Son and Euthanasia', *Age*, 13 April 1998; 'The Doctor, the Son and Euthanasia', *Age*, 15 April 1998, p. 15; 'Interpreting the Death of Jesus', *Age*, 15 April 1998, p. 14; 'Lifelines', *Australian Magazine*, 13–14 March 1999, p. 10. Whatever its theological merits, Syme's mischief radiates a measure of compassion that contrasts sharply with former Anglican Archbishop Hollingworth, who believes that euthanasia advocates show 'little awareness of the Christian experience that people may be redeemed and transfigured through their suffering': 'Euthanasia Rules Out', *Herald Sun* (Melbourne), 10 August 1998, p. 15.

27 'Right to Die Row Returns', *Age*, 2 November 1998, p. 1; 'Ending the Pain of Dying', *Age*, 2 November 1998, p. 15; 'Doctors Query Assisted-Death Claim', *Age*, 5 November 1998, p. 3; 'Specialist Protests at a Cruel End', *Age*, 30 August 1999, p. 3; R. Syme, 'Pharmacological Oblivion Contributes to and Hastens Patients' Deaths', 40.

28 'Mum Begs: Let Me Die', *Sun Herald*, 14 March 1999, p. 2.

29 'Euthanasia Mum Fights On', *Sunday Telegraph* (Sydney), 24 October 1999, p. 26.

30 Edmund Pellegrino, 'Ethics', 1675.

31 e.g. 'The Death Thing', *Sydney Morning Herald*, 18 December 1999, p. S9.

32 Cf. Charles H. Baron, Clyde Bergstresser, Dan W. Brock et al, 'A Model State Act to Authorize and Regulate Physician-Assisted Suicide', 21–2 (one prominent example of a model statute for assisted death, which only extends to assisted suicide and makes the treating physician's presence at the time of death optional).

33 Timothy E. Quill, Christine K. Cassel, Diane E. Meier, 'Care of the Hopelessly Ill: Proposed Clinical Criteria for Physician-Assisted Suicide', 1381.

34 See, e.g., Barbara Crouch, 'Toxicological Issues with Drugs used to End Life' in M. P. Battin & A. G. Lipman (eds), *Drug Use in Assisted Suicide and Euthanasia*, p. 211.

35 e.g. Guy Benrubi, 'Euthanasia—the Need for Procedural Safeguards', 197; Alfred Jonsen, 'To Help the Dying Die—A New Duty for Anesthesiologists?', 225; and resulting correspondence at 79: 402–5.

36 In *Compassion in Dying* v *Washington* 79 F.3d 790 (9th Cir. 1996), the Ninth Circuit Court of Appeal held that the prohibition on physician-assisted suicide in Washington State infringed the 'liberty' interest United States citizens enjoy under the Due Process Clause of the Fourteenth Amendment to the United States Constitution. In *Quill* v *Vacco*, 80 F.3d 716 (2d Cir. 1996), the Second Circuit Court of Appeal invalidated New York State's prohibition on physician-assisted suicide on the basis that it violated the Equal Protection Clause of the Fourteenth Amendment. Both decisions were subsequently reversed by the United States Supreme Court: *Washington* v *Glucksberg*, 521 US 702 (1997); *Vacco* v *Quill*, 521 US 793 (1997). Both decisions are on the internet: <http://supct.law.cornell.edu/supct/>.

37 As discussed below, the defence of 'necessity' in the Netherlands stems from the Dutch Supreme Court's interpretation of the defence of *force majeure*, which is recognised in Article 40 of the Dutch Criminal Code. Article 40 states 'Any person who was compelled by *force majeure* to commit an offence shall not be criminally liable'.

38 This defence was a particular application of the defence of *force majeure* (Article 40 of the Dutch Criminal Code), which applied to a doctor who was faced with conflicting duties; for further discussion, see Margaret Otlowski, *Voluntary Euthanasia and the Common Law*, pp. 392–404.

39 John Griffiths, Alex Bood, Heleen Weyers, *Euthanasia & Law in the Netherlands*, pp. 114–16; Margaret Otlowski, *Voluntary Euthanasia and the Common Law*, p. 442.

[40] Margaret Otlowski, *Voluntary Euthanasia and the Common Law*, pp. 409–16; John Griffiths, 'Recent Developments in the Netherlands Concerning Euthanasia and Other Medical Behavior that Shortens Life', 383.

[41] R. S. Magnusson, 'The Sanctity of Life and the Right to Die: Social and Jurisprudential Aspects of the Euthanasia Debate in Australia and the United States', 67.

[42] e.g. John Keown, 'Euthanasia in the Netherlands: Sliding Down the Slippery Slope' in J. Keown (ed.), *Euthanasia Examined: Ethical, Clinical and Legal Perspectives*, p. 265.

[43] Howard Brody, 'Assisted Death—A Compassionate Response to a Medical Failure', 1386, 1382.

[44] Gerrit van der Wal, Paul J. van der Maas, Jacqueline M Bosma et al, 'Evaluation of the Notification Procedure for Physician-Assisted Death in the Netherlands', 1707.

[45] John Griffiths, 'Assisted Suicide in the Netherlands: The *Chabot* Case', 238.

[46] Cf. I. Kennedy, 'The Right to Die', in C. M. Mazzoni (ed.), *A Legal Framework for Bioethics*, pp. 181–97.

[47] A. Caplan, L. Snyder & K. Faber-Langendoen, 'The Role of Guidelines in the Practice of Physician-Assisted Suicide', 476; J. Tulksy, R. Ciampa & E. Rosen, 'Responding to Legal Requests for Physician-Assisted Suicide', 494.

[48] L. Snyder & A. Caplan, 'Assisted Suicide: Finding Common Ground', 469.

[49] Commonwealth Department of Community Services and Health, *Legal Issues Relating to AIDS and Intravenous Drug Use*, February 1991, p. 7.

[50] See, generally, J. Godwin, J. Hamblin, D. Patterson & D. Buchanan, *Australian HIV/ AIDS Legal Guide*, p. 242ff.

[51] Mark Kleiman, 'AIDS, Vice and Public Policy', 337–9, 363–4; Paul Drielsma, 'AIDS Policy and Public Health Models: an Australian Analysis', 95–7.

[52] e.g. Kumar Amarasekara, 'Euthanasia and the Quality of Legislative Safeguards', 1; Timothy E. Quill, Christine K. Cassel, Diane E. Meier, 'Care of the Hopelessly Ill: Proposed Clinical Criteria for Physician-Assisted Suicide', 1380; Charles H. Baron, Clyde Bergstresser, Dan W. Brock et al, 'A Model State Act to Authorize and Regulate Physician-Assisted Suicide', 1; Raphael Cohen-Almagor, 'A Circumscribed Plea for Voluntary Physician-Assisted Suicide' in R. Cohen-Almagor (ed.), *Medical Ethics at the Dawn of the 21st Century*, p. 127.

[53] *Rights of the Terminally Ill Act* 1995 (NT) s. 4.

[54] This ensures that there is no prospect for improvement. See John Griffiths, Alex Bood, Heleen Weyers, *Euthanasia & Law in the Netherlands*, pp. 101–2. This position has not changed as a result of the November 2000 amendments to the Dutch Penal Code.

[55] *Death with Dignity Act* (Oregon) ss. 1.01, 2.01.

[56] 'If one accepts, as I do, that persistently suicidal patients are, indeed, terminal, then one must ask whether a persistently suicidal state can be as reliably diagnosed as an incurable illness. I believe in some cases, like that of my patient, it can', states Dr Boudewijn Chabot (in conversation with Arlene Klotzko: David C. Thomasma, Thomasine Kimbrough-Kushner, Gerrit K. Kimsma & Chris Cieslieski-Carlucci (eds), *Asking to Die: Inside the Dutch Debate about Euthanasia*, p. 378.

[57] Yale Kamisar, 'Physician-Assisted Suicide: the Last Bridge to Active Voluntary Euthanasia' in John Keown (ed.), *Euthanasia Examined: Ethical, Clinical and Legal Perspectives*, p. 234. Similarly, Callahan writes: 'If we really believe in self-determination, then any competent person should have a right to be killed by a doctor for any reason that suits him. If we believe in the relief of suffering, then it seems cruel and capricious to deny it to the incompetent. There is, in short, no reasonable or logical stopping point once the turn has been made down the road to euthanasia . . .': Daniel Callahan, 'When Self-Determination Runs Amok', 52.

58 John Griffiths, 'Assisted Suicide in the Netherlands: the *Chabot* Case', 238–9.

59 Dr Boudewijn Chabot (in conversation with Arlene Klotzko): David C. Thomasma, Thomasine Kimbrough-Kushner, Gerrit K. Kimsma & Chris Cieslieski-Carlucci (eds), *Asking to Die: Inside the Dutch Debate about Euthanasia*, pp. 376, 380, 381.

60 Kumar Amarasekara, 'Euthanasia and the Quality of Legislative Safeguards', 7.

61 'Dutch Parliament Introduces New Euthanasia Bill', 10 August 1999, Last Rights Information Centre, World News Bulletins (archives): <http://www.rights.org/death-net/bulletins>.

62 *Termination of Life on Request and Assisted Suicide (Review Procedures) Act* Article 2.2.

63 B. Kitchener & A. Jorm, 'Conditions Required for a Law on Active Voluntary Euthanasia: A Survey of Nurses' Opinions in the Australian Capital Territory', 28–9.

64 Some might argue that courts or hospital ethics committees should certify compliance with statutory safeguards. If this involved merely 'ticking off' compliance with procedures, no great harm would be done. If it involved substantive review, however, it would make the whole process needlessly cumbersome. Rarely could one justify substituting the views of lay persons or judges for the professional opinions of the treating physicians and specialists closest to the patient. Ultimately, doctors must be trusted when opting to act within a statutory framework. On the other hand, there are also benefits in retaining the Coroner's power to investigate euthanasia deaths: D. Ranson, 'The Coroner and the Rights of the Terminally Ill Act 1995 (NT)', 169.

65 Christopher Ryan, 'Velcro on the Slippery Slope: the Role of Psychiatry in Active Voluntary Euthanasia', 580.

66 Dworkin, Nagel, Nozick et al quote the Coalition of Hospice Professionals in their amicus brief to the US Supreme Court: 'removing legal bans on suicide assistance will enhance the opportunity for advanced hospice care for all patients because regulation of physician-assisted suicide would mandate that all palliative measures be exhausted as a condition precedent to assisted suicide': 'Assisted Suicide: The Philosophers' Brief', *The New York Review of Books*, 27 March 1997, p. 42.

67 Timothy E. Quill, Christine K. Cassel, Diane E. Meier, 'Care of the Hopelessly Ill: Proposed Clinical Criteria for Physician-Assisted Suicide', 1382.

68 Steven H. Miles, 'Physicians and their Patients' Suicides', 1787.

69 Christopher Ryan, 'Velcro on the Slippery Slope: the Role of Psychiatry in Active Voluntary Euthanasia', 584.

70 H. Chochinov, D. Tataryn, J. Clinch et al, 'Will to Live in the Terminally Ill', 818–19.

71 I. Maddocks, 'Hope in Dying: Palliative Care and a Good Death' in J. Morgan (ed.), *An Easeful Death? Perspectives on Death, Dying and Euthanasia*, p. 70.

72 Daniel Callahan, 'Good Stratgies & Bad: Opposing Physician-Assisted Suicide', 7.

73 Ronald Dworkin, Thomas Nagel, Robert Nozick et al, 'Assisted Suicide: The Philosophers' Brief', *The New York Review of Books*, 27 March 1997, p. 41.

74 M. Little, 'Assisted Suicide, Suffering and the Meaning of a Life', 290.

75 Steven Miles, 'Physicians and their Patients' Suicides', 1786.

76 Max Charlesworth, *Bioethics in a Liberal Society*, p. 4.

Appendix

1 R. Burgess, 'Elements of Sampling in Field Research' in R. Burgess (ed.), *Field Research: A Sourcebook and Field Manual*, p. 77; K. Eckhardt & M. Ermann, *Social Research Methods*, p. 253.

² The recruitment categories above were not entirely mutually exclusive. For example, a number of interviewees were present in the public presentations I gave, although the actual interview came about because of a specific referral.

³ J. Seidel & J. Clark, 'The Ethnograph: A Computer Program for the Analysis of Qualitative Data', 110–25; J. Seidel, J. Kjolseth & E. Seymour, *The Ethnograph: A Programme for the Computer Assisted Analysis of Text Based Data.*

⁴ A. Strauss, *Qualitative Analysis for Social Scientists*, p. 50.

Bibliography

Abbott, Tony, 'Act of Compassion or Merely Killing?', *Australian*, 27 September 1996, p. 13.

Ad Hoc Committee of the Harvard Medical School, 'A Definition of Irreversible Coma', *Journal of the American Medical Association*, vol. 205, 1968, pp. 337–40.

Alcorn, Gay, 'Marshall Law', *Age*, 24 May 1995, p. 13.

——, 'The Death Thing', *Sydney Morning Herald*, 18 December 1999, p. 9S (Spectrum Features).

Alfonso, Cesar, & Mary Adler Cohen, 'HIV-Dementia and Suicide', *General Hospital Psychiatry*, vol. 16, 1994, pp. 45–6.

Alfonso, C. C., M. A. Cohen, A. D. Aladjem et al, 'HIV Seropositivity as a Major Risk Factor for Suicide in the General Hospital', *Psychosomatics*, vol. 35, 1994, pp. 368–73.

Alpers, Ann, & Bernard Lo, 'Physician-Assisted Suicide in Oregon: A Bold Experiment', *Journal of the American Medical Association*, vol. 274, 1995, pp. 483–7.

Amarasekara, Kumar, 'Euthanasia and the Quality of Legislative Safeguards', *Monash University Law Review*, vol. 23, 1997, pp. 1–42.

Anderson, James G. & David P. Caddell, 'Attitudes of Medical Professionals Towards Euthanasia', *Social Science & Medicine*, vol. 37, 1993, pp. 105–14.

Andrews, Keith, 'Recovery of Patients after Four Months or More in the Persistent Vegetative State', *British Medical Journal*, vol. 306, 1993, pp. 1597–1600.

Andrews, Kevin, 'Are We Past Caring?', *Sunday Age*, 14 July 1996, p. 16.

——, Euthanasia Laws Bill 1996, Second Reading Speech, Australian House of Representatives, 28 October 1996.

Annas, George, 'The Long Dying of Nancy Cruzan', *Law, Medicine & Health Care*, vol. 19, 1991, pp. 52–9.

Aranda, Sancia, & Margaret O'Conner, 'Euthanasia, Nursing and Care of the Dying: Rethinking Kuhse and Singer', *Australian Nursing Journal*, vol. 3, 1995, pp. 18–21.

Areen, Judith, 'Advance Directives Under State Law and Judicial Decisions', *Law, Medicine & Health Care*, vol. 19, 1991, pp. 91–100.

Asch, David, 'The Role of Critical Care Nurses in Euthanasia and Assisted Suicide', *New England Journal of Medicine*, vol. 334, 1996, pp. 1374–9.

Australian Law Reform Commission 1977, *Human Tissue Transplants* (Report No 7), AGPS, Canberra.

Ballis, Peter, & Roger S. Magnusson, 'Treatment decision-making at the end of life: a survey of Australian doctors' attitudes towards patients' wishes and euthanasia' (Letter), *Medical Journal of Australia*, vol. 166, p. 562.

Barbour, Rosaline S., 'The Impact of Working with People with HIV/AIDS: A Review of the Literature', *Social Science & Medicine*, vol. 39, 1994, pp. 221–32.

Baron, Charles H., Clyde Bergstresser, Dan W. Brock et al, 'A Model State Act to Authorize and Regulate Physician-Assisted Suicide', *Harvard Journal on Legislation*, vol. 33, 1996, pp. 1–34.

Barthes, Roland, *Mythologies*, Vintage, London, 1993.

Battin, Margaret P., *Ethical Issues in Suicide*, Prentice Hall, New Jersey, 1995.

Battin, Margaret, & Arthur Lipman (eds), *Drug Use in Assisted Suicide and Euthanasia*, Pharmaceutical Products Press, Binghamton, New York, 1996.

Baume, Peter, 'Voluntary Euthanasia and the Liberal Tradition', 9th Lionel Murphy Memorial Lecture, 30 November 1995, Lionel Murphy Foundation.

Baume, Peter, & Emma O'Malley, 'Euthanasia: Attitudes and Practices of Medical Practitioners', *Medical Journal of Australia*, vol. 161, 1994, pp. 137–44.

Baume, P., E. O'Malley & A. Bauman, 'Professed Religious Affiliation and the Practice of Euthanasia', *Journal of Medical Ethics*, vol. 21, 1995, pp. 49–54.

Beauchamp, Tom L., 'Reversing the Protections (Public & Private: Redrawing Boundaries)', *Hastings Center Report*, vol. 24, 1994, pp. 18–20.

Beauchamp, Tom L., & James F. Childress, *Principles of Biomedical Ethics*, 4th edn, Oxford University Press, New York, 1994.

Beck, M., K. Springen, A. Murr et al, 'The Doctor's Suicide Van', *Bulletin* (*Newsweek* insert), 19 June 1990, p. 80.

Beckford, James A., 'Accounting for Conversion', *British Journal of Sociology*, vol. 29(2), 1978, pp. 249–62.

Bennett, Lydia, 'The Experience of Nurses Working with Hospitalized AIDS Patients', *Australian Journal of Social Issues*, vol. 27, 1992, pp. 125–43.

Bennett, L., P. Michie, & S. Kippax, 'Qualitative Analysis of Burnout and its Associated Factors in AIDS Nursing', *AIDS Care*, vol. 3, 1991, pp. 181–92.

Benrubi, Guy, 'Euthanasia—the Need for Procedural Safeguards', *New England Journal of Medicine*, vol. 326, 1992, pp. 197–9.

Billings, J. A., & S. Block, 'Slow Euthanasia', *Journal of Palliative Care*, vol. 12, 1996, pp. 21–30.

Bindels, Patrick J. E., Anneke Krol, Erik van Ameijden et al, 'Euthanasia and Physician-Assisted Suicide in Homosexual Men with AIDS', *Lancet*, vol. 347, 1996, pp. 499–505.

Black, B., J. Wallace, H. Starks et al, 'Physician-Assisted Suicide and Euthanasia in Washington State', *Journal of the American Medical Association*, vol. 275, 1996, pp. 919–25.

Bor, Robert, 'Counselling Patients with AIDS-Associated Kaposi's Sarcoma', *Counselling Psychology Quarterly*, vol. 6, 1993, pp. 91–8.

Brahams, Diana, 'Euthanasia: Doctor Convicted of Attempted Murder', *The Lancet*, vol. 340, 1992, pp. 782–3.

Branegan, Jay, 'I Want to Draw the Line Myself', *Time*, 17 March 1997, pp. 92–3.

Brody, Howard, 'Assisted Death—A Compassionate Response to a Medical Failure', *New England Journal of Medicine*, vol. 327, 1992, pp. 1384–8.

Burgess, J. A., 'The Great Slippery-Slope Argument', *Journal of Medical Ethics*, vol. 19, 1993, pp. 169–74.

Burgess, Robert G., 'Elements of Sampling in Field Research', in R. Burgess (ed.), *Field Research: A Sourcebook and Field Manual*, George Allen & Unwin, London, 1982, pp. 77–8.

Byock, Ira R., 'The Hospice Clinician's Response to Euthanasia/Physician Assisted Suicide', *Hospice Journal*, vol. 9, 1998, pp. 1–8.

Caddell, David P., & Rae R. Newton, 'Euthanasia: American Attitudes Toward the Physician's Role', *Social Science & Medicine*, vol. 40, 1995, pp. 1671–81.

Callahan, Daniel, 'When Self-Determination Runs Amok', *Hastings Center Report*, March-April 1992, pp. 52–5.

——, 'Good Strategies & Bad: Opposing Physician-Assisted Suicide', *Commonweal*, vol. 126, 3 Dec. 1999, p. 7.

Caplan, Arthur L, Lois Snyder, & Kathy Faber-Langendoen, 'The Role of Guidelines in the Practice of Physician-Assisted Suicide', *Annals of Internal Medicine*, vol. 132, 2000, pp. 476–81.

Cassel, Christine, 'Physician-Assisted Suicide: Progress or Peril?', in D. Thomasma & T. Kushner (eds), *Birth to Death: Science and Bioethics*, Cambridge University Press, Cambridge, 1996, pp. 218–30.

Chapman, Simon, & Stephen Leeder, *The Last Right? Australians take sides on the right to die*, Mandarin, Port Melbourne, Victoria, 1995.

Charlesworth, Max, *Bioethics in a Liberal Society*, Cambridge University Press, Cambridge, 1993.

Chochinov, Harvey, Douglas Tataryn, Jennifer Clinch et al, 'Will to Live in the Terminally Ill', *Lancet*, vol. 354, 1999, pp. 816–19.

Cleeman, M., & E. Crock, 'Nursing People with HIV/AIDS—A Way of Life', paper read at the Sixth Annual Australasian Society for HIV Medicine Conference, Manly, Sydney, 3 November 1994.

Cohen-Almagor, Raphael, 'Reflections on the Intriguing Issue of the Right to Die in Dignity', *Israel Law Review*, vol. 29, 1995, pp. 677–701.

——, 'A Circumscribed Plea for Voluntary Physician-Assisted Suicide', in R. Cohen-Almagor (ed.), *Medical Ethics at the Dawn of the 21ˢᵗ Century*, The New York Academy of Sciences, New York, 2000, pp. 127–49.

——, 'Language and Reality at the End of Life', *Journal of Law, Medicine & Ethics*, vol. 28, 2000, pp. 267–78.

Commonwealth Department of Community Services and Health 1991, *Legal Issues Relating to AIDS and Intravenous Drug Use* (Discussion Paper prepared for the Legal Working Party of the Inter-Governmental Committee on AIDS).

Concette, Gino, 'Life is not Ours to Choose', *Age*, 5 July 1996, p. A13.

Cook, Deborah J., Gordon H. Guyatt, Roman Jaeschke et al, 'Determinants in Canadian Health Care Workers of the Decision to Withdraw Life Support From the Critically Ill', *Journal of the American Medical Association*, vol. 273, 1995, pp. 703–8.

Cooke, Molly, Linda Gourlay, Linda Collette et al, 'Informal Caregivers and the Intention to Hasten AIDS-Related Death', *Archives of Inernal Medicine*, vol. 158, 1998, pp. 69–75.

Coté, T., R. Biggar, & A. Dannenberg, 'Risk of Suicide Among Persons with AIDS', *Journal of the American Medical Association*, vol. 268, 1992, pp. 2066–8.

Cotton, Paul, 'Medicine's Position is Both Pivotal and Precarious in Assisted-Suicide Debate', *Journal of the American Medical Association*, vol. 273, 1995, pp. 363–4.

Craig, Gillian, 'Is Sedation without Hydration or Nourishment in Terminal Care Lawful?', *Medico-Legal Journal*, vol. 62, 1994, pp. 198–201.

Crouch, Barbara, 'Toxicological Issues with Drugs used to End Life', in M. Battin & A. Lipman (eds), *Drug Use in Assisted Suicide and Euthanasia*, Pharmaceutical Products Press, New York, 1996, pp. 211–22.

Devettere, Raymond, 'Neocortical Death and Human Death', *Law, Medicine & Health Care*, vol. 18, 1990, pp. 96–104.

Devlin, Patrick, *Easing the Passing: The Trial of Dr John Bodkin Adams*, Bodley Head, London, 1985.

Dombrink, John, & Daniel Hillyard, 'Manifestations of Social Agency in the 1994 Reform of Oregon's Assisted Suicide Law', *Sociology of Crime, Law, and Deviance*, vol. 1, 1998, pp. 127–54.

Dow, Steve, 'Live & Let Die', *Australian Magazine*, 7–8 August 1999, pp. 30–3.

Drielsma, Paul, 'AIDS Policy and Public Health Models: an Australian Analysis', *Australian Journal of Social Issues*, vol. 32, 1997, pp. 87–99.

Dworkin, Ronald, *Life's Dominion: An Argument about Abortion and Euthanasia*, Harper Collins Publishers, Hammersmith, London, 1993.

Dworkin, Ronald, Thomas Nagel, Robert Nozick, John Rawls, Thomas Scanlon, & Judith Jarvis Thomson, 'Assisted Suicide: The Philosophers' Brief', *New York Review of Books*, 27 March 1997, pp. 41–7.

Dyer, Clare, 'Rheumatologist Convicted of Attempted Murder', *British Medical Journal*, vol. 305, 1992, p. 731.

Ebaugh, Helen, *Becoming an Ex.*, Chicago University Press, Chicago, 1989.

Eckhardt, K., & M. Ermann, *Social Research Methods*, Random House, New York, 1977.

Editorial, 'The Final Autonomy', *Lancet*, vol. 340, 1992, p. 757.

Emanuel, Linda L., 'Reexamining Death: The Asymptotic Model and a Bounded Zone Definition', *Hastings Center Report*, vol. 25, 1995, pp. 27–35.

Ewick, Patricia, & Susan S. Silbey, 'Subversive Stories and Hegemonic Tales: Towards a Sociology of Narrative', *Law and Society Review*, vol. 29, 1995, pp. 197–226.

Fagan, Denise, 'Euthanasia: Report on 1995 Survey of Attitudes and Practices of Doctors who are Members of The Australian Society for HIV Medicine', *Noah's ARC*, vol. 7, 1996, http://www.unsw.edu.au/clients/ashm/

Farsides, Bobbie, 'Palliative Care—a Euthanasia-Free Zone?', *Journal of Medical Ethics*, vol. 24, 1998, pp. 149–50.

Faust, Beatrice, 'Give Patients Free Will Over Life and Death', *Weekend Australian*, 10–11 June 1995, p. 26.

——, 'Bans on the Unbannable Devalue the Law', *Weekend Australian*, 7–8 June 1997, p. 25.

Ford, Norman, 'Killing and Caring Don't Mix', *Sunday Age*, 29 October 1994, p. 14.

Foucault, Michel, *The History of Sexuality: An Introduction*, Penguin Books, Harmondsworth (England), 1978.

Fox, Ellen, & Carol Stocking, 'Ethics Consultants' Recommendations for Life-Prolonging Treatment of Patients in a Persistent Vegetative State', *Journal of the American Medical Association*, vol. 270, 1993, pp. 2578–82.

Ganzini, L., H. Nelson, T. Schmidt et al, 'Physicians' Experiences with the Oregon Death With Dignity Act', *New England Journal of Medicine*, vol. 342, 2000, pp. 557–63.

Gawenda, M., 'Change of Heart on Euthanasia', *Age*, 27 May 1996, p. A15.

Gaylin, W., L. Kass, E. Pellegrino, & M. Siegler, 'Doctors Must Not Kill', *Journal of the American Medical Association*, vol. 259, 1988, pp. 2139–40.

Gee, James Paul, Glynda Hull, & Colin Lankshear, *The New Work Order: behind the language of the new capitalism*, Allen & Unwin, St Leonards, NSW, 1996.

Glare, Paul A., & Neil J. Cooney, 'HIV and Palliative Care', in G. Stewart (ed.), *Managing HIV*, Australasian Medical Publishing Company, Sydney, 1997, pp. 119–22.

Glover, R., 'Why the Vulnerable Flock to Dr Death', *Sydney Morning Herald*, 17 April 1999, p. S2.

Godwin, John, Julie Hamblin, David Patterson, & David Buchanan, *Australian HIV/AIDS Legal Guide*, 2nd edn, Federation Press, Sydney, 1993.

Goff, Robert, 'A Matter of Life and Death', *Medical Law Review*, vol. 3, 1995, pp. 1–21.

Griffiths, John, 'Assisted Suicide in the Netherlands: the *Chabot* Case', *Modern Law Review*, vol. 58, 1995, pp. 232–48.

——, 'Recent Developments in the Netherlands Concerning Euthanasia and Other Medical Behavior that Shortens Life', *Medical Law International*, vol. 1, 1995, pp. 347–86.

——, 'The Slippery Slope: Are the Dutch Sliding Down or Are they Clambering Up?', in D. C. Thomasma, T. Kimbrough-Kushner, G. K. Kimsma, & C. Cieslieski-Carlucci (eds), *Asking to Die: Inside the Dutch Debate about Euthanasia*, Kluwer Academic Publishers, Dordrecht, 1998, pp. 93–104.

Griffiths, John, Alex Bood, Heleen Weyers, *Euthanasia & Law in the Netherlands*, Amsterdam University Press, Amsterdam, 1998.

Hart, Bethne, Peter Sainsbury, Stephanie Short, 'Whose Dying? A Sociological Critique of the 'Good Death'', *Mortality*, vol. 3, 1998, pp. 65–77.

Harvard Program on Public Opinion and Health Care, 'Should Physicians Aid their Patients in Dying?', *Journal of the American Medical Association*, vol. 267, 1992, pp. 2658–62.

Hawkins, C., *Mishap or Malpractice?*, Blackwell Scientific Publications, Oxford, 1985.

Heilig, Steve, & Stephen Jamison, 'Physician AID-in-Dying: toward a "Harm Reduction" Approach', *Cambridge Quarterly of Healthcare Ethics*, vol. 5, 1996, pp. 113–20.

Henderson, Craig, Chris Ryan, & Tracey Aubin, 'A Fight to the Death', *Who*, 23 February 1998, pp. 34–5.

Hillyard, Daniel, & John Dombrink, *Dying Right: The Death With Dignity Movement*, Routledge, New York, 2001.

——, 'Using the Law to Redefine Killing in Medical Settings', unpublished paper.

Ho, Robert, 'Factors Influencing Decisions to Terminate Life: Conditions of Suffering and the Identity of the Terminally Ill', *Australian Journal of Social Issues*, vol. 34, 1999, pp. 25–41.

Ho, Robert, & Ronald K. Penney, 'Euthanasia and Abortion: Personality Correlates for the Decision to Terminate Life', *Journal of Social Psychology*, vol. 132, 1992, pp. 77–86.

Holden, J., 'Demographics, Attitudes, and Afterlife Beliefs of Right-To-Life and Right-To-Die Organization Members', *Journal of Social Psychology*, vol. 133, 1993, pp. 521–7.

Howard, Robin, & David Miller, 'The Persistent Vegetative State', *British Medical Journal*, vol. 310, 1995, pp. 341–2.

Humphry, Derek, *Final Exit*, Dell Publishing, New York, 1992.

Hunt, Roger, 'Euthanasia: An Issue that Won't Die', *General Practitioner*, vol. 2, 1994, pp. 8–9.

——, 'Palliative Care—the Rhetoric-Reality Gap', in H. Kuhse (ed.), *Willing to Listen, Wanting to Die*, Penguin Books, Ringwood, Victoria, 1994, pp. 115–37.

——, 'Legislative Reform is Needed', *Age*, 7 April 1995, p. 16.

Jamison, Stephen, 'When Drugs Fail: Assisted Deaths and Not-So-Lethal Drugs', in M. P. Battin & A. G. Lipman (eds), *Drugs Use in Assisted Suicide and Euthanasia*, Pharmaceutical Products Press, Binghamton, New York, 1996, pp. 223–43.

Jonsen, Alfred, 'To Help the Dying Die—A New Duty for Anesthesiologists?', *Anesthesiology*, vol. 78, 1993, pp. 225–8.

Kalichman, Seth, & Kathleen Sikkema, 'Psychological Sequelae of HIV Infection and AIDS: Review of Empirical Findings', *Clinical Psychology Review*, vol. 14, 1994, pp. 611–32.

Kamisar, Yale, 'Physician-Assisted Suicide: the Last Bridge to Active Voluntary Euthanasia', in J. Keown (ed), *Euthanasia Examined: Ethical, Clinical and Legal Perspectives*, Cambridge University Press, Cambridge, 1995, pp. 225–60.

Keizer, Bert, 'In Search of a Decent Death', *Guardian Weekly*, 13 April 1997, p. 24.

Kelly, Brian, Leonie Todhunter, & Beverley Raphael, 'HIV Care: the Impact on the Doctor', *Medical Journal of Australia*, vol. 165, 1996, p. 150.

Kennedy, Ian, 'The Right to Die', in C. M. Mazzoni (ed.), *A Legal Framework for Bioethics*, Kluwer Law International, The Hague, 1998, pp. 181–97.

Keown, John, 'Euthanasia in the Netherlands: Sliding Down the Slippery Slope?', in J. Keown (ed.), *Euthanasia Examined: Ethical, Clinical and Legal Perspectives*, Cambridge University Press, Cambridge, 1995, pp. 261–96.

——, 'Restoring Moral and Intellectual Shape to the Law After *Bland*', *Law Quarterly Review*, vol. 113, 1997, pp. 481–503.

Kirby, Justice Michael, 'AIDS: A New Realm of Bereavement', paper read at The Third International Conference on Grief & Bereavement in Contemporary Society, The University of Sydney, 4 July 1991.

Kissane, D., A. Street, & P. Nitschke, 'Seven Deaths in Darwin: Case Studies Under the Rights of the Terminally Ill Act, Northern Territory, Australia', *Lancet*, vol. 352, 1998, pp. 1097–1102.

Kitchener, Betty, & Anthony Jorm, 'Conditions Required for a Law on Active Voluntary Euthanasia: A Survey of Nurses' Opinions in the Australian Capital Territory', *Journal of Medical Ethics*, vol. 25, 1999, pp. 25–30.

Kleiman, Mark, 'AIDS, Vice and Public Policy', *Law and Contemporary Problems*, vol. 51, 1988, pp. 315–68.

Kleinman, Arthur, *The Illness Narratives: Suffering, Healing & the Human Condition*, Basic Books, New York, 1988.

Kuhse, Helga, & Peter Singer, 'Doctors' Practices and Attitudes Regarding Voluntary Euthanasia', *Medical Journal of Australia*, vol. 148, 1988, pp. 623–7.

Kuhse, Helga, & Peter Singer, 'Euthanasia: A Survey of Nurses' Attitudes and Practices', *Australian Nurses Journal*, vol. 21, 1992, pp. 21–2.

Kuhse, Helga, Peter Singer, Peter Baume et al, 'End-of-Life Decisions in Australian Medical Practice', *Medical Journal of Australia*, vol. 166, 1997, pp. 191–6.

Lanham, David, *Taming Death by Law*, Longman Professional, Melbourne, 1993.

——, & Belinda Fehlberg, 'Living Wills and the Right to Die with Dignity', *Melbourne University Law Review*, vol. 18, 1991, pp. 329–49.

Leiser, Roslyn, Thomas Mitchell, Judith Hahn et al, letter, *New England Journal of Medicine*, vol. 335, 1996, pp. 972–3.

Lewins, Frank, 'The Development of Bioethics and the Issue of Euthanasia: Regulating, De-Regulating or Re-Regulating?', *Journal of Sociology*, vol. 34, 1998, pp. 123–34.

Little, Archbishop Sir Frank, 'There is Nothing Compassionate in a Doctor's "Mercy" Killing', *Age*, 17 April 1995, p. 9.

Little, Miles, 'Assisted Suicide, Suffering and the Meaning of a Life', *Theoretical Medicine and Bioethics*, vol. 20, 1999, pp. 187–98.

——, Euthanasia and Assisted Suicide—Reflections on Suffering and the Meaning of a Life, unpublished paper.

Lundberg, George D., ' "It's Over, Debbie" and the Euthanasia Debate', *Journal of the American Medical Association*, vol. 259, 1988, pp. 2142–3.

Lupton, Deborah, *Moral Threats and Dangerous Desires: AIDS in the News Media*, Taylor & Francis, London, 1994.

——, 'Archetypes of Infection: People with HIV/AIDS in the Australian Press in the Mid 1990s', *Sociology of Health & Illness*, vol. 21, 1999, pp. 37–53.

McCall Smith, Alexander, 'Euthanasia: the Strengths of the Middle Ground', *Medical Law Review*, vol. 7, 1999, pp. 194–207.

McGarvie, R., 'Euthanasia and the Issue of Consent', *Age*, 21 April 1995, p. 12.

McGuinness, Padraic, 'Democracy and the Right to Die', *Sydney Morning Herald*, 6 July 1996, p. 33.

McInerney, F., ''Requested Death': A New Social Movement', *Social Science & Medicine*, vol. 50, 2000, pp. 137–54.

McInerney, Fran, & Carmel Seibold, 'Nurses Definitions of and Attitudes Towards Euthanasia', *Journal of Advanced Nursing*, vol. 22, 1995, pp. 171–82.

McKegney, F., & M. O'Dowd, 'Suicidality and HIV Status', *American Journal of Psychiatry*, vol. 149, 1992, pp. 396–8.

Maddocks, Ian, 'Hope in Dying: Palliative Care and a Good Death', in J. Morgan (ed.), *An Easeful Death? Perspectives on Death, Dying and Euthanasia*, Federation Press, Sydney, 1996, pp. 57–70.

Magnusson, Roger S., 'Privacy, Confidentiality and HIV/AIDS Health Care', *Australian Journal of Public Health*, vol. 18, 1994, pp. 51–8.

——, 'The Future of the Euthanasia Debate in Australia', *Melbourne University Law Review*, vol. 20, 1996, pp. 1108–42.

——, 'The Sanctity of Life and the Right to Die: Social and Jurisprudential Aspects of the Euthanasia Debate in Australia and the United States', *Pacific Rim Law & Policy Journal*, vol. 6, 1997, pp. 1–83.

——, 'A Matter of Life and Death', *Sydney Morning Herald*, 26 March 1997, p. 21.

——, & Peter H. Ballis, 'The Response of Health Care Workers to AIDS Patients' Requests for Euthanasia', *Journal of Sociology*, vol. 35, 1999, pp. 312–30.

Manne, Robert, 'The Slippery Slope is a Life and Death Argument', *Age*, 14 June 1995, p. 18.

——, 'Killing Made Easier', *Age*, 30 November 1998, p. 13.

Marzuk, Peter, 'Suicidal Behavior and HIV Illnesses', *International Review of Psychiatry*, vol. 3, 1991, pp. 365–71.

——, 'Suicide and Terminal Illness', *Death Studies*, vol. 18, 1994, pp. 497–521.

——, Helen Tierney, Kenneth Tardiff et al, 'Increased Risk of Suicide in Persons with AIDS', *Journal of the American Medical Association*, vol. 259, 1988, pp. 1333–7.

Meier, D. E., C. Emmons, S. Wallenstein et al, 'A National Survey of Physician-Assisted Suicide and Euthanasia in the United States', *New England Journal of Medicine*, vol. 338, 1998, pp. 1193–1201.

Meisel, A., *The Right to Die*, John Wiley & Sons, New York, 1989.

——, J. Jernigan, & S. Youngner, 'Prosecutors and End-of-Life Decision Making', *Archives of Internal Medicine*, vol. 159, 1999, pp. 1089–95.

Miles, Steven, 'Physicians and their Patients' Suicides', *Journal of the American Medical Association*, vol. 271, 1994, pp. 1786–8.

Multi-Society Task Force on PVS, 'Medical Aspects of the Persistent Vegetative State', *New England Journal of Medicine*, vol. 330, 1994, pp. 1499–1508 (Part 1), pp. 1572–9 (Part 2).

Name withheld by request, 'It's Over, Debbie', *Journal of the American Medical Association*, vol. 259, 1988, p. 272.

Nuland, S., 'Physician-Assisted Suicide and Euthanasia in Practice', *New England Journal of Medicine*, vol. 342, 2000, pp. 583–4.

O'Connor, Margaret, 'Nurses and Euthanasia—Some Issues', *Collegian* (Royal College of Nursing, Australia), vol. 3, 1996, pp. 34–7.

O'Connor, M., D. Kissane, & O. Spruyt, 'Sedation in the Terminally Ill— A Clinical Perspective', *Monash Bioethics Review*, vol. 18, 1999, pp. 17–27.

O'Donnell, Ian, Jose Catalan, & Richard Farmer, 'Suicidal Behaviour and HIV Disease: A Case Report', *Counselling Psychology Quarterly*, vol. 5, 1992, pp. 411–15.

O'Dowd, M., D. Biderman, & F. McKegney, 'Incidence of Suicidality in AIDS and HIV-Positive Patients Attending a Psychiatry Outpatient Program', *Psychosomatics*, vol. 34, 1993, pp. 33–40.

Ogden, Russel, *Euthanasia, Assisted Suicide & AIDS*, Peroglyphics Publishing, New Westminster, British Columbia, 1994.

——, 'Vancouver AIDS Suicides Botched', *New York Times*, 14 June 1994, p. C12.

——, 'Palliative Care and Euthanasia: A Continuum of Care?', *Journal of Palliative Care*, vol. 10, 1994, pp. 82–5.

——, 'Non-Physician Assisted Suicide: The Technological Imperative of the Deathing Counterculture', *Death Studies*, vol. 25, 2001, pp. 387–401.

Ognall, The Honourable Mr Justice, 'A Right to Die? Some Medico-Legal Reflections', *Medico-Legal Journal*, vol. 62, 1994, pp. 165–79.

Otlowski, Margaret, *Voluntary Euthanasia and the Common Law*, Clarendon Press, Oxford, 1997.

Palmer, Henry, 'Dr. Adams' Trial for Murder', *Criminal Law Review*, 1957, pp. 365–77.

Palys, T., & J. Lowman, 'Ethical and Legal Strategies for Protecting Confidential Research Information', *Canadian Journal of Law and Society*, vol. 15, 2000, pp. 39–80.

Parliament of the Commonwealth of Australia, Senate Legal and Constitutional Legislation Committee 1997, *Consideration of Legislation Referred to the Committee: Euthanasia Laws Bill 1996*, Canberra.

Pauer-Studer, Herlinde, 'Peter Singer on Euthanasia', *Monist*, vol. 76, 1993, pp. 135–57.

Pellegrino, Edmund, 'Compassion Needs Reason Too', *Journal of the American Medical Association*, vol. 270, 1993, pp. 874–5.

——, 'Ethics', *Journal of the American Medical Association*, vol. 273, 1995, pp. 1674–6.

Pence, G., 'Dr Kevorkian and the Struggle for Physician-Assisted Dying', *Bioethics*, vol. 9, 1995, pp. 62–71.

Perron, Marshall, First Reading Speech to the *Rights of the Terminally Ill Bill* 1995 (NT), Northern Territory Legislative Assembly, 22 February 1995.

——, former Chief Minister of the Northern Territory, speech given at 'Death and the State', a conference organised by the Centre for Public Policy, The University of Melbourne, 24 August 1995.

Pollard, Brian, Letter to the Editor, *Medical Journal of Australia*, vol. 161, 1994, p. 572.

——, *The Challenge of Euthanasia*, Little Hills Press, Crows Nest, New South Wales 1994.

——, 'Distracters in the Contemporary Debate on Euthanasia' in J. Morgan (ed.), *An Easeful Death? Perspectives on Death, Dying and Euthanasia*, Federation Press, Sydney, 1996, pp. 71–85.

——, & Ronald Winton, 'Why Doctors and Nurses Must Not Kill Patients', *Medical Journal of Australia*, vol. 128, 1993, pp. 426–9.

President's Commission for the Study of Ethical Problems in Medicine and Biomedical and Behavioural Research 1981, *Defining Death: A Report on the Medical, Legal and Ethical Issues in the Determination of Death*, US Government Printing Office, Washington DC.

Pugh, K., I. O'Donnell & J. Catalan, 'Suicide and HIV Disease', *AIDS Care*, vol. 5, 1993, pp. 391–400.

Quill, Timothy, 'Death and Dignity: A Case of Individualised Decision Making', *New England Journal of Medicine*, vol. 324, 1991, pp. 691–4.

——, Christine K. Cassel, & Diane E. Meier, 'Care of the Hopelessly Ill: Proposed Clinical Criteria for Physician-Assisted Suicide', *New England Journal of Medicine*, vol. 327, 1992, pp. 1380–4.

——, Bernard Lo, & Dan Brock, 'Palliative Options of Last Resort, *Journal of the American Medical Association*, vol. 278, 1997, pp. 2099–2104.

Rabkin, J., R. Remien, L. Katoff et al, 'Suicidality in AIDS Long-Term Survivors: What is the Evidence?', *AIDS Care*, vol. 5, 1993, pp. 401–11.

Ranson, David, 'The Coroner and the Rights of the Terminally Ill Act 1995 (NT)', *Journal of Law and Medicine*, vol. 3, 1995, pp. 169–76.

Reichel, William, & Arthur J. Dyck, 'Euthanasia: A Contemporary Moral Quandary', *Lancet*, 1989, vol. 2, pp. 1321–3.

Rupp, Michael, 'Issues for Pharmacists in Assisted Patient Death', in M. Battin & A. Lipman (eds), *Drug Use in Assisted Suicide and Euthanasia*, Pharmaceutical Products Press, New York, 1996, pp. 43–53.

Ryan, Christopher, 'Velcro on the Slippery Slope: the Role of Psychiatry in Active Voluntary Euthanasia', *Australian & New Zealand Journal of Psychiatry*, vol. 29, 1995, pp. 580–5.

Santamaria, B. A., 'Tacit Consent to Euthanasia', *Weekend Australian*, 1–2 April 1995, p. 28.

——, 'Euthanasia's Bell Tolls for Thee', *Weekend Australian*, 13–14 July 1995, p. 22.

Sargent, M., *The New Sociology for Australians*, Longman Cheshire, Melbourne, 1994.

Schmitz, Phyllis, 'The Process of Dying With and Without Feeding and Fluids by Tube', *Law, Medicine & Health Care*, vol. 19, 1991, pp. 23–6.

Schneider, Stephen, Shelley Taylor, Constance Hammen et al, 'Factors Influencing Suicide Intent in Gay and Bisexual Suicide Ideators: Differing Models for Men with and without Human Immunodeficiency Virus', *Journal of Personality and Social Psychology*, vol. 61, 1991, pp. 776–88.

Seale, Clive, 'Heroic Death', *Sociology*, vol. 29, 1995, pp. 597–613.

——, & Julia Addington-Hall, 'Euthanasia: Why People Want to Die Earlier', *Social Science & Medicine*, vol. 39, 1994, pp. 647–54.

Seidel, J., & J. Clark, 'The Ethnograph: A Computer Program for the Analysis of Qualitative Data', *Qualitative Sociology*, vol. 7, 1984, pp. 110–25.

Seidel, J., J. Kjolseth, & E. Seymour, *The Ethnograph: A Programme for the Computer Assisted Analysis of Text Based Data*, Version 3.00. Qualis Research Associates, Littleton, Colorado, 1988.

Silverman, Daniel, 'Psychosocial Impact of HIV-Related Caregiving on Health Providers: A Review and Recommendations for the Role of Psychiatry', *American Journal of Psychiatry*, vol. 150, 1993, pp. 705–12.

Singer, Peter, *Rethinking Life & Death*, Text Publishing Co, Melbourne, 1994.

——, 'Time Bids Farewell to the Politics of Fear', *Age*, 10 October 1996, p. 15.

Slome, L., J. Moulton, C. Huffine et al, 'Physicians' Attitudes Toward Assisted Suicide in AIDS', *Journal of Acquired Immune Deficiency Syndromes*, vol. 5, 1992, pp. 712–18.

Slome, L. R., T. F. Mitchell, E. Charlebois et al, 'Physician-Assisted Suicide and Patients with Human Immunodeficiency Virus Disease', *New England Journal of Medicine*, vol. 336, 1997, pp. 417–21.

Smith, George P., 'Terminal Sedation as Palliative Care: Revalidating a Right to a Good Death', *Cambridge Quarterly of Healthcare Ethics*, vol. 7, 1998, pp. 382–7.

——, *Human Rights and Biomedicine*, Kluwer Law International, The Hague, 2000.

Snyder, Lois, & Arthur L. Caplan, 'Assisted Suicide: Finding Common Ground', *Annals of Internal Medicine*, vol. 132, 2000, pp. 468–9.

Somerville, Margaret, 'Sentencing Society to Ethical Death', *Age*, 13 November 1995, p. 13.

——, 'Legalising Euthanasia: Why Now?, *Australian Quarterly*, vol. 68, 1996, pp. 1–14.

Sontag, Susan, *AIDS and Its Metaphors*, Penguin Books, London, 1990.

——, *Illness as Metaphor; AIDS and Its Metaphors*, Penguin Books, London 1991.

Span P., 'Philosophy of Death', *Washington Post*, 9 December 1999, p. C1.

Starace, Fabrizio, 'Suicidal Behaviour in People Infected with Human Immunodeficiency Virus: A Literature Review', *International Journal of Social Psychiatry*, vol. 39, 1993, pp. 64–70.

Steinberg, M. A., J. M. Najman, C. M. Cartwright et al, 'End-of-Life Decision-Making: Community and Medical Practitioners' Perspectives', *Medical Journal of Australia*, vol. 166, 1997, pp. 131–4.

Stewart, Graeme (ed.), *Managing HIV*, Australasian Medical Publishing Co Ltd, Sydney, 1997.

Strauss, A., *Qualitative Analysis for Social Scientists*, Cambridge University Press, Cambridge, 1987.

Sullivan, G., 'Ministering Death', *Oxford Journal of Legal Studies*, vol. 17, 1997, pp. 123–36.

Sulmasy, Daniel P., & Edmund D. Pellegrino, 'The Rule of Double Effect', *Archives of Internal Medicine*, vol. 159, 1999, p. 545.

Sundström, Per, 'Peter Singer and "Lives Not Worth Living"—Comments on a Flawed Argument from Analogy', *Journal of Medical Ethics*, vol. 21, 1995, pp. 35–8.

Syme, Rodney, 'A Patient's Right to a Good Death', *Medical Journal of Australia*, vol. 154, 1991, pp. 203–5.

——, 'Assisted Suicide is not a Synonym for Homicide', *Age*, 17 May 1995, p. 15.

——, 'An Act of Mercy for a Peaceful Exit', *Age*, 7 January 1997, p. A11.

——, 'Right to Die Row Returns', *Age*, 2 November 1998, p. 1.

——, 'Reply from Rodney Syme', *Monash Bioethics Review*, vol. 18, 1999, pp. 34–40.

——, 'Pharmacological Oblivion Contributes to and Hastens Patients' Deaths', *Monash Bioethics Review*, vol. 18, 1999, pp. 40–3.

Symposium, 'Family Privacy and Persistent Vegetative State: A Symposium on the Linares Case', *Law, Medicine & Health Care*, vol. 17, 1989, pp. 295–346.

Tallis, Raymond, 'Is there a Slippery Slope?', *Times Literary Supplement*, 12 January 1996, pp. 3–4.

Tännsjö, Torbjörn, 'Terminal Sedation—A Possible Compromise in the Euthanasia Debate?', *Bulletin of Medical Ethics*, November 2000, pp. 13–22.

Teichman, Jenny, 'Humanism and Personism', *Quadrant*, December 1992, pp. 26–9.

Thomasma, David C., Thomasine Kimbrough-Kushner, Gerrit K. Kimsma, & Chris Cieslieski-Carlucci (eds), *Asking to Die: Inside the Dutch Debate about Euthanasia*, Kluwer Academic Publishers, Dordrecht, 1998.

Thompson, Elaine, A/Professor of Public Policy, University of New South Wales, speaking to a conference entitled 'Death and the State', Centre for Public Policy, The University of Melbourne, 24 August 1995.

Tindall, B., S. Forde, A. Carr et al, 'Attitudes to Euthanasia and Assisted Suicide in a Group of Homosexual Men with Advanced HIV Disease', *Journal of Acquired Immune Deficiency Syndromes*, vol. 6, 1993, p. 1069.

Tobin, Bernadette, Letter, *Australian*, 24 May 1995, p. 10.

Tonti-Filippini, Nicholas, 'Some Refusals of Medical Treatment which Changed the Law of Victoria', *Medical Journal of Australia*, vol. 157, 1992, pp. 277–9.

——, 'Euthanasia Undermines Rights of Sick', *Australian*, 20 July 1994, p. 11.

Tulsky, James A., Ralph Ciampa, & Elliott J. Rosen, 'Responding to Legal Requests for Physician-Assisted Suicide', *Annals of Internal Medicine*, vol. 132, 2000, pp. 494–9.

Twycross, Robert, 'Where there is Hope, there is Life: A View from the Hospice', in J. Keown (ed.), *Euthanasia Examined: Ethical, Clinical and Legal Perspectives*, Cambridge University Press, Cambridge, 1995, pp. 141–68.

van der Maas, P., J. van Delden, L. Pijnenborg et al, 'Euthanasia and Other Medical Decisions Concerning the End of Life', *Lancet*, vol. 338, 1991, pp. 669–74.

van der Wal, Gerrit, Paul J. van der Maas, Jacqueline M. Bosma et al, 'Evaluation of the Notification Procedure for Physician-Assisted Death in the Netherlands', *New England Journal of Medicine*, vol. 335, 1996, pp. 1706–11.

van Reyk, Paul, 'HIV and Choosing to Die', in G. Stewart (ed.), *Managing HIV*, Australasian Medical Publishing Co Ltd, Sydney, 1997, p. 161.

The Vatican—Evangelium Vitae, *On the Value and Inviolability of Human Life*, 1995.

Vaux, Kenneth L., 'Debbie's Dying: Mercy Killing and the Good Death', *Journal of the American Medical Association*, vol. 259, 1988, pp. 2140–2.

Veatch, Robert, 'The Impending Collapse of the Whole-Brain Definition of Death', *Hastings Center Report*, vol. 23, July–August 1993, pp. 18–24.

Waddell, C., R. M. Clarnette, M. Smith et al, 'Treatment Decision-Making at the End of Life: A Survey of Australian Doctors' Attitudes towards

Patients' Wishes and Euthanasia', *Medical Journal of Australia*, vol. 165, 1996, pp. 540–4.

Walker, T., J. Littlewood, & M. Pickering, 'Death in the News: The Public Invigilation of Private Emotion', *Sociology*, vol. 29, 1995, pp. 579–96.

Walters J., 'Aid in Dying is Human, Humane', *Los Angeles Times*, 18 October 1992.

Ward B. J., & P. A. Tate, 'Attitudes Among NHS Doctors to Requests for Euthanasia', *British Medical Journal*, vol. 308, 1994, pp. 1332–4.

Werth, James, 'Rational Suicide Reconsidered: AIDS as an Impetus for Change', *Death Studies*, vol. 19, 1995, pp. 65–80.

Willis, Evan, *Medical Dominance*, Allen & Unwin, Sydney, 1989.

Winkler, Earl, 'Reflections on the State of Current Debate Over Physician-Assisted Suicide and Euthanasia', *Bioethics*, vol. 9, 1995, pp. 313–26.

Woodruff, Rodger, 'Facts Needed to Balance Doctors' Euthanasia Push', *Age*, 30 March 1995, p. 12.

Young, Roxanne K., 'It's Over, Debbie', *Journal of the American Medical Association*, vol. 259, 1988, p. 272.

Zalcberg, John R., & John D. Buchanan, 'Clinical Issues in Euthanasia', *Medical Journal of Australia*, vol. 166, 1997, pp. 150–2.

Zinn, C., 'Australian Doctors Go Public Over Euthanasia', *British Medical Journal*, vol. 310, 1995, p. 895.

Index

abandonment, 18–19, 46, 70, 269
Abbott, Tony, 265–6
advance directives, 59, 65–6
ambivalence, 83, 107, 111–13, 123, 208, 256
Andrews, Kevin, 32, 33, 48, 61, 62–3, 68, 264–5
anecdotes told in interview (nature of), 169–71
anger, 98
'anti-professionalism', 201, 229–30
assisted death: actions indirectly facilitating assisted death, 'lesser involvements', 112–13, 115, 193, 211; emotions of involvement, 114, 143–5, 189, 204–6, *see also* coping; factors motivating requests for assistance, 72–99 *passim*, 250, 252–3; forms of involvement in, 130, 132–4, 255, *see also* collaboration; how patients request assistance, 69–72; instructions by doctors to nurses, 192, 196, 221, 235–6; interviewees' criteria for involvement in assisted death, 105–6; methods of achieving death, 16, 28–9, 33, 62, 86–9, 111, 139–40, 192, 194–6 *passim*; motivations for involvement in, 150–1; patients with HIV but not AIDS, *see* 'prophylactic euthanasia'; 'personal' vs 'professional' involvement, 167, 243–4; quantitative research estimating levels of involvement in, 38–42, 115; verifying involvement in assisted death: specific reports, 131–4, 163–9; 'highest' level of involvement, 135–6; frequency of involvement, 134–8, 180–1, 185; where patients die, 138–9; who's involved?, 115, 253; *see also* collaboration in assisted death

assisted suicide: definition of, 24; legalisation of assisted suicide but not euthanasia, 268–9; *see also* assisted death; euthanasia

Battin, Margaret, 37, 51
Baume, Peter, 38–40, 43, 45, 101, 300
'botched attempts', 11, 112, 123, 139–40, 148–50, 157, 159–60, 166–9, 189, 202–10, 249, 254; reasons for failure, 202–4; suffocation and strangulation, 123, 140, 160, 166–7, 185, 205, 207, 215, 242–3
burn-out, 94, 104, 119, 241–4 *passim*, 251–2, 254

Callahan, Daniel, 100, 280, 293, 304
Catholic church: hierarchy, 2, 17, 45–6; nuns, 181; priests, 9, 74, 162, 223
Catholic hospitals (and health care workers), 16–17, 25, 89, 191, 193, 203
Chabot case (in the Netherlands Supreme Court), 213, 271, 275–6
Charlesworth, Max, 47, 281
Christian churches, 37, 42–3, 44–6, 61, 63, 141, 267
clinical discretion (role of, in assisted death), 103, 107–8, 266
collaboration in assisted death, 130, 174–99, 257; actions at the bedside, 188–90; assessment, 187–8; case study of collaboration: the 'angels of death', 183–6; collaboration in hospitals, 191–7; collaboration in specific accounts of assisted death, 178–80; collaboration in the community, 186–91; de-briefing after the event, 190; evidence of a 'euthanatic culture' in hospitals, 193–7; extent of knowledge of the wider 'euthanasia community', 180–2; ob-

322